GOOD FOOD

The Complete Guide to Eating Well

Margaret M. Wittenberg

The Crossing Press · Freedom, CA 95019

ACKNOWLEDGMENTS

Much love and thanks to...

Elaine Gill and Denny Hayes of The Crossing Press for their unwavering trust, understanding, and support.

My faithful four-legged companions, Mochi, Betty, Scooter, Kitten Marie, Junior, and Bud, whose ever-present vigil at my computer kept me motivated, inspired, and entertained.

And, especially my husband, Terry, for his love, humor, patience, and invaluable editing and cooking hints throughout the years, especially during the writing of this book.

© Copyright 1995 by Margaret M. Wittenberg
Cover Design by Mike Monteiro
Book Design by Sheryl Karas
Printed in the U.S.A.

Cautionary Note: The nutritional information, recipes, and instructions contained within this book are in no way intended as a substitute for medical counseling. Please do not attempt self-treatment of a medical problem without consulting a qualified health practitioner.

Library of Congress Cataloging-in-Publication Data

Wittenberg, Margaret M.
    Good Food : the complete guide to eating well / Margaret M. Wittenberg.
       p. cm.
    Includes bibliographical references and index.
    ISBN 0-89594-746-3 (paper)
    1. Food. 2. Nutrition. 3. Cookery. 4. Diet. I. Title.
TX354.W58 1995
641.3--dc20   95-67
                                       CIP

Contents

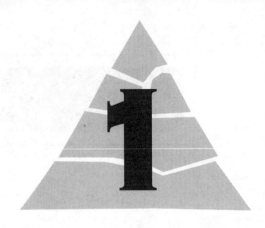

EXPLORING
YOUR OPTIONS

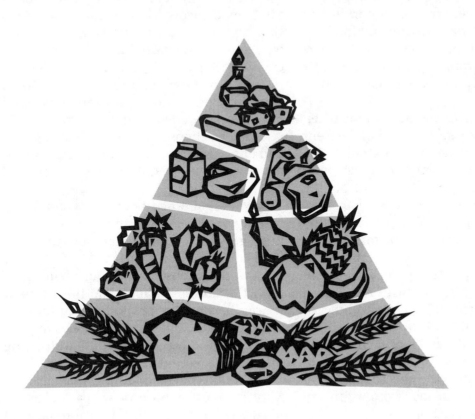

Making Choices

IN THE MIDST of busy lives, all too often meal preparation involves little more than adding water to a packaged mix or microwaving something out of the freezer. However, not only do you compromise flavor and nutrition, you also deprive yourselves of the more subtle benefits of cooking from scratch.

While it will be evident as you explore this book that I believe it is important for us to understand the nutrition and food science behind the foods we eat, I also believe it is equally important to appreciate the role food takes in helping us maintain balance in our lives.

It's amazing what happens to me when I allow myself the time to be totally present throughout the preparation of a meal. The simple rhythms involved with measuring, cutting, and stirring help me flow from the tensions of the day to the more relaxed atmosphere of my home. The palette of textures, colors, and flavors of the many foods from which I have to choose stimulate the more creative, expressive parts of my subconscious mind. The warmth of the oven and steam from the pots create feelings of security and comfort while the overall act of cooking with real, basic foods reminds me that the vegetables I cut, the grains I measure, the water I pour, the cheese I slice—all have their origins not just from a grocery store but from the earth itself.

A bit much to expect from the everyday reality of having to prepare three meals a day, 365 days of the year? Not when you consider that what we're talking about is simply experiencing the subtle grounding effects that emanate from a renewed respect for food and its effects on both body and mind.

We're continually faced with options in life: from the work we choose to do, the relationships we choose to cultivate, the lessons we choose to acquire, and the causes we choose to support. So, too, it is with foods.

We can choose to drink a glass of 100% apple juice or we can drink an apple-flavored beverage sweetened with corn syrup.

We can choose to limit our grains to rice and enriched white bread or we can experiment with millet, quinoa, spelt, teff, and crusty whole grain breads.

We can choose to buy foods simply according to price or we can actively seek out those grown according to methods that help sustain the environment.

We can choose to pick our menus simply by whatever is handy and fills us up or we can balance the proportions of protein, carbohydrates, and fat in our meals to positively impact our health and well-being throughout our entire lives.

We can choose to eat all our meals in front of the television or we can focus instead on pleasant conversation and the meal at hand.

In essence, exploring the options from which you can make choices about the foods you eat and how they fit into your diet is what this book is all about.

Good Food: The Complete Guide to Eating Well represents the information I have accumulated throughout the past 20 years of research, teaching, and consulting. Using the U.S. Department of Agriculture's Food Guide Pyramid as the organizational structure of the book, you'll learn basic principles of nutrition and how to incorporate them into your diet. You'll also learn about all the individual foods that comprise the various food groups highlighted in the Food Guide Pyramid, including background information, special features, how they are produced, buying and storage tips, and cooking guidelines.

In addition to applying the concepts of variety and moderation, knowing how to buy the highest quality will enable you to strike a healthy balance between taste and nutrition.

Open up to the possibilities of fresh, wholesome, artfully produced food simply prepared for optimum flavor, texture, and nutrients. Go ahead, explore your options.

—*Margaret Moothart Wittenberg*

Choosing a Healthy Diet

OPTIMUM HEALTH depends on a good, well-balanced diet. Epidemiological experts now estimate that up to 70% of all modern diseases have a dietary link. Culminating an exhaustive ten-year study by the Food and Nutrition Board of the National Academy of Sciences, the results, published in the landmark book, *Diet and Health: Implications for Reducing Chronic Disease Risk*, in 1989 finally corroborated what had been advocated for years: a reduction in fat and cholesterol intake and an increase in fruits, vegetables, and complex carbohydrates can dramatically reduce the incidence of chronic disease.

Accordingly, in 1990, the U.S. Department of Agriculture (USDA) and the U.S. Department of Health and Human Services (HHS) jointly issued seven basic suggestions for Americans aged 2 years and older to achieve a healthful diet.

THE DIETARY GUIDELINES FOR AMERICANS

•Eat a variety of foods.

There is no such thing as a "super food" that provides significant amounts of the more than 40 different nutrients we require for good health. Eating a wide spectrum of foods will satisfy the gaps in nutrition from one food to another.

•Maintain healthy weight.

Obesity increases the risk of chronic diseases such as high blood pressure, heart disease, stroke, certain cancers, and the most common kind of diabetes.

•Choose a diet low in fat, saturated fat, and cholesterol.

Eating leaner cuts of meat, poultry, and fish and increasing your consumption of cooked dried beans for protein will help reduce your risk of heart attack and certain types of cancer. It can also help you maintain a healthy weight.

•Choose a diet with plenty of vegetables, fruits, and grain products.

Foods such as these will provide needed vitamins, minerals, fiber, and complex carbohydrates while helping you lower your intake of fat.

•Use sugars only in moderation.

This includes not only white and brown sugars but also fructose, honey, and other "natural" sweeteners. A diet with too much sugar will supply too many calories for too few nutrients. It can also contribute to tooth decay.

•Use salt and sodium only in moderation.

Help reduce your risk of high blood pressure by learning how to flavor foods with herbs, spices, and lemon juice.

•If you drink alcoholic beverages, do so in moderation.

Investigate other modes of relaxation. Alcohol provides plenty of calories with little or no nutrients. It can also contribute to health problems as well as accidents.

THE FOOD GUIDE PYRAMID: A PRACTICAL APPROACH

To put the Dietary Guidelines into more practical terms, the USDA and HHS devised the Food Guide Pyramid as a visual outline of what to eat each day. The overall goal was to provide an outline for a diet that would contribute at least 60% of calories from carbohydrate, 10% from protein, and less than 30% of calories from fat. Suggested servings and servings sizes were used to spare people the need to calculate calories, grams of carbohydrate, protein, and fat, and their percentages as part of the total diet.

A major departure from the Basic Four Food Groups from the 1950s, the Food Guide Pyramid categorizes foods into five major groups plus another one which should be used sparingly. The groups are then represented as layers on a pyramid, situated according to the number of servings suggested for optimum health.

At the foundation of the pyramid is the **Bread, Cereal, Rice, & Pasta Group**, signifying that the highest proportion of our total calories should come from grain or grain products. Six to eleven servings are suggested each day. Your choices include 1 slice of bread, 1 ounce of ready-to-eat cereal, or 1/2 cup of cooked cereal, grains, or pasta.

The second building block of the Food Guide Pyramid is the **Vegetable Group**. Vegetables are major contributors of the vitamins, minerals, and fiber we need each day. Three to five servings are suggested each day. One cup of raw leafy vegetables, 1/2 cup of other vegetables (cooked or raw), or 3/4 cup of vegetable juice constitutes a serving.

The **Fruit Group** is located on the same level as vegetables, signifying that its nutrient contributions (vitamins, minerals, and fiber) are virtually the same but supplied in different proportions. Two to four servings are suggested each day. A serving can be a medium piece of fruit, 1/2 cup of freshly chopped, cooked, or canned fruit, 1 1/2 ounces of dried fruit, or 3/4 cup of fruit juice.

The protein group, situated on the next level up from vegetables and fruit, is dubbed the **Meat, Poultry, Fish, Dry Beans, Eggs, & Nut Group** to illustrate the many forms of protein available. Besides protein, this group contributes vitamins and minerals that are less plentiful in other food groups, such as iron and zinc. Two to four servings a day are suggested. Two to three ounces of cooked lean meat, poultry, or fish, 1/2 cup cooked dried beans, 1 egg, 2 tablespoons of peanut butter, and 1/3 cup nuts each constitutes a serving.

The **Milk, Yogurt, & Cheese Group** is located on the same level as the protein group, signifying that dairy products are also important sources of protein, vitamins, and minerals. Two to three servings per day are suggested. One cup of milk or yogurt or 1 1/2 ounces of natural cheese each constitute a serving. (Although the Food Guide Pyramid indicates that dairy products should be included in a well-balanced diet, if, either for physical or philosophical reasons, you cannot tolerate dairy products, you can use dairy substitutes instead, such as nut milk or soy milk, and concentrate on getting your calcium needs from calcium-rich foods and/or calcium supplements.)

At the very tip of the Food Guide Pyramid is the **Fat, Oils, and Sweets Group**. This

SERVING COMPARISONS BY THREE CALORIE LEVELS

Food Group	Sedentary women Some older adults Children About 1600 calories	Sedentary men Moderately active Women, teen girls About 2200 calories	Teen boys Active men Active women About 2800 calories
Bread Group	6 servings	9 servings	11 servings
Vegetable Group	3 servings	4 servings	5 servings
Fruit Group	2 servings	3 servings	4 servings
Meat Group	2-3 servings	2-3 servings	2-3 servings
Milk Group*	2-3 servings	2-3 servings	2-3 servings
Total Fat**	36 grams (20%) 53 grams (30%)	49 grams (20%) 73 grams (30%)	62 grams (20%) 93 grams (30%)
Total Added Sugars***	24 grams or 6 teaspoons	32 grams or 8 teaspoons	44 grams or 11 teaspoons

*Women who are pregnant or breast feeding, teenagers, and young adults to age 24 need 3 servings of milk or an appropriate substitute for calcium.

**Showing both 20% calories from fat as well as the 1990 U.S. Dietary Guidelines maximum of 30% fat, an amount which is generally considered too high. One gram of fat equals 9 calories.

***Using a maximum of 6% of total calories allotted to added sugars. Added sugars include those which are deliberately added to sweeten or foods/beverages which are primarily simple sugars such as soft drinks. It does not include naturally occurring simple carbohydrates in foods as found in fruits, dairy products, grains, and beans. One teaspoon equals 4 grams of sugar.

sixth grouping is considered to be expendable since they contribute calories and little else. Except for the general admonition to use them sparingly, no serving amounts or sizes are suggested. Beyond limiting your intake of obvious sources of fats, oils, and sugars that are normally considered a part of this sixth group, you should also choose lower fat and lower sugar foods from the other five food groups.

The number of servings you need depend on how many calories you need based on your age, sex, size, and activity level.

Several variations of the Food Guide Pyramid devised by other groups have emerged since its unveiling, including the Mediterranean Diet Pyramid developed and endorsed by the Harvard School of Public Health, Oldways Preservation & Exchange Trust, and the World Health Organization European Regional Office.

The Mediterranean Diet Pyramid emphasizes a diet consisting of daily servings of grains, potatoes and other vegetables, fruits, olive oil, cheese, and yogurt. While it's not necessarily low in overall fat, it's very low in animal fat. It is the type of fat that makes the difference, according to the developers of the Mediterranean version. In fact, considering that red meat is the largest source of saturated fats in our diet, they suggest that rather than viewing red meat as a regular protein option, it should be eaten no more than a couple of times a month. Fish and poultry are allowed a few times per week since they are lower in saturated fats.

Based on diets from regions with historically low chronic disease rates and high life expectancies, the Mediterranean Diet Pyramid is an interesting twist on the USDA's Food Guide Pyramid. No doubt, as more groups organize their ideas about diet and nutrition into a pyramid form, several more versions of the Food Guide Pyramid will emerge.

Still, the Food Guide Pyramid offers a good springboard from which to look at your diet. It covers the basic concepts of a good diet, the increased consumption of grains, fruits, and vegetables. It also suggests fewer amounts and servings of protein foods than many Americans are used to eating. And it's good advice to cut back on overall fat, especially saturated fat. More in-depth information concerning each of the food groups will be detailed in its corresponding section within this book.

A Day At The Pyramid

Setting a daily meal plan that fits within the guidelines of the Food Guide Pyramid is easier than you may imagine. While the system does not require the use of a calculator or food scale, initially it may be a good idea to use a measuring cup to get a good idea of what a 1/2-cup or 1-cup serving looks like. From there, you'll be able to approximate what you're eating by merely a glance. Once the Food Guide Pyramid becomes a habit, you'll probably only need to analyze your meals periodically to make sure that your diet remains close enough to good meal planning principles.

The chart below can be used to see how close your own meals are to the guidelines suggested by the Food Guide Pyramid.

FOOD/BEVERAGES CONSUMED	# SERVINGS PER FOOD GROUP					Grams	
	Bread	Vegetable	Fruit	Milk	Meat	Fat	Added Sugar
Breakfast							
Snacks							
Lunch							
Snacks							
Dinner							
Snacks							

Practice using the chart by considering two sample menus of a woman who exercises vigorously for an hour at least four times per week. According to the "SERVING COMPARISONS BY THREE CALORIE LEVELS" chart previously displayed in this chapter, a rough estimate would put this moderately active woman at the 2200 calorie per day level. At this level, she is advised to include at least 9 servings from the Bread Group, 4 servings from the Vegetable Group, 3 servings from the Fruit Group, 2-3 servings from the Meat Group, and 2-3 servings from the Milk Group.

Using the U.S. Dietary Guideline of 30% calories from fat, she could have up to 73 grams of fat per day. (At the preferred 20% calories from fat level, the grams of fat are reduced to a maximum of 49 grams.) Total added sugars, assuming no more than 6% of calories allotted for added sugars beyond the naturally occurring simple sugars in foods, are best limited to 32 grams or the equivalent of 8 teaspoons.

FOOD/BEVERAGES CONSUMED	# SERVINGS PER FOOD GROUP					Grams	
	Bread	Vegetable	Fruit	Milk	Meat	Fat	Added Sugar
BREAKFAST							
1 croissant	1					12 gr.	2 gr.
8 oz. orange juice			1				
8 oz. coffee/sugar/cream				1/8			9 gr.
SNACK							
8 oz. coffee/sugar/cream				1/8			9 gr.
1 piece chewing gum							4 gr.
LUNCH							
fish sandwich w/ tartar sauce	2				1	23 gr.	
french fries		1				12 gr.	
12 oz. cola soft drink							36 gr.
SNACK							
1 1/2 oz. chocolate bar w/ almonds						14 gr.	19 gr.
DINNER							
beef burrito	1	1/2		1	1	11 gr.	
8 oz. beer							
1/4 cup guacamole		1/2				6 gr.	
1/2 cup Spanish rice	1					2 gr.	
1/2 cup refried beans					1/2	1 gr.	
1 serving tortilla chips	1					8 gr.	
1/4 cup hot sauce		1/2					
SNACK							
1 scoop rich vanilla ice cream				1		11 gr.	14 gr.
TOTALS	7	2 1/2	1	2 1/2	2 1/2	100 gr.	93 gr.

The first sample menu features what could be expected if she ate the standard fast-food American diet. As you can see, while the number of servings per food group meets the suggestions for dairy and protein, this menu is lower than the suggested goals for bread, vegetable, and fruit—the food groups that should form the basis of her diet. Both fat and added sugars are significantly higher than they ideally should be for good health, a consequence of making choices within each of the food groups that are high in fat.

The second menu offers a more healthy alternative of the first sample. In this menu, suggested goals for bread, vegetable, milk, and meat have been met. One more serving of fruit would have been ideal, although It must be emphasized that the Food Guide Pyramid is a suggested meal plan, not a rigid guide. The amount of fat consumed is fairly close to the 20% calories from fat level of 49 grams. The amount of added sugars is much lower than the maximum suggested, an optimum situation.

FOOD/BEVERAGES CONSUMED	# SERVINGS PER FOOD GROUP					Grams	
	Bread	Vegetable	Fruit	Milk	Meat	Fat	Added Sugar
BREAKFAST							
1 buckwheat maple muffin	2				1/4	8 g	5 g
1/2 cup nonfat yogurt				1/2			
1/2 cup unsweetened applesauce			1				
1/2 cup cooked oatmeal	1					1	
1/4 cup raisins			1				
2 Tbsp. almonds					1/4	9 g	
LUNCH							
2 slices sourdough rye bread	2					2 g	
1/2 can water-packed tuna (3 1/2 oz.)					1	1 g	
2 tsp. olive oil						10 g	
1 tsp. balsamic vinegar							
1 small tomato		1/2					
1 cup lettuce mix		1					
handful whole wheat pretzels	1/2					1 g	
1 cup tea, unsweetened							
SNACK							
1 coconut walnut chip cookie	1/2					5 g	3 g.
1/2 cup low-fat milk				1/2		3 g	
DINNER							
1 cup pinto beans					1		
1 1/2 cups cooked rice	3						
1 1/2 oz. cheese				1		14 g	
1/2 cup green beans		1					
1/2 cup cooked carrots		1					
1/4 cup hot sauce		1/2					
1 whole wheat tortilla	1					1 g	
TOTALS	10	4	2	2	2 1/2	55 g	8 g

Now write down everything you eat and drink for three days. This will enable you to get an overall picture of the way you eat, allowing for normal fluctuations in appetite, activity level, and special occasions that will undoubtedly occur. For example, eating a gooey piece of cake during a birthday party at the office will make your sugar servings for the day escalate. The next day, your sugar servings may be very low. Averaging the two days will bring a more accurate picture of your diet.

To help you use the Food Guide Pyramid diet evaluation chart, each recipe within this book is nutritionally analyzed, with the data illustrated on the simplified version of the Nutrition Facts. The Appendix offers nutrition charts for commonly consumed foods.

A good diet can still include high-fat foods, sugar, and refined grains *if* in making these choices you fully acknowledge how often and how much of these foods you consume in relation to the rest of your diet. (Obviously, this is assuming that you have no major health problems that must be accounted for. Always follow your doctor's or health professional's suggestions that have been made specifically to meet your needs.)

It all involves the concept of "trading off" and a willingness to explore new foods and new cooking techniques. "Trading off" simply means that, for example, if you want to indulge in a high-fat food, you can balance it by combining it with lower-fat foods at the same meal, at any meal throughout the day, or even the next day. No fasting or bingeing is allowed; the "trading off" should be included within your regular meal schedule. The goal is to come out with an average ratio of protein, complex carbohydrates, and fat as recommended by the 1990 U.S. Dietary Guidelines.

If you can't imagine eating a baked potato without butter or sour cream, forego the dressing on the salad at the meal, the butter

Nutrition Facts		
Serving Size 1 piece (129 g)		
Servings Per Container 8		

Amount Per Serving		
Calories 190	Calories from Fat 45	
		% Daily Value*
Total Fat 5g		8%
Saturated Fat 0g		0%
Cholesterol 0mg		0%
Sodium 40mg		2%
Total Carbohydrate 31g		10%
Dietary Fiber 2g		8%
Sugars 8g		
Protein 5g		

Vitamin A 0%	•	Vitamin C 2%
Calcium 2%	•	Iron 4%

* Percent Daily Values are based on a 2,000 calorie diet. Your daily values may be higher or lower based on your calorie needs:

	Calories:	2,000	2,500
Total Fat	Less than	65 g	80 g
Sat Fat	Less than	20 g	25 g
Cholesterol	Less than	300 mg	300 mg
Sodium	Less than	2,400 mg	2,400 mg
Total Carbohydrate		300 g	375 g
Dietary Fiber		25 g	30 g

Calories per gram:
Fat 9 • Carbohydrate 4 • Protein 4

The New Food Label

or margarine on the bread or dinner roll, and choose a low-fat cut of meat, poultry without the skin, or minimal oil, dairy, or nuts in a vegetarian entrée. Spartan fare? Not if the salad is dressed with a flavorful vinegar, the bread so delicious that no butter is needed, and the main entrée is properly seasoned with herbs and spices.

READING LABELS

To compare nutrient values of similar foods in each of the Food Guide Pyramid food groups, take advantage of the information provided on the newly revised food labels.

Since 1994, the contents and design of the nutrition information panel have been completely revamped to reflect the switch in nutritional focus from concerns about vitamin/mineral deficiencies to the relationship between nutrition and chronic disease.

Starting with their new name, "Nutrition Facts," the rules require that labels on packaged and bulk foods show total calories, calories from fat, total fat, saturated fat, cholesterol, sodium, total carbohydrates, dietary fiber, sugars, protein, vitamin A, vitamin C, calcium, and iron. Other nutritional information, such as detailed analysis of fiber indicating the amounts of soluble and insoluble fiber, or the amount of monounsaturated and polyunsaturated fats included within the Total Fat, may be listed but is not required.

Daily Values

To help consumers see how the particular food fits into an overall daily diet, several key nutrients found in the food must be declared both in terms of the amount of weight per serving and as a percentage of the "Daily Value."

Daily Values is a new label reference tool used on food labels to indicate whether the food contributes just a little or a lot of a particular nutrient. Daily Values includes both the Reference Daily Intakes, the recommended daily amounts established for adults and children aged 4 and older of 19 vitamins and minerals, and Daily Reference Values.

Daily Reference Values (DRVs) are set for total fat, saturated fat, cholesterol, total carbohydrate, dietary fiber, sodium, potassium, and protein, assuming a daily intake of 2000 calories, an amount representative of the average amount of calories consumed by most adults and children aged 4 or older. Calculation of the DRVs are based on our country's dietary goals: 60% calories from carbohydrate, 10% calories from protein, less than 30% calories from fat with no more than 10% calories from saturated fat, and at least 11.5 grams of fiber per 1000 calories. Maximum limits for total fat, saturated fat, cholesterol, and sodium are suggested at the bottom of the label.

You won't find any information about fats or cholesterol on labels of infant and toddler foods made for children under the age of two. Adequate fat intake is vitally important during these years to ensure satisfactory growth and development.

There are a couple of ways you can use the Daily Values. If your daily caloric intake is approximately 2000 calories, you can add up the percentages of Daily Values for single nutrients in all foods you have consumed during the day with a total of 100% indicative that your diet fits within the government's dietary recommendations. If your calories vary from the 2000 calorie reference amount, you can calculate what the equivalent total percentage would be for your specific needs. For example, for a 1600 calorie diet, your total percentage of Daily Value can add up to 80%. A 2800 calorie diet could use 140% as the daily target amount.

You can also use the percentage of Daily Values listed on the label to compare like products, to quickly choose which one is more nutrient-dense.

Speaking the Same Language

The new standardized serving sizes make nutritional comparisons of similar products much easier. Rather than leaving it up to the discretion of the manufacturer who may be tempted to finagle the serving sizes to make its product look nutritionally superior, the serving sizes now reflect the amounts that people actually eat at one time.

Nutrient content claims like "low-fat," "low-cholesterol," "good source of," "high in" and "reduced" will mean the same for any product on which they appear.

Even the term **"healthy"** has regained believable status. Foods touted as "healthy" must have no more than 3 grams or less of fat (1 gram or less of saturated fat), no more than 480 milligrams (mg.) of sodium (360 mg. by 1998) and at least 10% of the Recommended Daily Intake (RDI) of either calcium, protein, fiber, or vitamins A or C. Foods packaged as meals, such as frozen dinners, are allowed a sodium limit of 600 mg. (480 mg. by 1998), but must contain at least 10% of the RDI for two or three of the six named nutrients.

"**Fresh**" may be used to distinguish a raw, unprocessed food. However, according to the FDA, "fresh" foods still include those that have been subjected to treatments routinely used in the distribution and handling of raw produce, including the post-harvest application of pesticides, waxes, coatings, mild chlorine or mild acid washes, and irradiation (ionizing radiation) under 1 kiloGray.

Not allowed to be labeled as "fresh" are foods that are treated with chemical treatments such as antioxidants, antimicrobial agents, or preservatives "that introduce chemically active substances that remain in or on the food to preserve or otherwise affect the food" (Federal Register, Vol. 58, No. 3. January 6, 1993).

"Fresh" can also be used to describe ingredients within otherwise processed foods. For example, a spaghetti sauce made with raw tomatoes that are subsequently cooked in the process of making the sauce can still be represented on the label as containing fresh tomatoes. However, if the sauce were made using tomatoes that are first processed and sold to the manufacturer in that form, such as tomato paste, "fresh" would not be an appropriate term to describe the tomatoes. "Fresh" frozen means food that has been quickly frozen while still in a fresh state.

Even though ready-to-eat bread is not a food that exists in a raw state, the FDA believes using the term "fresh" to describe bread will not confuse or mislead consumers as to what they are buying. Neither does

the phrase "fresh" milk present a problem. Even though, in some states, milk from healthy, clean cows is allowed to be sold as raw milk, in most people's minds fresh milk simply means milk that is not old, whether raw or pasteurized.

Regarding the term "**natural**," for the time being the FDA is staying with their current policy, restricting the term only when it involves added color, synthetic substances, and flavors. In these specific areas of concern, "natural" means that nothing artificial or synthetic, including color additives, regardless of their source, is included or added to the food.

The term "**organic**" will now be regulated by the U.S. government to ensure that any food that claims that some or all of the ingredients are "organic" abides by the regulations spelled out in The Organic Foods Production Act of 1990. Simply stated, organic ingredients are those which are produced without the use of toxic pesticides, herbicides, and fertilizers according to an agricultural method that improves and sustains the health of the environment. For more details on organic, refer to "The Organic Solution" found in the next chapter under the discussion of incidental additives.

Health Claims

Because it is recognized that what we eat can affect our risks for certain diseases, several claims are allowed to be used on food labels linking a nutrient or food to the risk of a disease or health-related condition. These include:

•calcium and a lower risk of osteoporosis
•fat and a greater risk of cancer
•saturated fat and cholesterol and a greater risk of coronary heart disease
•fiber-containing grain products, fruits, and vegetables and a reduced risk of cancer

NUTRIENT LABEL CLAIM DEFINITIONS*

LABEL CLAIM	DEFINITION
•Good Source, Contains, Provides	10-19% of the Daily Value
•High, Rich In, Excellent Source Of	20% or more of Daily Value
•Fortified, Enriched, Added	Contains at least 10% more of the Daily Value, compared to the reference food

Calorie-Related Claims

•Calorie-free	less than 5 calories
•Low calorie	40 calories or less
•Reduced calorie	At least 25% fewer calories
•Light or lite	At least 1/3 fewer calories or 50% less fat

Fat-Related Claims

•Fat-free	Less than 0.5 grams fat
•Low-fat	3 grams or less fat
•Reduced fat	At least 25% less fat
•Saturated fat-free	Less than 0.5 grams fat
•Low saturated fat	1 gram or less saturated fat and no more than 15% calories from fat
•Reduced saturated fat	At least 25% less saturated fat

Cholesterol-Related Claims

•Cholesterol-free	Less than 2 grams cholesterol and 2 grams or less saturated fat

*Per standard serving size. Some claims have higher nutrient levels for main dish products and meal products, such as frozen entrées and dinners.

NUTRIENT LABEL CLAIM DEFINITIONS

•Low cholesterol	20 mg. or less cholesterol and 2 grams or less saturated fat
•Reduced cholesterol	At least 25% less cholesterol and 2 grams or less saturated fat

Sodium-Related Claims

•Sodium-free	Less than 5 mg. sodium
•Very low sodium	35 mg. or less sodium
•Low sodium	140 mg. or less sodium
•Reduced sodium	At least 25% less sodium
•Light (or Lite) sodium	50% less sodium than normally used on the food
•Unsalted or No salt added	No salt added during processing

Sugar-Related Claims

(Sugars include table sugar (sucrose), milk sugar (lactose), honey, corn sweeteners, high fructose corn syrup, molasses, fruit juice concentrate, maple syrup, brown rice syrup, barley malt.)

•No added sugars	None of the above sugars is added during processing. It contains no ingredients that contain added sugar. The product it resembles and substitutes for normally contains added sugars.
•Sugar-free	Less than 1/2 gram sugars
•Reduced sugar	At least 25% less sugar

Lean/Extra Lean Meat and Poultry Claims

•Lean	Less than 10% total fat, less than 4 grams saturated fat, less than 95 mg. cholesterol per reference amount and 100 grams
•Extra Lean	Less than 5 grams total fat, less than 2 grams saturated fat, less than 95 mg. cholesterol per reference amount and 100 grams

•fruits, vegetables, and grain products that contain fiber and a reduced risk of coronary heart disease

•sodium and a greater risk of high blood pressure

•fruits and vegetables and a reduced risk of cancer

Criteria for use are quite strict. There are three basic criteria that must be met: 1) The food must not exceed set nutrient levels to qualify for a health claim. For example, per standard serving size for a food product, it must have no more than: 13 grams of fat, 4 grams saturated fat, 60 mg. cholesterol, and 480 mg. sodium.

2) The food must meet specific nutrient requirements for each of the health claims.

3) A food must contain at least 10% of the Daily Value of one or more of: protein, dietary fiber, vitamin A, vitamin C, calcium, or iron.

Full Disclosure

The new food labels also require more detailed information.

All FDA-certified color additives must now be listed by name rather than the nondescript, all-inclusive term "color." Previously, only Yellow #5 was required to be specifically listed, due to the number of people allergic to the additive.

Sources of hydrolyzed vegetable proteins, a flavor enhancer used in many foods, must now be specifically named.

Foods that claim to be nondairy, such as coffee whiteners and soy cheese, but include caseinate as an ingredient must now indicate that caseinate is derived from milk.

Beverages that claim to contain juice are required to declare their total percentage of juice on the label.

Exemptions

But don't expect everything you eat to sport a label. Foods served in restaurants, airplanes, from vending machines, sidewalk vendors, cookie and candy counters, or ready-to-eat food prepared and sold primarily on-site such as bakery, deli, or candy store items, are not required to be sold with a nutritional label. Foods produced by small businesses are also exempt.

If the food package has less than 12 square inches available for labeling, they are exempt from printing the nutritional data on the label but they must provide an address or telephone number to enable consumers to obtain the information, if so desired.

Additives and Alternatives

A FOOD ADDITIVE is a substance that is not normally consumed as a food by itself but added either intentionally or indirectly. Indirect or incidental additives are those that are the result of contact with the food during growing, processing, packaging, or storing before the food is consumed.

INTENTIONAL ADDITIVES

Relatively innocuous food additives such as salt, smoke, and spices have been used for thousands of years, primarily as a means to maintain a steady supply of food through times of scarcity.

As rural populations moved to the cities and relinquished their previous control over the growth and preparation of basic foods, the role of food additives changed dramatically. Substances were intentionally added to extend available food sources, to cut manufacturing costs, and to manipulate the characteristics of a food.

By the late 19th century, it wasn't uncommon for cocoa to contain brick dust, cheese and candy to be contaminated with copper and lead salts, and bread to include chalk and bone ashes. Often the same batch of dye used to color textiles would be used to color foods.

Thanks to concerned consumers, journalists, and especially Dr. Harvey Washington Wiley, the chief of the U.S. Department of Agriculture's Bureau of Chemistry from 1883-1912, the safety of food additives was ardently challenged. Through their efforts, The Pure Food and Drug Act was enacted in 1906. The Act defined pure and adulterated food and prohibited the manufacture and shipment of adulterated or misbranded foods and drugs. Further refinements occurred in the 1938 Food, Drug, and Cosmetic Act.

Responsibility for proving the safety of an additive lay with the U.S. Food and Drug Administration (FDA). During and after World War II, hundreds of new compounds were introduced as a means to protect and enhance foods, particularly for military purposes. This dramatic increase in additives soon overwhelmed the capacity of the FDA to monitor and adequately test the chemicals in foods.

The Food Amendment of 1958 attempted to remedy the situation in a number of ways. For the first time, the burden of proof concerning the safety of a food additive switched from the FDA to the food manufacturer who petitioned its use. The Amendment's **"Delaney Clause"** mandated that no substance that is known to cause cancer in animals or human beings at any dose level could be used in any food. And a new category regarding the safety of food additives was introduced: **GRAS (Generally Recognized as Safe)**.

Generally, recognition of safety is based on proven safety through scientific testing or, in the case of substances introduced and used prior to January 1, 1958, through experience based on extended, common use in food. Both synthetic and naturally derived substances are included. Unlike other food additives, no limits were specifically set for the amount that could be added to foods. Rather, they are allowed to be used in accordance with good manufacturing practices (GMPs) in which the quantity does not exceed the amount reasonably required to accomplish its intended function.

Many of the most widely used and suspect food additives used today are found on the GRAS list. The artificial sweetener, saccharin, and the preservative, BHT, are just two of the GRAS substances which are now steeped in controversy. Even when under investigation, these substances are allowed to be used.

Safety Doubts

Children are particularly vulnerable to additives in foods. Because they have special needs for high-quality, nutrient-dense foods to fuel continued growth spurts, poor-quality, additive-laden foods severely compromise their ability to maximize both mental and physical potential. Children's immune systems are less developed than adults' and are less capable of dealing with even moderate amounts of artificial colors, flavors, and preservatives. Behavior problems, insomnia, apathy, listlessness, and fatigue are often consequences of marginal malnutrition.

Unfortunately, the use of food additives remains a grand experiment. Scientific analysis is only as reliable as currently accepted testing methodology. Repeatedly, more sophisticated techniques have exposed problems with previously approved substances.

Artificial colors are a good example. The 1960 Color Additives Amendment forbids the use of colors shown to induce cancer in laboratory animals. Since that time, many previously accepted certified colors have, one by one, been shown to be toxic or carcinogenic. New labeling laws require that certified color additives must be declared by their common/usual name, not collectively as previously allowed under the general term "colorings."

Noncertified colors, those from natural rather than synthetic sources such as annatto extract, caramel, grape skin extract, and paprika oleoresin, are considered GRAS substances. They may be declared collectively as "color added" or even under the potentially confusing phrase "artificial color." No doubt, most foods that contain naturally derived colors will be declared by their common/usual name.

Critics of the above-mentioned Delaney Clause claim that sophisticated testing can make it look like everything causes cancer and that its continued acceptance inhibits research and development towards scientific progress.

Although common in the early 1900s, food chemicals cannot be tested on humans before the substances are subjected to extensive animal studies. Now, animals such as rats, mice, and dogs are subjected to huge doses of an additive, many times the normal human dose, in hopes that the effects will be detected in a few hundred animals in a matter of months rather than decades.

However, results in animal studies, either pro or con, don't constitute absolute proof that a human being will react accordingly. Neither can we test to see the synergistic effect between the additive in question and other components of a diversified diet. As a result, once an additive is approved or maintained on the GRAS list, all we can do is hope that the FDA's interpretation of their studies and those given by the manufacturer are conclusive.

Then, are all food additives harmful? Should they be avoided entirely? Not at all. Many additives offer beneficial results without harmful consequences. For instance, vitamin C is often used as a natural antioxidant to keep foods from spoiling. Ferrous gluconate provides a source of iron and also gives black olives their characteristic color. Sodium bicarbonate (baking soda) is used to react with acids in quick bread batters to make baked goods rise.

Unfortunately, however, the most widely used additives are those intended merely to make food look and taste "better," including coloring agents, flavoring agents, and flavor enhancers. A case in point is the use of monosodium glutamate.

Monosodium Glutamate

Monosodium glutamate (MSG) is a flavor enhancer that is commonly found in commercially prepared frozen dinners, snacks, spice mixes, soups, casseroles, and sauces. MSG is also sold to consumers to be used as a seasoning added during cooking.

MSG was originally isolated in 1908 as the component, specifically glutamic acid, in kombu seaweed that was responsible for the flavor-enhancing properties of dashi, the Japanese broth made with kombu that forms the basis of Japanese cuisine. MSG is now synthetically produced from a fermentation process of starch or molasses. The end product is a pure, white, crystalline form of MSG, much more concentrated that what is naturally occurring in kombu.

In its "bound" form when linked with other amino acids to form proteins, glutamic acid (glutamate) does not provide any special flavor-enhancing benefits. It's only in its "free" form, unbound to protein, that its flavor-enhancing properties and potential risks arise. Free glutamic acid occurs naturally at low levels in foods such as soy sauce, kombu seaweed, mushroom, tomatoes, and Parmesan cheese. It's a well-known fact that cooks have traditionally used these foods as ingredients in recipes to help enhance flavors of various entrees without any harmful side effects. In contrast, pure, concentrated forms of free glutamic acid as present in synthetic MSG have been shown to cause some serious reactions in sensitive individuals. Problems with synthetic MSG were first identified in 1968 and originally linked to soup served in Chinese restaurants, hence MSG's infamous nickname, "Chinese Restaurant Syndrome." Although many people can ingest MSG without any apparent effects, several people have reported symptoms including headaches, tightness in the chest, burning sensations in the forearms and the back of the neck, asthma attacks, migraine headaches, and skin rashes.

Some people are concerned that "natural flavors" may hide the presence of MSG. However, by law, foods purchased from the grocery stores that contain concentrated, isolated MSG are labeled as such. On the other hand, no labeling is required for restaurant foods that contain MSG. The only way you'll know is if you ask.

Contrary to popular belief, hydrolyzed vegetable protein, a flavor enhancer derived from wheat, soybeans, or milk, does not contain isolated MSG. In the process of manufacturing MSG, some free glutamate is formed from the interaction of sodium with the glutamic acid derived from protein. There's always the possibility that sensitive individuals could react to foods that contain hydrolyzed vegetable protein; however, the sensitivity could just as easily be from the protein source used in manufacture. To alleviate any fears many manufacturers have replaced the hydrolyzed vegetable protein found in some of their foods with substances like nutritional yeast.

New food labeling requires that hydrolyzed vegetable protein added to foods must be listed as a separate ingredient rather than being included as a natural flavoring. The identity of its protein source must be revealed on the label. Acceptable names include hydrolyzed wheat gluten, hydrolyzed soy protein, autolyzed yeast extract, and hydrolyzed casein.

Food Irradiation

Although including food irradiation along with intentional additives may not seem like a right fit, the FDA classifies it as such because its use affects the characteristics of a food.

Food irradiation is a process in which food is exposed to gamma radiation from radioactive materials such as cobalt-60 or cesium-137 or through linear accelerator electron beams to kill bacteria, insects, or parasites that may be present in food. Cobalt-60, the material used in most irradiation facilities, is a radioactive isotope manufactured in the Canadian Candu nuclear reactors from cobalt metal. Cesium-137 is a waste product from the reprocessing of spent fuel from other nuclear reactors. Even though the doses are too weak to actually make the food radioactive, they are strong enough to disrupt the chemical bonds that hold molecules together, thus killing or inhibiting the growth of organisms that cause disease and spoilage.

A typical chest X-ray delivers a dose of 1/100 of one rad (radiation absorbed dose). In contrast, the amount of energy used in food irradiation is considerably higher, measured in units called "Grays" where 100,000 rads= 1000 Grays= 1 kiloGray (1kGy). One kilogray increases the shelf life of some fruit and vegetables by changing the chemistry

of their cells to slow ripening and rotting. Higher doses, 4.75 to 8 kilograys, kill salmonella. (Poultry is allowed to undergo irradiation at 3 kGy.) Very high doses, up to 30 kGy used to irradiate herbs and spices, renders foods sterile.

History of Irradiation

Food irradiation in the United States has been developed primarily at government expense. It all started with the U.S. Army's post-World War II research to create good-tasting, economical, shelf-stable field rations for the troops. Interest in food irradiation research and development further expanded in both the government and private sectors during the early to mid-1950s.

Progress slowed after the passage of the Food Additives Amendment to the Federal Food, Drugs, and Cosmetic Act of 1958 when Congress and administrative agencies classified irradiation as a food additive rather than a process. Companies wishing to use irradiation were required to petition the FDA with appropriate toxicological studies proving that the proposed use was safe.

The first approved use of irradiation occurred in 1963 with canned bacon, wheat, and wheat products. When further evaluation of the data raised doubts that the safety of radiation-sterilized bacon had been demonstrated, approval for its use on bacon was revoked in 1968.

The FDA established the Bureau of Foods Irradiated Food Committee in 1979 to review the agency's policies regarding irradiation and to recommend how to test more accurately for the effects of food irradiation.

The committee estimated that 1 kGy irradiation dose would form 30 parts per million of "radiolytic products," a class of molecules formed when the ions produced by radiation react with other molecules in the food. They also acknowledged that 10% of these molecules could likely be new unknown compounds of which there would be no prior knowledge of their specific type or effect. Despite the fact that it takes only one mutant molecule to start cancer, the committee concluded that at doses below 1kGy, any single "unique" radiolytic product of unusual toxicity would be negligible.

Because it is impossible to test a food for the amount of radiation administered, the Committee based their evaluation of irradiation primarily on theoretical estimates extrapolated from radiation chemistry. Unbelievably, in 1981, the FDA completely reversed its testing policy, concluding that an adequate margin of safety had been demonstrated for foods irradiated below 1 kGy. Without the burden of testing, new uses of food irradiation were approved more quickly.

To date, approval has been given to irradiate pork, fresh fruits and vegetables, dry or dehydrated enzyme preparations, herbs and spices, and poultry. Irradiation of ground beef is also being considered.

More Concerns

Besides the introduction of unique radiolytic products whose effects are unknown and, therefore, suspect, several questions and concerns about irradiation cannot be ignored.

Significant nutrient losses occur during the process, particularly vitamins C and A, beta carotene, and the B vitamins.

While high doses of irradiation can kill bacteria like salmonella and other potentially dangerous microorganisms, both the FDA and the World Health Organization emphasize that irradiation is not a substitute for careful handling, storage, and cooking of food—the primary way foods are contaminated with salmonella in the first place.

Botulism also remains a major concern. Doses above 1 kGy irradiation can significantly retard microbial spoilage but not eliminate it. At the same time, the irradiation process kills the odorous bacteria whose bad smell we depend upon to warn us that contamination has taken place.

And there's evidence that some foods are actually more vulnerable to fungi and insects *after* irradiation. Likewise, irradiation causes several fruits, including pears, apples, citrus fruits, and pineapples to spoil faster than normal.

Environmental Impact

Increased transport and handling of dangerous radioactive materials, danger of exposure to workers, and increased production of radioactive wastes with no place to put them, make irradiation a major cause for concern.

Contamination of the environment due to accidents and safety violations is also a very real possibility. Results of an eight-month study commissioned by the Environmental Protection Agency (EPA) released in April 1992 indicated that more than 45,000 locations nationwide that use radiation, including factories and hospitals, are potentially contaminated by radioactivity. With more food irradiation plants, the risks naturally increase.

Labeling

Careful label reading won't guarantee you'll be able to avoid irradiated food. The FDA currently requires single-ingredient foods that are irradiated, such as a bag of flour, a piece of produce, etc., to be labeled with the phrase "treated by irradiation" as well as the flower-like international irradiation logo. However, a multiple-ingredient food product which may contain one or more irradiated ingredients does not require labeling, such as a packaged pilaf mix that contains irradiated dried mushrooms.

And, although it's hard to believe, new labeling regulations now allow the word "fresh" to describe foods that have been irradiated at levels no higher than 1 kGy.

As many manufacturers are waiting to see how consumers react to the reality of irradiation, the strongest statement you can make is to avoid buying irradiated foods.

What To Do About Food Additives

It's actually very easy to avoid questionable food additives. Just read food labels and buy accordingly. Since manufacturers will produce only what they know will sell, responsibility for safe foods now and in the future depends on us, the consumers. Already, in response to the renewed interest in nutrition and safe foods by consumers, manufacturers have modified numerous products. Many breakfast cereals and vegetable oils are now manufactured without preservatives. Natural alternatives are replacing artificial flavorings. Ironically, many manufacturers have repeatedly claimed that certain foods couldn't be made without an additive and that the world would starve due to the increased expense of manufacturing foods without it. Interestingly enough, once manufacturers decided that more consumers wanted to avoid these additives, the technology to produce foods without them "magically" appeared.

Even so, the typical American diet is amply laced with foods that are little more than additives, so you need to read food labels carefully. Avoid products that contain artificial colors, flavors, sweeteners, and preservatives. Support the many manufacturers who have removed harmful additives completely from their products or have never used them in the first place. Familiarize yourself with additives you may not recognize.

ADDITIVES ROASTING ON AN OPEN FIRE

Today's typical holiday menu at Grandmother's house may appear similar to those of yesteryear, but, unfortunately, that's often where the similarity ends.

Instead of basting the turkey throughout the day with its natural juices, Grandmother may opt for a self-basting turkey that is injected with a blend of both partially hydrogenated and liquid soybean oil, highly saturated coconut oil, water, salt, sodium phosphate, emulsifiers, and artificial flavor.

Instead of stuffing the turkey with a mixture of bread, giblets, onion, celery, and sage, she may use a prepared dry stuffing mix based on enriched, bromated wheat flour embellished with corn syrup, salt, partially hydrogenated oils, seasonings, flavor enhancers such as disodium inosinate and disodium guanylate and preserved with calcium propionate, sodium sulfite, BHA, BHT, TBHQ, citric acid, and propyl gallate.

Even more lamentable is the indignity that has been cast on our hallowed pumpkin pie. Instead of making the traditional homemade flaky pie crust, Grandmother may depend on chilled prepared pie crusts made from wheat starch, hydrogenated lard preserved with BHA and BHT, bleached flour, water, wheat gluten, salt, xanthan gum, sodium propionate and potassium sorbate as preservatives, citric acid, and artificial color, including FD & C Yellow #5.

And, more often than not, usual the crowning touch of freshly whipped cream has been replaced by nondairy whipped topping fabricated from corn syrup, hydrogenated coconut and palm kernel oils, natural and artificial flavors, emulsifiers, thickeners, and artifical color.

Is nothing sacred?

Exploring Intentional Food Additives

Several types of food additives are detailed throughout the book in connection with their use in specific foods. Refer to the list below to find particular food additives that may be of interest.

Grains (in general)—nutrient enrichment and fortification

Breakfast Cereals—additives that decrease cooking time

Flour—bleaching and maturing agents

Breads—emulsifiers, enzymes, dough conditioners, fermentation accelerators, preservatives, chemical leaveners

Meats—preservatives (including nitrates), binders, fillers

Poultry—preservatives

Fish—preservatives

Fruits—sulfur dioxide

Milk, Yogurt, & Cheese—emulsifiers, thickening agents, fat substitutes, animal and vegetable rennet, calcium caseinate (imitation cheeses)

Sweets—artificial sweeteners and other sweetening agents, sulfur dioxide

INCIDENTAL ADDITIVES

Incidental additives include residues from packaging chemicals, pesticide residues, and fumigants applied during transportation and storage, and drugs administered to farm animals.

Packaging materials for foods may be treated with fungicides, fumigants, and insecticides to protect the packaging and, therefore, the product itself, from moisture, mold, and insects. It may also be treated with preservatives to increase product shelf-life. However, none of these are inert. Unfortunately, as an incidental additive, the type of treatment it has been subjected to doesn't need to be listed on the package. Microwavable packaging is also suspect. Plasticizers and other components of packaging have the potential to leach into the food contained within.

The incidental additives of most concern are agricultural chemicals.

Agricultural Chemicals

In the past twenty-five years, farmers have dumped over 5 billion pounds of insecticides onto their crops, more than 11 billion pounds of herbicides into the soil, and almost 2 billion pounds of fungicides—all in the hopes of a good harvest. While thirty years ago, the health effects of pesticides were rarely considered, no longer is there any doubt that agricultural poisons pose health risks to farm workers. What we don't know are the long-term chronic effects of pesticide exposure on the general population, in particular, our children.

History of Farm Chemicals

Our reliance on fertilizers and pesticides developed as an outgrowth of the successful application of pesticides to control malaria-bearing mosquitoes and head lice during World War II.

In the quest for greater agricultural productivity and prosperity, cheap chemicals based on petroleum and oil were substituted for higher-priced labor-intensive weed and insect control methods. Fertilizers and pesticides made it possible to switch from a diversified system of agriculture to intensive, one-crop (monoculture) farming, increasing yields of picture-perfect crops on less acreage. Annual pesticide use today totals approximately 470 million pounds.

Although defenders of pesticides continually claim the benefits outweigh the risks involved, any risk/benefit analysis must include the assessment of their overall effect and expense to growers, consumers, taxpayers, public health, and the environment.

The Environment

While most of the talk about food and pesticides has focused on the effects of pesticides on human health, their impact on our environment and our economy is devastating. Water pollution is the most damaging and widespread environmental effect of agricultural production. More than 50% of suspended sediments reaching lakes, rivers, and streams originate from agricultural land in the form of runoff from fertilizers, pesticides, and animal waste. Herbicides are being detected in drinking water samples from intensely farmed states in the Midwest, despite conventional water treatment and more sophisticated carbon-filtration systems.

Detectable levels of organo-chlorine pesticides, such as DDT, are found in several fish, shellfish, and bird species and in water-borne sediments, particularly in the Great Lakes area of the country. Even though the use of most persistent organo-chlorine pesticides has been phased out of the United States, they continue to enter the environment as inert ingredients that are used in a few currently used pesticides and through their continued use worldwide.

Until the late 1970s, it was generally accepted that groundwater was protected from agricultural chemical contamination by impervious layers of rock, clay, and soils. However, since agencies increased their monitoring efforts in the late 1970s, pesticides have been detected in the groundwater of twenty-six states, not from the misuse of agricultural chemicals but as a result of normal agricultural activities.

A 1985 U.S. geological survey projected that at least 20% of the nation's wells are contaminated with nitrate from excessive amounts of nitrogen fertilizers in the soil. As high levels of nitrates can potentially interfere with the ability of the blood of infants to absorb oxygen, infants under the age of six months and pregnant or lactating women are especially at risk.

Soil erosion is another source of water pollution. Instead of utilizing crop rotation and conservation tillage methods, modern agriculture since the 1940s has emphasized continuous planting of a single crop in the same field year after year. As a result, soil has been depleted of its nutrients and is more susceptible to increased risk of erosion. In fact, the nation as a whole has lost over 1/3 of its topsoil, losing it eighteen times faster than it is being replaced. Since the nutrients and water-holding capacity of the soil have been reduced, causing rooting depth to be restricted, crop productivity has been adversely affected, requiring the use of even more fertilizers.

Are Pesticides Effective?

Although the eradication of pests is one of the major reasons for using pesticides, over a third of our food crop is lost before harvest. In fact, crop losses inflicted by insect pests have nearly doubled from 7% to 13% since the early 1940s, despite a tenfold increase in pesticide usage.

The modern practice of intensive monoculture is contrary to natural ecosystems which normally consist of a variety of compatible plant communities. Altering the soil nutrients, especially through depletion resulting from monoculture, can influence the density of pests feeding on it. Pesticides are also responsible for killing some of the natural predators of destructive pests. It is also estimated that 428 insects and mites are now resistant to pesticides, requiring the development of new, more effective pesticides. And, oddly enough, the use of pesticides can alter the physiology of crops and make them more susceptible to pest attack.

About 2/3 of all insecticides and fungicides are applied aerially while herbicides in row crops are applied by spray rigs pulled by tractors. A particularly disturbing fact is that except for direct spraying of weeds and trees, very little of applied pesticides even reaches the target pests—in some cases, less than 1%. Most of what is applied moves into the ecosystems to contaminate the land, water, and air, affecting not only wildlife, but our own health as well.

Exploring Incidental Additives

In the succeeding chapters you'll find detailed information on specific production and processing methods that are contributors of incidental additives. Refer to the list below to find particular subjects that may be of interest.

Whole Grains—lime-processing of corn
Breads—sodium hydroxide (pretzels)
Meat—growth hormones, antibiotics
Poultry—antibiotics, salmonella
Fish—environmental pollutants, microbiological hazards, parasites, antibiotics, dyes
Eggs—salmonella
Nuts—aflatoxins
Milk, Yogurt, & Cheese—growth hormones (including BST), antibiotics
Fats & Oils—hydrogenation and trans-fats, solvent extraction, oil refining

THE ALTERNATIVE TO CHEMICAL FARMING

Many waves were created in the agricultural community following the 1989 publication of *Alternative Agriculture*, the results of the National Academy of Science's landmark four-year study concerning the scientific and economic viability of adopting alternative agricultural systems. The committee appointed to thoroughly analyze the situation were convinced that if widely adopted, alternative methods of agriculture would produce an ample food supply with a corresponding reduction of our nation's environmental problems and health concerns due to pesticide residues.

Alternative systems more deliberately integrate and take advantage of naturally occurring, beneficial interactions. Instead of depending on chemical intensive farming methods, alternative agricultural systems emphasize management, biological relationships between pest and predator, and natural processes such as nitrogen fixation from cultivated legumes which are then plowed under.

Included under the auspices of alternative agriculture are integrated pest management (IPM) and certified organic food production techniques.

Integrated Pest Management (IPM) production methods minimize dependence upon chemicals through physical, cultural, biological, genetic, and preventative means. Alternative practices include setting up traps and barriers to discourage insects, rotation of crops, the introduction of natural predators to kill target pests, the breeding of naturally resistant plant strains, and quarantines when necessary. Pesticides and herbicides remain an option. While IPM is a step in the right direction, it's still no guarantee that the product is grown without agricultural chemicals.

The Organic Solution

Certified organic agriculture is a management-intensive production method designed to achieve a balance in the agricultural system similar to that found in natural systems to produce healthy soils and, therefore, high-quality crops and livestock.

While it's true that organic foods are produced without the use of toxic pesticides and fertilizers and minimally processed without artificial ingredients, preservatives, or irradiation, the best way to describe the basic precepts of organic agriculture is to repeat what is written in the Organic Foods Production Act of 1990.

"Organic farming practices are based on a common set of principles that aim to encourage stewardship of the earth. Organic producers:
•Seek to provide food of the highest quality, using practices and materials that protect the environment and promote human health
•Use renewable resources and recycle materials to the greatest extent possible, within agricultural systems that are regionally organized
•Maintain diversity within the farming system and in its surroundings, including the protection of plant and wildlife habitat
•Replenish and maintain long-term soil fertility by providing optimal conditions for soil biological activity
•Provide livestock and poultry with conditions which meet both health and behavioral requirements
•Seek an adequate return from their labor, while providing a safe working environment and maintaining concern for the long-range social and ecological impact of their work."

The Organic Foods Production Act of 1990 was passed in order to ensure consumers that anything they buy labeled as certified organically grown has been produced according to federally approved, nationwide standards.

Under the auspices of the U.S. Department of Agriculture, the National Organic Standards Board, composed of individuals representing all facets of agriculture, developed the guidelines and procedures which will regulate all crops from produce, grains, meat, dairy, eggs, and processed foods. Beginning in 1995, it will be a federal offense to sell or label an agricultural product as organically produced, or to affix a label or provide any other market information that implies directly or indirectly that the product is organically produced, unless the product is produced and handled in accordance with the requirements established by the program.

Farms wishing to be certified must complete an Organic Farm Plan, a written document, to be updated annually, that details how the organic farm is managed. It must address the key elements of organic crop product, including soil and crop management, resource management, crop protection, and maintenance of organic integrity through growing, harvesting, and post-harvest operations.

In addition to certifying farms as organic, processors, distributors, shippers, packers, and retailers who process organic agricultural products must also be certified as handlers of organic product. They, too, must present a yearly plan which details procedures that prevent commingling of the organic with nonorganic products, pest management systems that are within the guidelines of the 1990 Organic Food Production Act, and the establishment of an audit trail. A key component to assuring organic integrity, an audit trail is a lot number or serial number system that can trace all raw materials from the supplier, through the entire plant process, and on through the distribution system to the retailer.

Meat, poultry, and dairy products can also be certified as organically grown. Their own Organic Farm Plan must address livestock health, care, and breeding practices without depending on the use of antibiotics, manure management, sourcing of animals, certified organic feed sources, feed contigency plans for shortages and emergencies, maintenance of organic feed integrity from field to feeding, housing and living conditions, record keeping, animal handling practices, pasture and grazing land management, ecosystem oversight to reduce the environmental impact of animal production practices, and, if applicable, appropriate details for ensuring integrity of organic animals if animals raised along conventional practices are also present on the farm.

And, finally, manufacturers and processors of organic products must be certified that they use only accepted ingredients and processing methods.

The percentage of organic ingredients must be declared on the information panel above the ingredient listing. To be labeled as an organic product, it must be made of 95% certified organic ingredients. A product containing a minimum of 50% certified organic ingredients may be labeled as "made with organic ingredients." Each organic ingredient must be identified in the ingredient declaration with the words "organic" or "organically grown". The name and address of the certifying agent must also appear on the label.

Buy organic and dramatically reduce the sources of incidental additives in your diet. Support alternative, sustainable agriculture. It's a safe investment.

BIOTECHNOLOGY

Biotechnology is the application of new technologies of genetic modification to bacteria, plants, and animals to improve specific characteristics of these organisms. Although it is not considered a food additive, the increasing number of processing aids, foods, and animal drugs developed in this manner warrant a discussion of what it means and why some people are concerned.

Genetically engineered foods are produced by removing the specific genes or group of genes responsible for a certain trait and splicing in other genes that are seen as more desirable. In some cases, genes containing unwanted traits are blocked and not replaced. The overall purpose of genetic manipulation is to develop new varieties more resistant to insects, better in flavor, texture, or color, more durable to the rigors of shipping, or able to stay "fresh" longer. The replacement genes can originate from bacteria, plants, insects, fish, animals, or possibly even humans.

While there's no denying that today's plants and animals bear little resemblance to their wild ancestors, their evolution has occurred gradually and systematically through both natural selection and selective breeding. Commonly referred to as "survival of the fittest," modification of species through natural selection requires thousands of generations. Those plants and animals with certain characteristics best adapted to the environment tend to survive longer and produce similarly adapted offspring.

In traditional breeding methods, specific plants or animals with desired traits are interbred until that trait becomes part of a new variety. Recent breeding has developed cows to produce more milk and chickens with more breast meat. Quicker than natural selection, selective breeding still requires several generations to get the desired results.

In contrast, genetic engineering enables humans to manipulate genes much more effectively and precisely than had been possible before. However, unlike the slow processes of natural selection and selective breeding which stay within the confines of a species, many believe that genetic engineering steps outside those boundaries, going completely contrary to the laws of nature.

Since the 1970s more human-compatible forms of insulin as well as human growth hormone were developed from genetically altering bacterial DNA to replace animal-derived sources. And while, at least in theory, the beneficial aspects of genetic engineering seem boundless, several safety and ethical questions come up with the use of genetic engineering in food development.

The FDA requires labeling of bioengineered foods only if the transferred gene is from a food known to be a common allergen. Other bioengineered foods may be sold without informing consumers of their origin, therefore compromising the ability of individuals who wish to avoid certain foods either for personal, cultural, or religious reasons to choose foods that correspond to their own belief system.

Other concerns include the possibility of changes in the foods, otherwise natural nutritional value, as well as the bioavailability of the nutrients themselves; the possibility of producing plants with higher levels of natural toxins than normal which may cause adverse reactions in humans and other animals that eat the plants; and the introduction of unknown substances into the food supply.

The FDA claims that genetically engineered foods are just as safe as those conventionally bred. While the agency has always required approval of bioengineered foods if the nutritional value or level of toxins has significantly changed or if developed from a known allergen, it has relied on the companies themselves to make the decisions whether they needed to consult with the FDA about their new product. Fortunately, the FDA has revised its original guidelines to require all companies to at least describe the safety tests they've done before they can proceed to market.

Perhaps it's just that it just sounds so bizarre. Or maybe it's because introducing these products into the food system seems too premature, lacking the assurance of foods bred over the course of time. At the very least, it makes sense to require that all bioengineered foods be labeled as such so that consumers can decide for themselves whether they want genetically engineered foods on their table.

BREAD, CEREAL, RICE & PASTA GROUP

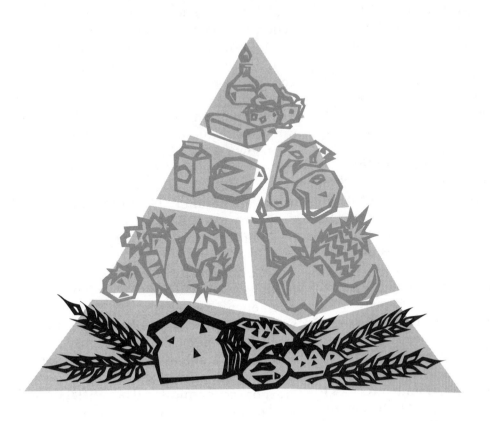

Whole Grains

UNTIL YOU'VE eaten a grain in its whole form, you'll have never experienced the full flavor and texture inherent in the grain. Although this is not a form of grain most people are accustomed to cooking, renewed interest in nutrition and traditional cuisines has revitalized the art of cooking whole grains.

But there's another benefit beyond taste, one a bit more esoteric. More than any other food, whole grains contribute a stabilizing effect on both body and mind. Perhaps it's because the preparation of some grains takes a little extra time or maybe it's because they take longer to chew. Whatever the case, eating whole grains may just help you to slow down, even for just a few minutes, and reintroduce some simplicity into your life.

So what can you do with cooked whole grains? They can be the focal point of the meal served with a simple sauce or light sprinkling of nuts or seeds; topped Chinese-style with a variety of vegetables; prepared as a side dish with beans, meat, or poultry; cooked with dried fruit for breakfast; tranformed into casseroles, croquettes, salads, or stuffings; or appreciated for its texturizing attributes in soups.

You've probably used rice in preparation of many of these dishes. Now try substituting other whole grains in familiar recipes to experience new dimensions of tastes and textures. Then let your creative juices go wild.

NUTRITION

As the richest source of complex carbohydrates, grains contain both starch and fiber. Starch is a polysaccharide comprised of hundreds to thousands of glucose units. As it slowly digests in the body, its glucose units are released into the blood to fuel both muscles, nervous system, and the brain, what many people refer to as "blood sugar." When the body has more glucose than it needs for immediate energy, extra glucose is stored in muscles and in the liver as glycogen, a long polymer composed of many glucose units.

In addition to its fame as promoter for intestinal regularity, the fiber in grains helps slow down the digestion of starch to encourage sustained blood sugar levels. Fiber also fills us up faster. Combined with the fact that grains are naturally low in fat, a diet based on grains will help keep your weight to its optimum level without much work on your part.

Another major role for complex carbohydrates is to spare protein from being used as an energy source so it can do the work it was meant to do. Unlike grains, protein foods are an inefficient and expensive source of energy. Meals based on grain supplemented with moderate amounts of protein are more economical and beneficial towards achieving peak stamina and performance in whatever we do.

While even refined carbohydrates contain energy-producing starch and some protein, whole grains are significantly higher in fiber as well as B-vitamins and trace minerals. A look at the basic structure of a whole grain will explain why.

Consider a whole grain as a seed waiting to germinate into a plant. The germ at the base of the seed is the life force of the grain, the part that sprouts when sown. It contains vitamin E, unsaturated fats, B vitamins, and protein—all the nutrients needed to get the sprout going during its initial growth phase.

The endosperm, comprising 80% of the weight of the seed, consists of starch and protein as stored fuel to nourish the sprouted grain during its early growth.

The bran protects the germ and the endosperm until conditions are right for germination. As the outer covering of the grain, it contains the highest concentration of fiber and is rich in B vitamins and minerals.

Cooking a grain in its whole seed form will provide us all the nutrients originally stored for germination of the seed into a plant. On the other hand, refined grains are processed to remove the bran and germ, leaving only the endosperm. So, while white flour, white pasta, white bread, and refined breakfast cereals contain the complex carbohydrates and protein found in the endosperm, you'll miss out on 22 various nutrients found in the bran and germ.

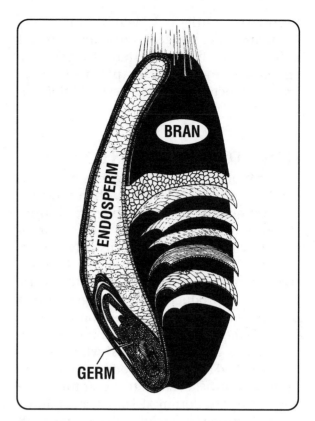

ENRICHMENT

Enrichment of refined wheat flour, breads, macaroni products, cornmeal, and white rice, as well as milk, margarine, and salt, came about as a result of health surveys in the late 1930s which revealed alarming nutritional deficiencies in B vitamins, iron, and iodine. The American Medical Association, the National Research Council, the National Academy of Sciences, and several public health authorities decided a good ploy would be to fortify commonly consumed refined foods.

In 1941, the FDA set standards for the use of the term "enriched" used on grain products as the addition of three B vitamins: thiamine (B_1), riboflavin (B_2), and niacin (B_3) as well as iron. In response to research showing that adequate intake of folic acid prior to conception dramatically reduces the incidence of the neural tube defects (spina bifida and anencephaly), folic acid was added to the enrichment list in 1993.

While not required to by Federal law, most states have accepted the enrichment standards. As a consequence of interstate commerce, regardless of state standards, most refined flour and flour products are enriched to ensure their wide distribution.

Considering that only four out of the

twenty-two nutrients depleted during refinement are being replaced, enrichment is just a drop in the bucket. Perhaps programs to encourage higher consumption of whole grain products would have been a better suggestion.

HOW TO BUY AND STORE

Look for plump, unbroken grains with uniform size and color, organic when possible. For best quality and flavor, buy grains from stores that have a high turnover of products. Buying grain in bulk is usually less expensive, but only buy bulk if the bins are tightly covered and constructed to ensure rotation of product. Bulk packages should be nitrogen-flushed to prevent rancidity.

The more whole the grain, the more resistant it is to rancidity. Most whole grains can be stored at moderate room temperature up to 6 months, even up to a year for barley and rolled oats. Cornmeal, kamut, and quinoa are more prone to rancidity due to their high oil content. Along with cracked grains, they should be stored at cool room temperatures (below 70° F) or refrigerated. Refined grains lack the natural oils found in bran and wheat germ, so they can be stored up to a year.

Grain pests such as weevils and mealworm moths can be avoided by storing grains in clean, airtight containers. Do not keep grains in plastic or cellophane bags bound with a twist-tie or rubberbands. Instead, use glass jars or rigid plastic containers with good seals.

PREPARATION GUIDELINES

All whole grains should be rinsed prior to cooking to remove dirt and dust which may have settled during processing or storage. For best results, place the grain in the cooking pot, add approximately twice the amount of cool water, and swish the grain to allow grit to rise to the top. Carefully strain off the water to remove the grit, repeating the process one or two more times to ensure that all the dirt is washed away.

Just as there are many varieties of grains, there are many ways to prepare them. Each cooking method contributes a special quality and texture.

Boil/Simmer

Appropriate year-round in any climate, the boil and simmer method is most commonly used. Depending on the amount of water added, the texture of simmered grain can range from somewhat dry and dense to moist or almost soupy.

To cook, bring the liquid to a boil in the pot and add the grain and a pinch of salt (optional). Allow the liquid to return to a boil, cover, and reduce the heat to a low simmer until the grain is cooked and the liquid is absorbed. To prevent a sticky texture, avoid stirring or removing the lid during cooking. Allow the pot to stand undisturbed for 5-10 minutes before fluffing with a fork to separate the grains.

Pre-roasting, Boil/Simmer

Dry-toasting or oil-sautéing the grain before cooking enhances the flavor of the grain. Dry-toasted grain cooks up dry, and light and fluffy. Oil-sautéed grain, generally used when making a pilaf, results in a soft, moist texture with more separate individual grains.

Over medium heat, toast the grain in a dry skillet or sauté it in 1-3 teaspoons of oil or butter. With either method, stir constantly until slightly browned and fragrant, taking extra care not to burn the grain. Next, add the appropriate proportion of boiling water or stock plus a pinch of salt to the grain. Return the water to a boil, reduce the heat, cover, and simmer until the grain is cooked.

Pressure Cooking

Pressure cooking yields a softer, sweeter, more densely textured grain. Due to its concentrated nature and warming effect on the body, pressure cooking is more appropriate during autumn or winter months.

In general, use 1/2 cup less water than normal per 1 cup dry grain as required, unless a softer consistency is desired. Add the washed grain, salt, and water to the pressure cooker and bring to full pressure. Place a flame deflector under the pressure cooker to distribute the heat evenly and to prevent burning. Reduce the heat to medium low and start gauging the cooking time.

When done, remove the pressure cooker from the heat and let the pressure come down naturally. If pressed for time, place the pressure cooker in the sink and run cold water over the lid until the pressure comes down. With either method, let the grain sit in the unopened pressure cooker for 5 to 10 minutes before serving.

Baking

Cooking grain in an oven is a handy method to use when all the burners on your stove are already in use. Since hot ovens generate plenty of heat in the kitchen, you'll probably want to limit use of the baking method to colder months of the year.

In a 400° F. oven, the grain will cook somewhat longer than grain that is boiled and simmered. First, sauté 1 cup of grain with 1 tablespoon of oil or butter in a stove- and ovenproof pot. (Another alternative is to use a regular saucepan for the stovetop operations while preheating a covered baking dish in the oven.) Add water and bring to a boil, cover, and place the grain in the oven for approximately an hour until the water is absorbed and the grain is tender.

Sprouting

Whole grains can also be sprouted. During the process of sprouting, protein and vitamin content increases. Enzymes convert the stored complex carbohydrates into simpler sugars.

Although technically any grain can be sprouted, barley, buckwheat, and wheat are usually easiest to grow. Buckwheat is usually grown in soil and eaten like lettuce. Barley and wheat sprouts are steamed and eaten like cereal. They can also be dried and ground for use as a sweetener to improve flavor and texture in breads. Some breads are made from 100% sprouted grain.

For detailed instructions about how to sprout, refer to the Vegetable Group chapter.

Seasoning Grains

Adding a pinch of salt per cup of grain enhances the grain's naturally sweet flavor. Salt's flavor permeates the food while cooking, helping reduce or eliminate the tendency to add more salt or soy sauce at the table.

Cooking grain with salt may also improve its digestibility. Chlorine, one of the main minerals found in salt (sodium chloride), is an important component of our body's digestive juices.

Another way to vary the flavor of the grain is with fresh or dried herbs. Add fresh herbs during the last few minutes of cooking. Dried herbs can be added at the start of the cooking process.

Consider using liquids other than water to cook grains such as vegetable, meat, and fish stocks or diluted fruit and vegetable juices.

COOKING TIMES AND LIQUID PROPORTIONS

Depending on appetite and accompaniments to the meal, one cup raw whole grain yields enough cooked grain to serve 2-4 people. When cooking more than 1 cup of grain at a time, use slightly less liquid than would normally be used if multiplied proportionally. For example, if 1 cup millet requires 21/2 cups water, for 11/2 cups millet use 31/2 cups water instead of 4 cups. To shorten cooking time by approximately one-third, presoak grains 6-8 hours.

Grain (1 cup)	Water	Cooking Time	Yield
Amaranth	21/2-3 cups	20-25 minutes	21/2 cups
Barley, pearled	3 cups	60 minutes	31/2 cups
Barley, whole soaked	3 cups	60 minutes	31/2 cups
Barley flakes	3 cups	25 minutes	31/2 cups
Barley grits	2 cups	10 minutes	2 cups
Buckwheat	2 cups	20 minutes	21/2 cups
Bulgur	2 cups	15-20 minutes	21/2 cups
Cornmeal (polenta)	4 cups	25 minutes	3 cups
Couscous	11/2 cups	15 minutes	3 cups
Cracked Wheat	2 cups	25 minutes	21/3 cups
Kamut, whole soaked	3 cups	30-40 minutes	3 cups
Kamut, flakes	2 cups	15-18 minutes	21/2 cups
Millet	21/2 cups	35 minutes	31/2 cups
Oats, rolled	2 cups	10 minutes	21/2 cups
Oats, steel-cut	2 cups	30 minutes	3 cups
Oats, whole	3 cups	90 minutes	3 cups
Quinoa	2 cups	15 minutes	31/2 cups
Rice, Brown	2 cups	45 minutes	3 cups
Rice, White Aromatic	13/4 cups	15 minutes	21/2 cups
Rice, Arborio	3 cups	20-25 minutes	3 cups
Rice flakes	3 cups	25-30 minutes	3 cups
Rye, whole soaked	4 cups	45 minutes	31/2 cups
Rye flakes	3 cups	25-30 minutes	3 cups
Spelt, whole soaked	3 cups	30-40 minutes	3 cups
Spelt flakes	2 cups	15-18 minutes	21/2 cups
Teff	4 cups	15-20 minutes	3 cups
Triticale flakes	2 cups	15-20 minutes	2 cups
Wheat berries soaked	3 cups	45 minutes	3 cups
Wheat flakes	3 cups	30 minutes	3 cups
Wild Rice	3 cups	60 minutes	4 cups

Exploring Your Options

AMARANTH

Facts and Features

Amaranth, referred to as "the grain of the future," is actually a rediscovered ancient Aztec seed harvested from a broad leaf plant. Although it is difficult to plant and hard to harvest, amaranth is naturally resistant to weeds and can grow in poor soil and drought conditions, making it a promising crop for otherwise unproductive areas. It is a high-yield crop with each plant producing up to 500,000 seeds about the size of poppy seeds. Ranging in color from purple-black to buff yellow, golden-colored seeds are the ones most often used for food. Amaranth is commonly available organically grown.

Amaranth is high in fiber and rich in calcium, iron, and phosphorus, offering superior nutrition. It is especially noted for its high concentration of lysine, the amino acid usually found in limited proportions in grains. Since the extra lysine makes its protein of higher quality than any other grain except quinoa, it is included in recipes to improve the protein balance. And because amaranth is gluten-free, it is also a favorite with individuals allergic to wheat and/or other gluten-containing grains.

Varieties and Cooking Guidelines

Whole Amaranth can be prepared by itself, like any other whole grain, but its strong and nutty, mildly spicy flavor and unusual sticky gelatinous texture is self-limiting in some recipes. However, once you begin to incorporate amaranth into your recipes, you will appreciate not only these unique character-istics, but amaranth's versatility as well.

To prepare amaranth, combine 1 part amaranth and 3 parts water, add a pinch of salt, bring to a boil, reduce heat and simmer for 20-25 minutes. Plain cooked amaranth

POPPED AMARANTH

1 Tbsp. whole amaranth

Heat a wok or deep heavy skillet until very hot. Add 1 tablespoon amaranth and move the seeds constantly with a pastry brush to prevent them from burning. Remove popped amaranth into a bowl and, if more is desired, add another tablespoon and continue popping.

Makes 1/4 cup.
(Pyramid Servings: 1/2 Bread/Grain Group)

Nutrition Facts

Serving Size 1/4 cup (12 g)
Servings Per Container 1

Amount Per Serving	
Calories 45	Calories from Fat 5

	% Daily Value*
Total Fat 1g	1%
Sodium 0mg	0%
Total Carbohydrate 8g	3%
Dietary Fiber 2g	7%
Protein 2g	

Calcium 2%	•	Iron 6%

Not a significant source of Saturated Fat, Cholesterol, Sugars, Vitamin A and Vitamin C.
* Percent Daily Values are based on a 2,000 calorie diet.

congeals as it cools, so eat it immediately or keep it warm until ready to eat.

However, amaranth is best when cooked in a 1:3 proportion with another grain. Cook according to the predominant grain's instructions.

Amaranth can also be popped like popcorn. It turns rancid quickly so make only what you'll use immediately. Use popped amaranth as a snack, as a substitute for bread crumbs, or in granola, soups, stews, and cakes for added texture and flavor.

For extra crunch in cookies, muffins, and quick breads, add a tablespoon of raw amaranth along with the basic batter ingredients.

Flavor Enhancers: onion, garlic, parsley, cumin, bell peppers, lemon, and olive oil.

Menu Companions: Amaranth blends well with brown rice, buckwheat, and millet.

BARLEY

Facts and Features

Barley is an old soul. It was one of the first grains grown and cultivated to provide food for both humans and animals. During the early Roman empire and the Middle Ages, barley was associated with poverty since coarse, heavy breads made with it were typically consumed by the poor.

Whole hulled barley is a good source of protein, potassium, calcium, iron, B vitamins, and fiber. Due to its two hard inedible husks, most barley except for high beta-glucan barley, is milled to some degree in order to be usable. The term "pearling" is used to describe the gradual process of refining barley down to the grain's endosperm layer. After the husks, bran, and germ are completely removed, the remaining grain looks very much like a pearl. Depending on the extent of the processing, pearled barley contains significantly less of these nutrients. Some brands of barley are pearled up to six times more than other brands. For the highest protein, fiber, vitamins, and minerals, look for the largest kernels, pearled only enough to remove some of the tough outer layers.

Recently a substance that inhibits cholesterol production in the blood has been found in barley. Fortunately the cholesterol-inhibiting substance in barley is found in the nonfibrous portion of the grain, so even pearled barley can make this claim.

In addition to its fame for thickening soups and stews, barley is an excellent hot breakfast cereal and a base for warming pilafs or cooling summer salads. When roasted and ground, barley is also an ingredient in many coffee substitutes. When sprouted, dried, and ground, it has been used to make malt for use both as a sweetener and as an ingredient in making beer.

Barley contains small amounts of gluten.

Varieties and Cooking Guidelines

Whole hulled barley is lightly pearled to remove its tough outer hull. With the delicate aleurone layer (which includes the germ and the bran) left intact, whole hulled barley is the most nutritious form of barley.

However, because it is only minimally processed, whole barley requires the longest cooking time. To cook, add barley to cold water, add a pinch of salt, bring to a boil, reduce heat, and continue cooking for 90 minutes. Presoaking the barley for about six hours decreases the cooking time to 60 minutes and produces a softer grain. To pressure cook 1 cup barley, use 2 cups water and cook 25 minutes. When cooked, barley expands fourfold.

CREAMY BARLEY SALAD

1 cup pearled barley
3 cups water
1/2 tsp. dillweed
1 green pepper, diced
3 ribs celery, diced
4 oz. mushrooms, medium
   thick sliced
1 bunch green onions,
   thinly sliced
2 teaspoons canola oil
1/2 cup cooked fresh peas
   or frozen, thawed
2 Tbsp. white miso
3 Tbsp. brown rice
   vinegar
4 Tbsp. water

Combine barley, water, and dillweed in a pot. Bring to a boil, reduce heat to low and cook 45 minutes to an hour. Meanwhile, prepare vegetables. Sauté all vegetables except peas in oil until crisp/tender. Blend miso, vinegar, and water. When barley is done, mix in sautéed vegetables, peas, and miso dressing while the barley is still warm. Allow to cool and let flavors meld before serving.

Serves 6.
(Pyramid Servings: 1 Bread/Grain Group, 1/2 Vegetable Group, 2 grams Fat)

Nutrition Facts

Serving Size 1/6 recipe (246 g)
Servings Per Container 6

Amount Per Serving

Calories 160   Calories from Fat 20

	% Daily Value*
Total Fat 2g	3%
Sodium 110mg	4%
Total Carbohydrate 32g	11%
Dietary Fiber 7g	28%
Sugars 2g	
Protein 5g	

Vitamin A 4%	•	Vitamin C 25%
Calcium 4%	•	Iron 10%

Not a significant source of Saturated Fat and Cholesterol.
* Percent Daily Values are based on a 2,000 calorie diet.

Barley flakes are produced from lightly toasted pearled barley rolled into flakes. Use like oatmeal in casseroles, cookies, breads, or as a thickening agent in soups and stews. To make a hot cereal, add 1 cup barley flakes to 3 cups boiling water and a pinch of salt. Lower heat, cover, and simmer for 25 minutes or until water is absorbed.

Barley grits are made from toasted and cracked scotch barley, reducing cooking time down to about 20 minutes. Use as a hot cereal, for puddings, or to thicken soup. A tasty breakfast "bread" can be made by spreading cooked barley grits in an oiled baking dish. When cool, it can be cut into individual pieces and topped with nut butters and apple sauce or fried like cornmeal mush and topped with syrup.

Fine pearled is the most extensively pearled barley and, therefore, the whitest, smallest, and least nutritious. Using 3 cups water per 1 cup barley, cook for about 35-40 minutes.

Hato mugi or "Job's Tears" has a teardrop shape that resembles barley. Since only the outer husk is removed it is a good source of dietary fiber. The seed of a wild grass cultivated for over 4000 years in China, hato mugi has been used extensively in Oriental medicine to strengthen the stomach and nervous system and purify the blood.

Like wild rice, its pleasant nut-like flavor permeates the dish. Generally, it is cooked along with other grains, soups, or stews rather than prepared alone. For a good balance of flavor and texture, use one part hato mugi to four parts of another grain. Cook about 10 minutes longer than is usually required for the primary grain.

High beta-glucan hulless barley is a new hybrid of barley that does not require pearling and, therefore, has more of the soluble fiber, called beta-glucan. Most of the inedible hull comes off during combining and harvesting. The remaining hull is removed as the barley is run through an aspirator.

Unlike conventional barley, the starch in high beta-glucan hulless barley remains relatively stable during freezing and thawing—a plus if you freeze casseroles or barley-based soups. Its flavor is also significantly more full-bodied and earthy.

Like whole hulled barley, high beta-glucan hulless barley takes longer to cook than pearled barley. Soak 1 cup grain in 4 cups of water for 6-8 hours or overnight. Using the same water, cook 45 minutes or until done. If the barley is left unsoaked, plan on simmering hulless barley 90 minutes.

Medium pearled is the most commonly packaged barley, pearled longer than scotch barley, just until the grains are white. Cook for about 45 minutes using 3 cups water per 1 cup barley.

Scotch or pot barley is pearled somewhat longer than whole hulled barley, leaving it with the distinction of being the largest variety of pearled barley. To cook 1 cup dry barley, combine with 3 cups water and cook for approximately 60 minutes.

Flavor Enhancers: onions, mushrooms, parsley, thyme, garlic, chives, cilantro, basil, dill, and peas. Add salad dressings, oils, and vinegars when the barley is still warm.

Menu Companions: Both regular barley and hato mugi combine well with rice.

BUCKWHEAT

Facts and Features

Despite its name, buckwheat is not related to wheat or to any other grain. Instead, it is the edible fruit seed of a plant related to rhubarb. Brought by Dutch and German settlers to the United States, the name "buckwheat" is a variation on its Dutch name, "bockweit," and the German "Bucheweizen" (beechwheat). Both peoples named it as such since its three-cornered kernels resembled beechnuts in appearance while its nutritional qualities seemed more similar to wheat.

Buckwheat is rarely grown with agricultural chemicals since fertilizer tends to encourage too much leaf growth and pesticides destroy the bees needed for buckwheat's pollination.

With its high proportion of all eight essential amino acids, especially lysine, buckwheat is close to being a complete protein. It also contains good amounts of calcium, iron and B vitamins.

Buckwheat is gluten-free.

Varieties and Cooking Guidelines:

Kasha or **roasted buckwheat** has undergone extensive roasting, giving it an assertive flavor and drier texture when cooked. Traditional foods such as kasha varnishkes, stuffed cabbage rolls, or dumplings are based on kasha.

To prepare kasha the traditional way, coat 1-2 cups grain with one beaten egg prior

BUCKWHEAT PILAF

1 Tbsp. safflower or corn oil
1 1/2 cups buckwheat groats, raw or toasted
1 small onion, diced
3 medium potatoes, cut in 1-inch chunks
3 stalks celery, cut in 1-inch diagonals
3 cups boiling water
1/2 tsp. dried thyme
1 tsp. tamari soy sauce
Parmesan cheese (optional)

To prepare this recipe with untoasted buckwheat groats, first roast the groats in oil over low heat for 5 minutes. Add remaining ingredients, bring to a boil, cover, reduce heat, and simmer 20 minutes.

Serve this savory pilaf with fish, tofu, or a dash of Parmesan cheese. Make instant knishes by wrapping some of the pilaf in tortillas.

Serves 6.
(Pyramid Servings: 1 Bread/Grain Group, 1 Veg. Group, 3.5 grams Fat)

Nutrition Facts

Serving Size 1/6 recipe (265 g)
Servings Per Container 6

Amount Per Serving

Calories 230   Calories from Fat 30

	% Daily Value*
Total Fat 3.5g	5%
Sodium 75mg	3%
Total Carbohydrate 48g	16%
Dietary Fiber 6g	23%
Sugars 2g	
Protein 7g	

Vitamin C 20% • Calcium 6%

Iron 10%

Not a significant source of Saturated Fat, Cholesterol and Vitamin A.
* Percent Daily Values are based on a 2,000 calorie diet.

---

to cooking. Over medium heat, stir the egg/kasha mixture constantly until toasted. The egg coating serves to seal each groat, preventing the kasha from becoming mushy. Then add the toasted grain to 2 cups boiling water with a pinch of salt. Reduce the heat and simmer 15-20 minutes until the water is absorbed.

Unroasted whole white buckwheat has a mild flavor and soft texture, making it the variety of buckwheat to use if serving with delicately flavored foods. If a more nutty flavor is desired, white buckwheat can be dry-roasted or sautéed in butter or oil, stirring constantly for 2-3 minutes. To cook, add 1 cup buckwheat to 2 cups boiling water. Add a pinch of salt, reduce heat, cover, and simmer for 15-20 minutes. Unlike kasha, white buckwheat does not require or benefit from

the egg treatment.

To make buckwheat "polenta", combine 1 1/2 cups white or roasted buckwheat with 4 cups water. Bring to a boil, reduce heat, and simmer about 25 minutes or until the buckwheat becomes so thick that a spoon can stand upright in it. Transfer the buckwheat into an oiled baking dish and allow to cool one hour. Cut into polenta strips, slices, or cubes. Or leave it uncut, spread with pesto or pizza sauce and veggies, and bake at 400°F for 15 minutes.

Buckwheat grits or **"cream of buckwheat"** is cracked from unroasted white buckwheat. Requiring only 10-12 minutes cooking, buckwheat grits make a delicious, very digestible hot cereal similar to cream of wheat.

To cook, bring 2 1/2 cups water to a boil. Add a pinch of salt and 1/2 cup cream of buckwheat. Reduce heat and simmer 10-12 minutes. When spread in a baking dish and allowed to cool, buckwheat grits can be sliced and reheated or fried like savory polenta or breakfast instead of pancakes.

Sprouting: With its hard, inedible black three-cornered shell intact, buckwheat can also be sprouted.

Flavor Enhancers: onions, parsley, sage, poultry seasoning, garlic, red bell pepper, thyme, mushrooms, black pepper, and potatoes.

Menu Companions: Traditional kasha varnishkes blends kasha with bow tie pasta. For a lighter dish, cook quinoa with buckwheat using the same water proportions and cooking time.

CORN

Facts and Features

Corn is one of the few native grains of the Western Hemisphere. Unlike most grains, corn is rarely cooked and served in its whole grain form. Instead, it is usually ground and then cooked or further processed into such forms as tortillas, cornbread, corn flakes, polenta, tamales, corn chips, and, especially, popcorn. As the basis for corn starch, corn syrup, and even fructose, corn also is a major component found in many convenience foods.

Corn is the only grain that contains vitamin A, with yellow corn containing more than white. In its whole, undegerminated form, corn is also a good source of B vitamins, vitamin C, potassium, and fiber.

However, it also has significant nutritional deficiencies. Besides being low in two essential amino acids, tryptophane and lysine, most of its niacin (50-80%) is bound by another molecule, making it unavailable to the body.

In the past, whole regions and cultures, including the southern United States, Spain, and Italy have suffered devastating epidemics of pellagra, a serious disease caused by niacin deficiency, from eating a primarily corn-based diet. The disease manifests itself in the four "D's": diarrhea, dementia, dermatitis, and, if not controlled, death.

Fortunately, many native cultures instinctively cooked whole corn with slaked lime (calcium hydroxide), wood ashes (potassium hydroxide), or lye (sodium hydroxide). Today, slaked lime is most often used.

Slaked lime is related to limestone, that is, calcium carbonate. Heating limestone to decomposition will yield quicklime or calcium oxide. When quicklime is added to water, it bubbles wildly and creates a great deal of heat, forming a powerful alkali. Slaked lime is formed from the aftermath of quicklime's reaction with water, creating a less caustic alkali.

Not only does this alkalinizing treatment with slaked lime help remove the corn's tough outer hull for easier eating and processing, it improves the amino acid balance, liberates the bound niacin, and, in the case of slaked lime, provides calcium, as well.

The distinctive slightly sour flavors of corn tortillas, corn chips, hominy, and masa harina can also be attributed to their manufacture from alkaline-treated corn.

Aflatoxin concerns

It is also important to buy corn products from reputable suppliers and manufacturers. Field corn is especially vulnerable to aflatoxin, a carcinogenic toxin produced by a fungus called Aspergillus flavus. This mold grows best on plants that are weakened by insects or stressed from the lack of moisture during drought.

The last major aflatoxin outbreak occurred in 1988 when a significant amount of the Midwest's drought-stricken corn harvest was shown to contain dangerous levels of aflatoxin.

Like other molds produced in nature, the fungus that produces aflatoxin is impossible to completely eliminate. No hybrid varieties of corn have been found to be resistant to the mold and there is no safe way to rid crops of aflatoxin once the mold's growth has begun. However, there are precautionary steps that farmers and manufacturers can do to minimize the amount in our food. Strong, healthy plants, irrigated when necessary, naturally resist the mold which produces aflatoxin. Because of the emphasis on growing methods which regenerate the land, organically grown plants resist aflatoxin best, making them less vulnerable to the stress conditions of drought. After-harvest outbreaks of aflatoxin can be avoided by proper drying and storage in cool, dry environments from the farm to the manufacturer.

Your best bet is to buy organic whenever possible and support companies with high integrity who routinely analyze their corn for aflatoxin as soon as it arrives at their dock or manufacturing plant.

Corn is gluten-free.

Varieties and Cooking Guidelines

Stone-ground cornmeal is made from corn kernels crushed under millstones. Since the nutritious corn germ is retained in the process, fresh stoneground corn has a rich corn flavor. Keep stoneground cornmeal refrigerated and use within 3 months.

To cook, use 4 parts water to 1 part cornmeal. Bring water to a boil, slowly whisk in cornmeal, and cook for 25-30 minutes. Cornmeal is also a natural in breads, muffins, and pancakes.

Blue corn has been used for thousands of years by Hopi and Navajo Indians of the Southwestern United States. A longer growing season, lower yields, and manual harvesting contribute to its higher price. Blue corn's deep, purplish-blue kernels turn pale grey when ground, and lavender when mixed with water. Sweet, nut-like in flavor, its texture is more coarse than yellow or white cornmeal. Nutritionally it contains 21 percent more protein, twice the manganese and potassium, and up to 50 percent more iron than other varieties of corn.

To cook, use 4 parts water to 1 part blue cornmeal. Bring water to a boil, slowly whisk in cornmeal, and cook for 25-30 minutes. Be adventurous and use blue cornmeal to make purple pancakes, muffins, and cornbread.

Corn germ is especially rich in B vitamins, minerals, and vitamin E. Like wheat germ, corn germ can be sprinkled on cereal, salads, or yogurt, or added to breads and muffins before baking. Due to its high oil content, corn germ should be refrigerated and used quickly.

Corn grits are a coarse cereal made from cornmeal from which the bran and usually the germ are removed. Stone-ground grits, processed to retain the bran and germ, are preferable. Unlike true hominy grits, corn grits are not processed with lime.

To cook, use 4 parts salted water to 1 part corn grits. Bring water to a boil, add grits, and cook for 25-30 minutes.

Degerminated cornmeal is ground between massive steel rollers that separate out the fiber and corn germ, leaving a nutrient-depleted and less flavorful grain. Because all the natural oils are removed, degerminated cornmeal is more shelf-stable than stoneground, making it a common ingredient in

COOKED HOMINY

1 cup whole dry corn or whole dry hominy

To cook hominy, you'll first need to obtain a source of slaked lime (calcium hydroxide) or clean wood ashes. Ethnic markets and local tortilla factories will probably sell lime. If you're planning to use your own wood ashes, they must be from clean hardwood (no paint or preservative-impregnated wood) burned without the help of newspapers or chemical firestarters. Sift the ashes before use to get rid of small pieces of wood that may remain.

Soak 1 cup of whole dry corn overnight or 8 hours in a stainless steel pressure cooker with 2 cups water.

If using wood ashes, add 2 more cups water and 1/4 cup wood ashes. Bring the cooker to pressure and cook 1 1/2 hours until corn has softened and the hulls have loosened. Drain the liquid and thoroughly rinse the corn of the ashes. Add 2 cups fresh water and 1/4 tsp. salt (if desired), return the cooker to pressure, and cook for another 1/2 hour.

If using slaked lime, drain soaking water, put corn in a saucepan with fresh water to cover, bring to a boil and add 1/4 tsp. slaked lime. Boil 10 minutes, uncovered, and then set aside for 1/2 hour, covered with a lid. Rinse the corn well and remove any loose outer skin from the kernels. When using lime instead of wood ashes, you have your choice of doing the remaining cooking in a pressure cooker or in a regular pot on the stove. Pressure cook for 1 hour or stovetop cook for 1 1/2 hours until the corn is tender.

Serves 4.

(Pyramid Servings: 1 1/2 Bread/Grain Group)

Nutrition Facts

Serving Size 3/4 cup cooked (219 g)
Servings Per Container 4

Amount Per Serving

Calories 150   Calories from Fat 20

	% Daily Value*
Total Fat 2g	3%
Sodium 20mg	1%
Total Carbohydrate 31g	10%
Dietary Fiber 6g	22%
Protein 4g	

Vitamin A 4%	•	Iron 6%

Not a significant source of Saturated Fat, Cholesterol, Sugars, Vitamin C and Calcium.
* Percent Daily Values are based on a 2,000 calorie diet.

---

low-quality quick cornbread and pancake mixes.

To cook, use 4 parts water to 1 part cornmeal. Bring water to a boil, slowly whisk in cornmeal, and cook for 25-30 minutes.

High-lysine corn is a hybrid that contains up to 70% more than ordinary corn, along with higher levels of tryptophan, isoleucine, threonine, and other amino acids. The cornmeal ground from this strain has an exceptionally nutty, sweet, delicious flavor.

To cook, use 4 parts water to 1 part cornmeal. Bring water to a boil, slowly whisk in cornmeal, and cook for 25-30 minutes. It is exceptional in breads, muffins, and pancakes.

Hominy, whole flint or dent corn processed in slaked lime (calcium hydroxide) or wood ashes, is also known as **posole**, or **samp** (broken hominy). The whole, cooked kernels are very chewy with a slightly sweet, slightly sour, not very corn-like flavor. Hominy is used whole in soups and stews, as a grain side dish, or ground in a food processor or hand-operated steel mill to make masa.

Precooked, canned whole hominy is available in many grocery stores. Home-made hominy takes about 21/2 hours to cook, but the difference in flavor makes up for the inconvenience. At the very least you'll appreciate all the work it takes to make those corn tortillas and chips you likely devour without a second thought.

Hominy grits are from ground, dried hominy, available in coarse, medium, or fine grinds. In addition to being served as a hot cereal or as the basis for soufflés and puddings, they are a familiar side dish topped with butter and gravy in traditional Southern-style meals.

To cook, use 4 parts water to 1 part hominy grits. Bring water to a boil, slowly whisk in grits, and cook for 25-30 minutes. Quick-cooking grits are ground finer than regular grits, reducing the cooking time from 20 minutes to 5 minutes.

Masa is whole corn dough made from ground, freshly cooked hominy, typically used to make tamales, tortillas, arepas, and dumplings. It can also be served like mashed potatoes topped with butter or cheese.

Masa harina is the dried and finely ground form of hominy. The only cornmeal used to make tamales, tortillas and corn chips, it is the result of lime processing, which provides its characteristic flavor and improved protein, niacin, and calcium profile.

Polenta, Italy's culinary contribution to corn-cooking, is best made with coarse-ground cornmeal either imported from Italy or domestically grown. Made similarly to cornmeal mush, polenta is used as an appetizer, grain accompaniment, or as a main course made with or topped with herbs, cheeses, or sumptuous sauces.

To make polenta, bring 3 cups water to a boil, add a pinch of salt, and slowly add 1 cup coarsely ground cornmeal, stirring constantly. Continue stirring until the polenta thickens and stiffens, about 20 minutes. Spoon onto plates or an oiled platter and top with a sauce. Or transfer it to an oiled baking dish and allow it to cool. Slice and then bake, broil, or fry.

Popcorn is derived from another variety of corn that has a hard protein outer layer sealing inner starch layers with a moisture content between 11-14%. Under high heat the interior starch layers explode under pressure, yielding the cooked and dried light crisp kernel.

Yellow popcorn, with its corny flavor and crunchy firm texture, pops up the most, expanding 40-46 times its original size. In contrast, white popcorn has a slightly sweet taste, crisp yet tender kernels and expands 35-40 times.

Popcorn is one of the more healthy snack foods around. It contains 2 grams fiber and only 69 calories per 3 cups popped if left unadorned.

One quarter cup of popcorn kernels will yield 8 cups popped corn.

Store dry popcorn in a tightly sealed jar or plastic container, preferably in the refrigerator, to retain the moisture inside the kernels.

Flavor Enhancers: onions, chives, tomatoes, cilantro, cumin, cheese, garlic, hot and sweet peppers, chili powder, and parsley.

Menu Companions: Hominy is often cooked with dried beans. As a hot cereal, corn grits strikes a good blend with coarsely ground grains such as wheat, rye, rice, and barley.

KAMUT

Facts and Features

Kamut is a recently rediscovered, unhybridized variety of wheat believed to have originated in Egypt around 4000 B.C. Named after the ancient Egyptian word for wheat, kamut is about 2-3 times the size of a normal wheat kernel. Kamut is higher in nutrition as well. It is 20-30% higher in protein than wheat and contains more magnesium, zinc, and vitamin E.

Most noteworthy is its successful use by many wheat-sensitive individuals—despite the fact that kamut contains gluten. It may be because kamut is an ancient form of durum wheat (Triticum durum) containing only 28 chromosomes, quite different from our common variety of wheat (Triticum sativum) which has 42 chromosomes. Nonetheless, anyone severely allergic to wheat should consult with a doctor or health practitioner before trying kamut.

Kamut's flavor is rich and buttery and its texture is pleasantly chewy. Hot or cold, it makes a terrific breakfast cereal, with or without milk or soymilk. Marinated in salads it provides an interesting contrast to crisp veggies. It's also an excellent extender for soups, stews, chilis, meat loaves, and meat or grain patties.

Kamut's expanding popularity is reflected in the increased variety of kamut products available, including kamut flakes, pasta, and, especially, ready-to-eat kamut cereals.

ANCIENT GRAINS PANCAKES

1 1/2 cup teff flour
1/2 cup whole cooked kamut
1/2 cup spelt flour
1/2 cup kamut flour
2 tsp. baking powder
1/2 tsp. salt
2 eggs
1 3/4 cup milk or soymilk
3/4 cup water
1 tsp. orange extract
2 Tbsp. oil or pitted prune purée or applebutter

Preheat pancake griddle over medium heat. Stir together all the dry ingredients. Beat the eggs lightly and combine with the milk, water, extract, and oil. Add mixture to the dry ingredients and stir briefly. Ladle batter onto a lightly oiled griddle. Cook over medium heat, turning once when bubbles come to the surface and the edges are slightly dry.

Makes 18 average-sized or 8 jumbo sized
(Pyramid Servings: 1 Bread/Grain Group, 3 grams Fat)

Nutrition Facts

Serving Size 1 pancake (62 g)
Servings Per Container 18

Amount Per Serving	
Calories 100	Calories from Fat 25

	% Daily Value*
Total Fat 3g	4%
Saturated Fat 0.5g	3%
Cholesterol 25mg	8%
Sodium 85mg	4%
Total Carbohydrate 17g	6%
Dietary Fiber 3g	11%
Sugars 1g	
Protein 4g	

Vitamin A 2%	•	Calcium 4%
Iron 6%		

Not a significant source of Vitamin C
* Percent Daily Values are based on a 2,000 calorie diet.

Varieties and Cooking Guidelines

Whole grain kamut looks like a giant, soft, white humpbacked kernel of wheat. With a texture and appearance similar to pine nuts, cooked whole grain kamut is excellent in baked goods, salads, cereals, or pilafs.

Whole kamut is best soaked in cold water overnight, drained, and cooked in boiling salted water (3 parts water/1 part kamut) for 30-40 minutes until the grains are plumped and a few have burst. To pressure cook 1 cup kamut, use 21/2 cups water and cook 50 minutes.

If making more kamut than immediately needed, refrigerating extra kamut in its cooking liquid will help keep the cooked grain soft. Excess liquid should be reserved for stock.

Kamut flakes, similar to oatmeal, can be made into a hot breakfast cereal or added to casseroles and baked goods, including cookies. Combine 1 cup kamut flakes with 2 cups water, bring to a boil, and cook 15-18 minutes.

Flavor Enhancers: onion, garlic, parmesan cheese, parsley, basil, pepper, mushrooms, raisins, and lemon. For a terrific hot cereal, cook kamut flakes with vanilla extract and dried apples. Top with roasted pecans just before serving.

Menu Companions: Combine cooked kamut with rice, barley, or quinoa for appealing texture contrast in side dishes and grain-based salads. Cooked whole kamut enhances both flavor and texture in pancake batter and muffins.

MILLET

Facts and Features

Millet looks like tiny yellow round birdseed and, unfortunately in the United States, most millet is used for that very purpose. However, millet is now rising from its humble position. Interest in traditional African and Indian cooking and appreciation for its delicious, delicate flavor and soft, cohesive texture make it a favorite, quick-cooking grain perfect for basic side dishes, stuffings, "burgers," and casseroles. Small amounts cooked with stews and soups provide body. Leftover millet splashed with your favorite dressing is exceptional as a basis for a grain and vegetable salad.

In addition to phosphorus, B vitamins, and iron, millet is rich in lysine, making it a high-quality protein. Even though the outer hull is removed, the bran remains intact. It is also very alkaline, making it soothing and very easy to digest.

Always buy bright, golden-colored millet sold specifically for human consumption. Millet from feed stores or pet shops still contains the indigestible outer hull.

Millet is gluten-free.

Varieties and Cooking Guidelines:

To cook 1 cup raw millet, bring 21/2 cups water to a boil, cover with a lid, reduce heat to medium, and cook for 15 minutes. Remove from heat and let sit uncovered for 20 minutes for optimum texture and flavor. To pressure cook 1 cup millet, use 21/4 cups water and cook 20 minutes.

For a softer-textured millet similar to mashed potatoes, increase the water to 31/2 cups and simmer, covered, 45 minutes to 1 hour until the water is absorbed. Use 5 cups water or a combination of water and apple

BAKED MILLET CROQUETTES

1 Tbsp. safflower or
   sesame oil
1 cup millet
3 cups water
1/2 teaspoon salt
1/2 small onion, finely
   chopped
3/4 lb. fresh spinach
1/8 teaspoon chili powder
1 tsp. fresh dillweed or
   1/2 tsp. dried dill
1/3 cup whole wheat flour
1/3 cup walnuts or pecans

Preheat oven to 375°F. Heat oil in a large saucepan and add millet. Stir for 3 minutes until millet gives off a nutlike fragrance. Add water and salt. Bring to a boil, reduce heat to medium and cook for 20 minutes or until liquid is absorbed. Meanwhile, thoroughly wash spinach and place immediately in a hot skillet. Cover and steam over medium heat until spinach wilts. Remove spinach, drain, and finely chop. When millet is ready, stir in spinach and remaining ingredients. When cool enough to handle, form millet mixture into golf ball-sized croquettes. Place on an oiled cookie sheet and bake for 20 minutes. Serve warm with your favorite sauce or creamy salad dressing.

Serves 6
(Pyramid Servings: 1 Bread/Grain Group, 1/2 Veg. Group, 7 grams Fat)

Nutrition Facts

Serving Size 1/6 recipe (233 g)
Servings Per Container 6

Amount Per Serving

Calories 220   Calories from Fat 70

                            % Daily Value*

	% Daily Value*
Total Fat 7g	**11%**
Saturated Fat 1g	**4%**
Sodium 240mg	**10%**
Total Carbohydrate 33g	**11%**
Dietary Fiber 6g	**23%**
Sugars 1g	
Protein 7g	

Vitamin A 80% • Vitamin C 30%
Calcium 8% • Iron 15%

Not a significant source of Cholesterol
* Percent Daily Values are based on a 2,000 calorie diet.

---

juice to transform millet into a rich, creamy hot cereal or snack.

Warm cooked millet can be pressed into an oiled baking dish and allowed to cool to make sliceable polenta-like strips. Use muffin cups to make millet timbales.

Flavor Enhancers: Curry, chili powder, orange, rosemary, onion, chives, parsley, black pepper, bay leaf, thyme, garlic, ginger. To enhance millet's nutty flavor, toast it in a skillet with or without oil or butter, stirring constantly for 3-4 minutes.

Menu Companions: Quinoa, brown rice, or basmati rice are exceptionally good when cooked with millet.

OATS

Facts and Features

Of all the grains, oats is the ultimate "comfort" food, bringing soothing warmth whether cooked into a bowl of hot, steaming oatmeal, a chewy raisin-studded oatmeal cookie, or as the substantial basis for meat loaf or casserole. Some of this esteem may simply be connected to memories of enjoying oats in less complicated times. Much of it may be due to its chewy, moist texture that is appreciated not only in hot cereals, but also in breads, soups, and stews. In its more whole-grain forms, steel-cut-oats and oat groats are terrific substitutes for rice at lunch or dinner.

Only the outer indigestible husk is removed during milling, leaving oat's bran and germ intact. All forms of oats are good sources of seven B vitamins, vitamin E, nine minerals, including calcium and iron, and high quality protein. Oats contain about three times more fat than wheat.

In the 1980s, oatbran gained instant fame as a major cholesterol-lowering agent. Now it is known that whole oat groats, steel-cut oats, and oatmeal all contain the same cholesterol-lowering soluble fiber found concentrated in oat bran.

Because oats contain a natural antioxidant, when stored at moderate room temperature, it has a shelf life of up to one year, and even longer if kept under cooler conditions.

Oats contain small amounts of gluten.

Varieties and Cooking Guidelines:

Whole oat groats provide the true full-bodied slightly sweet flavor found in oats—exceptional at breakfast or as a pilaf at lunch or dinner. Whole oats absorb a great deal of water while cooking.

For 1 cup groats bring 3 cups of water to a boil, lower the heat, and simmer about 90 minutes, adding more water if necessary. To pressure-cook, use 3 cups water and cook 30 minutes.

Oat bran is high in soluble fiber. Its lighter color, texture, and pleasant flavor make oat bran more appealing to many people than wheat bran. It can also be added to breads, casseroles, and soups, and made into a delicious hot cereal ready to eat in only 2 minutes.

Oatmeal comes in several forms, varying only in size and cut.

Rolled oats are made by steaming oat groats and pressing them flat between steel rollers. To cook, add 1 cup oatmeal to 2 cups boiling water and simmer over low heat for 15 minutes.

Oatmeal also makes a delicious, creamy base for dairy-free soups. To serve four, add 3 cups vegetables cut into chunks, 1/2 cup dry oatmeal, 1 teaspoon of any herb or spice, and water to cover. Bring to a boil, reduce heat, and simmer 1/2 hour. Puree in a blender or food processer to desired consistency.

Quick cooking oats have been cut into pieces before they are rolled to make a thinner flake suitable for cooking in 3-5 minutes. Unlike regular rolled oats, quick oats tend to lose their chewy texture upon standing.

Instant oatmeals are precooked, rolled from oat groats into extremely thin oat flakes that require only boiling water and 1 minute standing time. New processes have been devised to produce an instant oatmeal with no additives, preservatives, or synthetic fortification for those who want convenience without chemicals.

Steel-cut or scotch oats are whole oat groats that have been steamed and cut into small, coarse pieces with sharp steel blades to reduce cooking time from 90 minutes for whole oat groats to 30 minutes. Steel cut oats make a remarkable hot cereal or a flavorful addition to breads.

To cook, add 1 cup steel-cut oats to 2 cups boiling water. To pressure-cook, use 21/2 cups water to 1 cup oats and cook 20 minutes.

"CREAM" OF ASPARAGUS SOUP

1 tsp. sesame oil
4 green onions, minced
    (including greens)
2 stalks celery, cut into
    1/2" slices
3/4 lb. asparagus, trimmed
    and peeled
4 1/2 cups water
1/2 cup rolled oats
1/4 tsp. salt
2 Tbsp. fresh dillweed

In a saucepan, sauté green onions and celery for 2 minutes. Cut tips off asparagus and set aside. Slice stalks into 1" pieces. Combine all ingredients except asparagus tips and dill with the onions and celery. Bring to a boil, reduce heat, and simmer 30 minutes. Purée soup in a blender or food processor and return to the saucepan. Add asparagus tips and fresh dill, simmering 3 minutes over low heat. Adjust seasonings and serve.

Serves 4
(Pyramid Servings: 1/2 Bread/ Grain Group, 1 1/2 Veg. Group,

Nutrition Facts

Serving Size 1/4 recipe (404 g)
Servings Per Container 4

Amount Per Serving

Calories 80   Calories from Fat 20

                              % Daily Value*

Total Fat 2g   3%

Sodium 190mg   8%

Total Carbohydrate 12g   4%

    Dietary Fiber 4g   14%

    Sugars 3g

Protein 4g

Vitamin A 10%   •   Vitamin C 25%

Calcium 4%   •   Iron 8%

Not a significant source of Saturated Fat and Cholesterol.
* Percent Daily Values are based on a 2,000 calorie diet.

Flavor Enhancers: dried fruits, cinnamon, honey, and maple syrup. For a savory flavor, cook steel-cut oats and oat groats with sage, Parmesan cheese, dill, nutmeg, parsley, and celery.

Menu Companions: For an interesting texture contrast, try combining cooked oat groats with quinoa or rice.

QUINOA

Facts and Features

Cultivated for centuries by Inca tribes in the Andes Mountains of South America, quinoa (pronounced keen-wa) has regained its popularity now in modern times. Not only does it have a delicious, uniquely nutty flavor and light, semi-chewy texture, quinoa also has the highest amount of protein and protein quality found in any grain.

And then there's its quick-cooking attribute and versatility. In only 15 minutes, quinoa can be transformed into an outstanding main grain, side dish, breakfast cereal, or dessert.

Although prepared as a grain, quinoa is actually the fruit of an herb related to lamb's quarters, a common native plant found in the United States.

Its nicknames, "supergrain" and "the mother grain" refer to quinoa's amazing nutritional profile. Quinoa is high in pro-

WALNUT ROSEMARY QUINOA

1 Tbsp. safflower or
 sesame oil
1 small onion, diced
1¼ cup quinoa,
 thoroughly rinsed
1 small red bell pepper,
 diced
3 cups water
1 tsp. tamari soy sauce
1 tsp. fresh rosemary or
 1/2 tsp. dried
1 cup fresh or frozen peas
1/3 cup walnuts, chopped

Preheat oven to 350°F. Heat oil in a saucepan and add onion and quinoa. Sauté over medium heat, stirring constantly for 3 minutes. Add red bell pepper and sauté an additional 2 minutes. Add water, soy sauce, and rosemary. (If using fresh peas, add them now.) Bring contents to a boil, cover and simmer 15 minutes. Meanwhile, roast walnuts in 350°F oven for 5 minutes. Once quinoa is cooked, turn off heat and mix in walnuts and frozen peas. Let sit an additional 10 minutes and serve.

Nutrition Facts

Serving Size 1/4 recipe (318 g)
Servings Per Container 4

Amount Per Serving

Calories 340 Calories from Fat 120

	% Daily Value*
Total Fat 13g	20%
Saturated Fat 1.5g	7%
Sodium 130mg	5%
Total Carbohydrate 47g	16%
Dietary Fiber 7g	26%
Sugars 4g	
Protein 11g	

Vitamin A 25%	•	Vitamin C 70%
Calcium 6%	•	Iron 35%

Not a significant source of Cholesterol
* Percent Daily Values are based on a 2,000 calorie diet.

Serves 4
(Pyramid Servings: 2 Bread/Grain Group, 1 Veg. Group, 13 grams Fat)

tein, containing twice as much as rice or barley. Unlike other grains that are deficient in lysine, quinoa's amino acid profile shows it to be an unusually complete protein, close to ideal. Combine it with other grains or beans to boost their protein values.

A good source of phosphorus, iron, magnesium, vitamin A, vitamin E, and the B vitamins, quinoa contains more fat as well as more calcium than any other grain: 41 mg. per 1/2 cup cooked. Quinoa contains more fat than other grains, so it is particularly important to store it in a relatively cool area in clean, airtight containers.

Quinoa is gluten-free.

Varieties and Cooking Guidelines

Quinoa's texture, flavor, and color can vary depending on where the it was grown. Dark tan-colored grains grown at sea level impart a somewhat bitter flavor. Yellowish grains from the valley regions vary in quality. Quinoa that contains a lot of black or colored wild quinoa grains may not cook fully, regardless how long one attempts to cook it. For best flavor and texture results, buy the largest, whitest grains, grown high in the mountain regions.

Quinoa has a naturally occuring, bitter tasting coating called saponins that repels insects while it grows. Although most of this is removed before packaging, it's still a good idea to rinse quinoa thoroughly before cooking.

For a richer flavor, toast quinoa in a dry or oiled skilled before cooking. Then combine 2 cups water, 1 cup quinoa, a pinch of salt, and cook 15-20 minutes. To pressure cook, use 13/4 cups water and cook 10 minutes. During the cooking process, quinoa expands almost five times in volume.

Flavor Enhancers: curry, onion, parsley, cilantro, cumin, coriander, and orange are particularly appealing. Cook leftover plain quinoa with apple juice, dried fruit, nuts, and vanilla for a tantalizing breakfast or unique dessert.

Menu Companions: For flavor and texture variety, combine quinoa with grains that have similar cooking times such as millet, white basmati rice, bulgur, and buckwheat. Use 1 part grain combination with 2 cups water. Substitute quinoa for bulgur wheat in your favorite tabouli recipe.

RICE

Facts and Features
Over 7000 varieties of rice are grown throughout the world. While in comparison only a small percentage are commercially available, interest in ethnic cooking has introduced us to the wide array of colors, flavors, and textures of rices, easily shattering the common belief that the only difference between rice is whether it is white or brown.

Long-grained, short-grained, and medium-grained rice all have similar nutrient values. Rice is fairly low in protein but its exceptional balance of amino acids makes its protein of very high quality.

Whole grain brown rice, processed with only its inedible hull removed, is also a good source of fiber, phosphorus, B vitamins, potassium, and vitamin E.

However, when milled into white rice, nutrient levels decrease significantly. White rice is denuded of its bran and germ by machines that rub the grains together under pressure, leaving only the starchy endosperm. In an effort to try to replace some of the nutrients lost through processing, several brands of white rice are enriched with thiamine (B_1), riboflavin (B_2), niacin, and iron.

Converted or parboiled rice is white rice that has been soaked, steamed, and dried before the hull and bran layers are removed. In the process, about 70% of the B vitamins and iron from the bran and germ and 85% of the protein are sealed in the grain. Nutritionally, it lies between brown and white rice.

Given its depleted nutrient levels, should white rice never be consumed? In a well-rounded healthy diet, occasional use of refined grains such as white rice is generally considered acceptable. While there is no question brown rice is more nutritious, in certain recipes and situations white rice may be more appropriate. Some individuals may also have difficulty digesting the high fiber of brown rice. And, during hot summer temperatures lighter-textured white rices may seem more appropriate than brown rice.

Varieties and Cooking Guidelines:
The primary difference between the various rices is the predominant type of starch in the grain. Within these classifications lie several varieties of rice which differ according to flavor and cooking characteristics.

Long Grain Rices
Long grain rice is more fluffy, flaky, and separate. It is often the rice of choice for pilafs,

curries, paellas, rice salads, and warm weather cooking.

Enriched, nonconverted white rice is coated with thiamin, niacin, and iron to replace a few of the nutrient losses from milling. (Because it would make the rice appear yellow, riboflavin (B_2) is not added.) To retain these added ingredients, do not rinse enriched white rice before cooking. To prepare, use 2 cups water to 1 cup rice and cook 15 minutes.

Long-grain brown rice adds plenty of fiber, nutrition, and distinctively nutty flavor to any dish. Unlike white rice which depends on several seasonings or a well-seasoned accompaniment to make up for its relatively bland flavor, brown rice can easily stand on its own. To cook, combine 2 cups water and 1 cup rice. Bring to a boil, reduce heat, and cook 45 minutes. Don't peek until the rice is completely done.

Parboiled or converted rice has a mild, pleasant flavor and fluffy texture. As a result of the special steam pressure process it undergoes before milling, not only are nutrients sealed within, the starch is gelatinized in the grain, making the grain resistant to becoming sticky. To cook, use 2 cups water to 1 cup rice and cook 15 minutes.

Aromatic rices are special long-grain rices known for their fragrant, nutty flavor and aroma.

Basmati rice is named after a very fragrant Southeast Asian flower. Grown in northern India and Pakistan, true basmati must always be imported into the United States for two reasons. Unlike the subtropical climates found in U.S. rice-growing areas, basmati rice is more productive in cooler temperatures. And, due to its characteristic 5-to 6-foot height, basmati rice could not withstand the windy conditions commonly found in U.S. rice country.

After harvest, basmati is aged for a year to develop its full flavor and to decrease its moisture content. While generally sold in its white form refined of its bran and germ, brown basmati is also available. Like typical brown rice, brown basmati takes almost three times to cook and has a chewier texture and more intense, nutty flavor.

A unique charactistic of basmati rice is that it doubles its length during cooking. To keep the kernels from breaking or splitting apart in the process, rinse basmati several times prior to cooking. The rinsing also releases excess starch that would otherwise make for very sticky rice.

To cook white basmati, bring 13/4 cup water to a boil, add a pinch of salt and 1 cup rice, reduce heat and cook 15 minutes. Brown basmati requires 2 cups water to 1 cup rice and 45 minutes cooking time.

Black japonica rice has a somewhat sticky texture and good but grassy flavor. Because of its striking, shiny black color, it can be found in several gourmet rice blends along with brown rice. When cooked on its own, it is often made into a salad with a Thai-seasoned marinade or combined with coconut for Asian-inspired desserts. Cook 1 cup black japonica rice in 11/2 cups water for 25 minutes. Allow it to stand 10 minutes before serving. Salt after cooking.

Instant white rice is partially cooked and dried, creating a porous structure that allows for rapid rehydration. Although quick, flavor and texture tend to suffer in the process. Instant white rice is often enriched.

Jasmine rice, traditionally grown in Thailand, is now grown in the United States, thanks to a new variety introduced in 1989. Delicately flavored and very white in color, jasmine rice is known for its soft, slightly sticky texture that remains as such even after refrigeration. While not traditionally eaten in this form, whole grain jasmine rice is also available. To cook, combine 13/4 cup water and 1 cup rice. Bring to a boil, add salt, reduce heat, and cook 15 minutes. Brown jasmine rice requires 2 cups water to 1 cup rice and 45 minutes cooking time.

Popcorn rice is a very white, flavorful, long-grain aromatic rice grown in Louisiana. As the name suggests, this rice has an aroma remarkably similar to cooked popcorn. To cook, combine 13/4 cup water and 1 cup rice. Bring to a boil, add salt, reduce heat, and cook 15 minutes.

Quick-cooking brown rice provides a quick 15 minute option for making brown rice, leaving virtually the same nutrients as found in conventionally prepared brown rice. By briefly exposing individual whole grains of rice to dry heat, the moisture inside the grain turns to steam and exits the grain by creating tunnels within the rice. This effect gives the rice its quick-cooking properties while retaining its rich natural nutrition. Like instant white rice, given the trade-off in time, the texture of quick-cooking brown rice is acceptable but doesn't quite match unprocessed brown rice cooked to its longer required time.

Texmati rice was developed to provide a less expensive aromatic alternative to basmati that could be grown in the United States. As its name implies, Texmati is grown primarily in Texas, a variation of a strain introduced by USDA researchers in 1971 by cross-breeding basmati with long-grain rice.

While similar to basmati, Texmati rice is milder in flavor, making it a more all-purpose type of aromatic rice. Texmati is most widely marketed in its white refined form; however, like basmati, an unrefined brown Texmati is also available.

To cook white Texmati, combine 13/4 cup water and 1 cup rice. Bring to a boil, add salt, reduce heat, and cook 15 minutes. Brown basmati requires 2 cups water for 1 cup rice and 45 minutes cooking time.

Wehani rice is a chewy, sweet, russet-colored basmati hybrid developed by the Lundberg Family Rice Farms in California. Only available in its whole-grain version, wehani rice gets its color from the rice's red outer bran layer. For a striking color contrast, try it in grain salads and pilafs made with celery, peas, and yellow squash. To cook, combine 2 cups water and 1 cup rice. Add salt after cooking the grain for 45 minutes.

Wild pecan rice, another variation of the same strain used to develop Texmati rice, has a very nutty flavor and aroma. Unlike what its name implies, it does not contain pecans nor is it wild. Grown in Louisiana, wild pecan rice is amber-colored and contains some of the bran. To cook, combine 13/4 cup water and 1 cup rice. Bring to a boil, add salt, reduce heat, and cook 15 minutes.

Medium Grain Rices

Medium-grain rice takes the middle road, featuring the sweet nutty flavor of short grained rice with the fluffy texture of a long grain. It's perfect for stuffings and as a thickening agent for soups.

Golden Rose Rice is an especially flavorful variety of medium brown rice. To cook, combine 1 cup rice with 2 cups water and simmer for 50 minutes. To pressure-cook, use 11/4 cups water and cook 50 minutes.

Short Grain Rices

Short-grain rice is more moist and sticky in texture and sweeter in flavor. Use it for rice

PERFECT RISOTTO

1 Tbsp. olive oil or butter
1 cup arborio rice
3 cups hot stock or broth
   (vegetable, poultry,
   meat, or fish)
1/2 tsp. salt (only if stock
   isn't salted)
Parmesan cheese (opt.)

Sauté the rice in oil or butter until translucent. Then over medium-high heat, add 1/2 cup of hot stock, stirring constantly until the liquid is completely absorbed (about 1 minute). Repeat with the remaining stock, adding 1/2 cup at a time. Gradual additions of stock allow the rice to release starch, producing a creamy texture with chewy individual grains. The rice is done when the grains become creamy and just tender, about 20-25 minutes. For added richness, sprinkle Parmesan cheese on top just before serving.

Nutrition Facts

Serving Size 1/3 recipe (309 g)
Servings Per Container 3

Amount Per Serving

Calories 270   Calories from Fat 45

	% Daily Value*
Total Fat 5g	8%
Saturated Fat 0.5g	3%
Sodium 210mg	9%
Total Carbohydrate 52g	17%
Dietary Fiber 3g	12%
Protein 6g	

Vitamin A 8%	•	Vitamin C	15%
Calcium 2%	•	Iron	2%

Not a significant source of Cholesterol and Sugars.
* Percent Daily Values are based on a 2,000 calorie diet.

Serves 3
(Pyramid Servings: 2 Bread/Grain Group, 5 grams Fat)

puddings, croquettes, casseroles, and for general colder weather cooking. Short-grain rice absorbs flavors more readily than long- or medium- grain rices.

Arborio rice is an Italian short-grain rice that is shorter and rounder than American short-grain rice. With its ability to absorb large amounts of liquid to provide a creamy but slightly chewy texture, arborio is the rice of choice for making risotto.

The quality of arborio rice is determined by its size and rate of absorption. Arborio Superfino indicates a large short-grain variety. Smaller-kerneled Vialone Nano is classified a semifino. Superfino, fino, and semifino can all be used to make risotto and desserts. Soups, salads, or desserts can be made with the lesser-quality comune variety.

Arborio rice can also be used to make quick and delicious stove-top rice dessert or breakfast puddings by cooking it with diluted fruit juice, raisins, vanilla or ginger. For extra creaminess, increase the liquid to about 31/2 cups. Top with chopped almonds before serving.

California Pearl is a domestically grown short-grain rice that is very absorbant, soft, and sticky. Use for risotto, paella, and Spanish rice.

Christmas Rice is a reddish-brown whole short-grain rice developed by California-based Lundberg Farms from an Asian strain.

WAYS TO PREPARE MOCHI

Baked: Preheat oven or toaster oven to 450°F. Place individual squares of mochi on a cookie sheet. Bake 10 minutes or until mochi has "puffed up". Remove from the oven before the surface of the mochi cracks and exposes the insides. Cut in half and stuff or spread with your favorite filling. Eat immediately.

Pan-fried: Brush both sides of mochi with oil and place it in a heavy skillet preheated over a medium flame or setting. Cover with a lid and cook approximately 4 minutes on each side. Watch it carefully to avoid burning. Serve as above.

Waffled: Place one or two pieces in a lightly oiled waffle iron, close the lid, and wait, approximately 10 minutes, until the "jaws" of the waffle iron touch.

Simmered: Add pieces directly in soups or stews. The smaller the pieces, the shorter the simmering time. For pieces approximately 2 inches square, plan on adding them during the last 15 minutes of cooking. If cooked too long, the mochi will dissolve and thicken the soup.

Melted: Grate mochi and sprinkle on top of vegetables, casseroles, or pizza. Cover with a lid or foil and steam or bake as normal. Serve immediately.

(Pyramid Servings: 2 Bread/Grain Group)

Nutrition Facts

Serving Size 1 piece (45 g)
Servings Per Container 8

Amount Per Serving	
Calories 110	Calories from Fat 10

	% Daily Value*
Total Fat 1g	2%
Sodium 0mg	0%
Total Carbohydrate 24g	8%
Dietary Fiber 2g	8%
Protein 2g	

Iron 4%

Not a significant source of Saturated Fat, Cholesterol, Sugars, Vitamin A, Vitamin C and Calcium.

* Percent Daily Values are based on a 2,000 calorie diet.

Its flavor is similar to wild mushrooms. To cook, combine 21/4 cups water with 1 cup rice. Bring to a boil, season with salt, reduce heat, and cook for 50 minutes.

Granza rice whose name means short, thick, and plump, is grown in Spain. Use for risotto and paella.

Mochi is a traditional Japanese food made from steamed and mashed sweet rice dried in shallow pans and cut into squares. When baked in a 450° F. oven, broiled, or pan-fried for 10 minutes, mochi puffs up into delicious, chewy "biscuits."

Symbolizing longevity and wealth, mochi is featured at several Japanese festivals, especially on New Year's Day. It is also highly regarded as a natural way to increase stamina and to promote lactation in nursing mothers. Although extremely digestible, mochi is best consumed during colder months due to its hearty, warming nature.

The centuries-old method of making mochi is to pound the steamed rice with wooden mallets in a large wooden mortar or hollowed-out log. Modern commercially-made mochi is ground in extrusion machines that imitate the process. While both are delicious and can be used interchangeably in recipes, traditionally made mochi is more gooey while the mechanically extruded mochi has a more crisp exterior. Depending on the brand, flavor varieties include plain, sesame/garlic, cinnamon/raisin, vanilla/almond, date/sesame, and mugwort (a plant with high calcium and iron content with a flavor similar to spinach).

Although, given plenty of time and energy, sweet brown rice can be cooked and pounded to make mochi from scratch at home, ready-made whole-grain mochi can be found in the refrigerated or frozen food cases in natural food stores. Imported Japanese whole grain mochi is sometimes available vacuum packed, requiring no refrigeration during storage. Oriental markets also sell mochi, however, it may be made with refined white sweet rice and contain additives, preservatives, or sugar.

Mochi can be served muffin- or pita-style, split and stuffed with nut butter and apple sauce or jam, sandwich spreads, dips, beans, or salad fixings. It can be flattened into waffles or expanded into dumplings. When grated and sprinkled on steamed vegetables or casseroles just before cooking or baking, it transforms into a "cheesy" topping. The possibilities are endless.

Once prepared, mochi should be eaten immediately since it hardens upon cooling. Keep extra pieces of mochi covered during the meal to retain heat. Hardened mochi can be refreshed in a steamer or tortilla warmer.

Short grain brown rice is a hearty, somewhat sticky whole grain rice particularly appealing during the colder months. Pressure cooking enhances its sweet flavor and compact texture. To cook short grain brown rice use 21/4 cups water to 1 cup rice and 50 minutes cooking time. To pressure cook, use 13/4 cups water and cook 50 minutes.

Short grain white rice cooks in much less time than brown rice but is more bland in flavor. Cook 1 cup with 11/4 cup water for 15 minutes.

Sushi rice is a semi-polished white, very sticky short-grain rice traditionally used to make nori-wrapped sushi rolls. Before cooking, rinse and drain the rice several times until the rinse water is almost clear. Allow it to drain for 30-60 minutes. When the rice is ready, combine equal amounts of water to rice, bring to a boil over medium heat, and cook for 1 minute. Then reduce heat to low and cook for 8-10 minutes. Reduce the heat once again to very low and cook an additional 10 minutes, making sure to keep the cover on at all times during cooking. Remove from heat and let the rice stand, covered, for 10 minutes more before fluffing and using for sushi or vegetarian nori maki. For a soft version, cook 20 minutes using twice as much water to rice.

Sweet rice or oriental glutinous rice is a short, round-shaped rice that cooks up very sticky due to its extremely high carbohydrate content. Typically it is used to make amasake, mochi, and desserts. Despite being called glutinous rice, it contains no gluten. For more nutrients and flavor, choose sweet brown rice over the more refined white version. To cook 1 cup sweet brown rice, combine with 11/2 cups water and cook 30 minutes. To pressure cook, use 1 cup water and cook 20 minutes.

Miscellaneous Rice Products

Cream of Rice is a delicious hot cereal made from dry roasted finely ground rice or rice grits. For best nutrition and flavor, look for brands made from brown rice. Follow manufacturers' suggested cooking times.

Rice bran, containing nearly twice the fiber as oat bran, is also considered beneficial in lowering cholesterol. Add small amounts to

NORI MAKI SUSHI

1 cup short grain brown
    rice or sushi rice
2 cups water
1-2 Tbsp. brown rice
    vinegar
1 Tbsp. grated ginger or
    pickled ginger
1 carrot, cut into 3"-long
    matchstick shapes
1 bunch green onion, cut
    into lengthwise strips
1 Tbsp. umeboshi paste or
    prepared mustard
1 package sushi nori
bamboo sushi mat

Rinse and drain rice three times or until the rinse water is clear. Add water, soak for 45 minutes, and bring to a boil. Cover, cook for 45 minutes over low heat, and let rice sit for 10 minutes before removing lid.

Stir in vinegar. Squeeze juice from ginger and add juice to rice. While rice cools, boil water in a small pot. Drop carrot matchsticks into the boiling water for 1 minute. Remove carrots and rinse under cold water to stop cooking. Drop green onions into boiling water for 30 seconds, remove, and rinse under cold water.

Lay 1 sheet of nori, shiny side down, on a bamboo sushi mat. Lightly spread umeboshi paste or mustard over the nori. Wet hands and spread cooked rice about 3/8 inch thick over nori, covering all but a one-inch strip at both the top and bottom. Place strips of carrot and green onion horizontally in the middle of the rice. Sprinkle with sesame seeds.

Lift the sushi mat with your fingers on top of the rice and your thumbs beneath the mat. Roll the mat forward as tightly as you can, pushing with your fingers and guiding with your thumbs. Be sure not to roll the mat inside with the filling! When you reach the end of the rice, moisten the edge of the nori to seal. Squeeze the roll gently and firmly and then remove the mat. Slice the roll into 6 slices with a very sharp knife. Rinse the knife with water to prevent sticking.

Makes 6 rolls
(Pyramid Servings: 1 Bread/Grain

Nutrition Facts

Serving Size 1 roll (140 g)
Servings Per Container 6

Amount Per Serving	
Calories 130	

	% Daily Value*
Total Fat 0g	0%
Sodium 45mg	2%
Total Carbohydrate 27g	9%
Dietary Fiber 2g	6%
Sugars 1g	
Protein 3g	

Vitamin A 70%	•	Vitamin C 6%
Calcium 2%	•	Iron 4%

Not a significant source of Calories from Fat, Saturated Fat and Cholesterol.
* Percent Daily Values are based on a 2,000 calorie diet.

breads, pancakes, and muffins. Remember, however, that the benefits of rice bran are automatically included when whole-grain brown rice is consumed.

Rice Flakes can be cooked into a hot cereal or used as the basis for a casserole. Combine 1 cup rice flakes with 3 cups boiling salted water and cook for 25-30 minutes.

Packaged rice pilaf mixes abound in every supermarket and specialty store. On the positive side, they are generally quick-cooking and they illustrate the various ways rice can be seasoned. On the other hand, you can add your own seasonings to either regular rice or plain quick rice for a lot less money and significantly less sodium.

Wild rice is neither a rice nor a grain. Instead its long, dark-brown kernel is the seed of a grass which grows in the marshy areas of northern Minnesota, Wisconsin, and southern Canada.

State laws regulate the length of the picking season and protect the rights of Chippewa and Winnebago tribes who are considered wild rice's "official" harvesters. Harvesting is done manually, using only a canoe and "ricing sticks." While one person guides the canoe, another person uses one stick to pull the head of rice over his/her lap. The other stick is used to knock the ripe seeds loose. The rice is parched in a drum over a fire to dry it to about 8% moisture and to give the wild rice its characteristic flavor. The chaff is then removed in a thresher and fanning mill.

Often rice listed as "wild" rice is actually cultivated and harvested in rice paddies in Oregon and California, a practice that started years ago when the demand for wild rice exceeded the wild supply. While its nontraditional growing and harvesting methods yield a less expensive rice, its flavor is not as robust or nutty as true wild rice. Also, cultivated rice is more likely to be grown with fertilizers, herbicides, and insecticides. All in all, your best bet is to insist on traditional, organically grown wild rice.

Different grades of wild rice are on the market. For special dishes, use "Giant" wild rice featuring 1"-long uniform grains. For salads, soups, and stuffings, medium-sized "Fancy" wild rice is most commonly used. Least expensive "Select" wild rice, generally including broken, uneven lengths and sizes of kernels, can be used in muffins, pancakes, soups, and stuffings where uniform appearance doesn't matter.

Both wild rice and cultivated wild rice can be combined with brown rice without sacrificing its hearty flavor. Use in side dishes, salads, soups, and stuffings. To cook, use 3 parts water to 1 part wild rice and cook for 60 minutes or until done.

Flavor Enhancers: onion, mushrooms, garlic, curry, bay leaf, raisins, dill, roasted red bell peppers, parsley, basil, ginger, and grated lemon zest. Try an exotic combination suggested by natural gourmet chef and health educator Annemarie Colbin: 1/2 cinnamon stick, 4 whole cloves, and 6 cardamom seeds. It tastes terrific and helps lighten the character of the rice.

Menu Companions: Cook equal parts of brown rice with barley using 21/2 cups water per 1 cup mixed grain for 45 minutes. White aromatic rices are perfect grain companions when cooked with shorter-cooking grains such as millet, quinoa, bulgur, and buckwheat. Plan on cooking the same amount of time as its companion grain but use less water to compensate for the small amount usually required for the white aromatic rices.

RYE

Facts and Features

Rye has bluish-brown kernels that are longer and thinner than wheat. Many people falsely equate rye's flavor with caraway seeds as several rye breads and crackers are seasoned with them. Rye, however, has a delicious, hearty flavor of its own.

Rye continues to be popular in Northern and Eastern Europe, especially for bread. In the United States, most rye is made into whiskey, but interest in more rye-based food products such as breads, crackers, and hot cereals seems to be increasing.

Rye grows well in poor soil and moist climates, conditions also favorable for a fungus called ergot. In fact, contaminated rye is now blamed for epidemics, hysteria, and even mass riots during the 11th to 18th centuries, manifesting in progressive gangrene, mental derangement, hallucinogenic effects, and uncontrollable muscular spasms. Fortunately, modern storage methods have eliminated problems with ergot.

Whole rye is higher in protein, phosphorus, iron, potassium, and B vitamins than wheat, thus verifying the old saying: "Rye builds muscle; wheat builds fat." It also contains a significant amount of fiber, specifically long chains of 5-carbon sugars called pentosans. Pentosans digest slowly and retain moisture very well, so food made with rye tends to be more satisfying, giving the sensation of fullness.

Rye contains a small amount of gluten.

Varieties and Cooking Guidelines

Whole rye has only the outer hull removed. It can be cooked alone or with other grains and added to soups, salads, breads, or served as a grain side dish. For a chewy consistency, use 4 parts water to 1 part rye and cook for 1 hour. For a softer grain, soak 6 hours and simmer 2-3 hours or pressure-cook in the soaking water for 45 minutes.

Rye flakes are made from whole rye steamed, pressed, and rolled into thick flakes. Use as a hot cereal or add to breads for flavor and texture. To cook, add 1 cup rye flakes to 3 cups boiling salted water and cook for 25-30 minutes.

Rye grits is whole rye cracked in small pieces. It is ideal as a hot cereal or added to casseroles. For each cup of rye grits, add to 31/2 cups boiling salted water and cook for 35-40 minutes.

Flavor Enhancers: caraway seeds, fennel, anise, orange zest, and raisins.

Menu Companions: Combine small amounts with brown rice or barley, using 3 cups water per 1 cup grain mixture.

SORGHUM

Facts and Features

Whole-grain sorghum looks similar to a large seeded millet. There are many varieties with just as many colors. Its flavor is pleasantly sweet. Although still a major food grain in Africa and Asia to make porridge, flat breads, and beer, sorghum (also known as milo) is currently grown in the United States almost exclusively for animal feed.

Fortunately, sweet, mineral-rich sorghum syrup produced from concentrating the juice in sorghum stalks can still be found on grocery store shelves. Occasionally you'll find whole-grain sorghum in some specialty stores or food mail-order companies.

Sorghum is similar nutritionally to corn but with a slightly higher tryptophan content. Sorghum is gluten-free.

Varieties and Cooking Guidelines:

Whole grain sorghum can be cooked like rice, using a proportion of 1 cup sorghum to 2 cups water. Cook for about 45 minutes.

Cracked sorghum can be made into porridge or mush. Follow directions on the package.

Flavor Enhancers: curry, chili powder, orange, rosemary, onion, chives, parsley, black pepper, bay leaf, thyme, garlic, and ginger.

Menu Companions: Cook sweet whole-grain sorghum with brown rice or barley.

SPELT

Facts and Features

Known as "farro" in Italy and "dinkel" in Germany and Switzerland, spelt has been grown commercially for thousands of years in several parts of Europe as a major bread wheat. Until the Third Reich outlawed its cultivation to force production of higher-yielding varieties of wheat, spelt was Germany's premier grain. Today it is experiencing a resurgence, so much so that German farmers can't keep up with the supply.

With the exception of its reddish color, spelt closely resembles a typical grain of wheat in appearance, flavor, and starch properties. As an unhybridized grain, spelt retains its distinctive flavor and spectrum of nutrients, characteristics often sacrificed in modern varieties of wheat that are developed for high crop yields, versatility, and pest resistance. Spelt is very high in complex carbohydrates, B vitamins, and contains 30% more protein than wheat.

Like wheat, spelt contains gluten. Nevertheless, individuals severely allergic to wheat should proceed with caution when experimenting with spelt under the guidance of a doctor or qualified health practitioner, as intolerance to any degree remains a possibility.

Varieties and Cooking Guidelines:

Whole spelt can be cooked and added to casseroles, salads, breads, pilafs, and cereals. To cook, soak whole spelt 6-8 hours or overnight. Drain, add to 3 cups water for each 1 cup dry and cook 50-60 minutes until tender. To pressure-cook 1 cup whole spelt, use 21/2 cups water and cook 50 minutes.

Spelt flakes can be used like any other flaked grain for hot cereals, granolas, cookies, and casseroles. For a hot cereal, combine 1 cup spelt flakes with 2 cups water, bring to a boil, and cook 15-18 minutes.

Flavor Enhancers: onion, chives, dill, mushrooms, pepper, garlic, curry, parsley, and cilantro. Sweet seasonings include cinnamon, pumpkin pie spices, apple pie spices, ginger, and allspice.

Menu Companions: To add texture to other whole grains, combine cooked whole spelt to quinoa, bulgur, millet, and barley. Spelt flakes can be combined with other flaked grains to add extra flavor.

TEFF

Facts and Features

The name teff means "lost," an appropriate name considering its seeds are so minute that if any dropped on the ground, it would be difficult to find them.

Introduced to the United States during the 1980s, teff is the most commonly cultivated grain in Ethiopia. It is traditionally made into soup, porridge, beer, and especially into injera, a crêpe-like Ethiopian bread that is used as plate, fork, and food during the meal. In fact, 92% of the rural diet is comprised of this giant bread, measuring up to 2 feet in diameter.

Teff is only available in its whole-grain form since it would be impossible to refine away the bran or germ on each tiny seed. It is particularly high in minerals including calcium, magnesium, boron, copper, phosphorus, zinc, and manganese. Most significant is teff's iron content, containing two to three times more than wheat, barley, or sorghum. Teff is gluten-free.

It contains a naturally occurring yeast which easily ferments when moisture is added, resulting in a sweet and malty flavor. White teff has the most delicate and mild flavor while red and brown teff have a more nutty flavor.

When cooked as a cereal, pudding, or prepared like polenta, its texture is sticky and slightly crunchy.

Varieties and Cooking Guidelines:

To make basic cooked teff cereal combine 1 cup whole teff with 4 cups water and cook 15 minutes. For a richer flavor, lightly toast the teff before cooking.

If making "polenta", rinse an 8" X 8" baking dish in cold water. Spread the cooked teff into the dish and set aside for about an hour to cool and solidify.

A small amount of whole, uncooked teff can be added to baked goods to substitute for sesame seeds.

Flavor Enhancers: cinnamon, allspice, dried fruits, or maple syrup in teff cereals and puddings. Savory herbs, onions, or curry powder.

Menu Companions: For added texture in fa-miliar grains, add 2 Tbsp. of teff when cooking 1 cup of rice, millet, or barley.

TRITICALE

Facts and Features

Triticale has grayish-brown, oval-shaped kernels larger than wheat and plumper than rye. Hailed as a new superfood in the 1960s, triticale was developed to merge the nutty flavor and high yields exhibited in wheat with the hardiness and better balance of amino acids found in rye. Pronounced trit-i-kay'-lee, its name is derived from combining the scientific names of wheat (Triticum) with rye (Secale). It is also high in fiber and magnesium. Like wheat and rye, triticale contains gluten.

For some reason, triticale never really caught on. Although it may occasionally be found in its whole-grain or flaked form, most often triticale is sold as flour.

Varieties and Cooking Guidelines:

Whole grain triticale can be sprouted or cooked for use in pilafs, salads, or breads. Soak 1 cup whole triticale for 6-8 hours or overnight. Drain, add to 3 cups boiling water or broth, and cook for 50 minutes until tender.

Triticale flakes can be added to granolas, cookies, and meat or bean loaves for flavor and bulk. It also makes a delicious hot cereal. When cooking 1 cup triticale flakes, add to 2 cups boiling water and simmer for 15-20 minutes.

Flavor Enhancers: onions, sage, pepper, garlic, dill, basil, oregano, and thyme. Sweet seasonings include cinnamon, ginger, raisins, and dates.

Menu Companions: Whole triticale adds flavor, texture, and nutrition to any grain. Cook along with long-cooking grains such as brown rice and barley. If adding to quinoa, millet, or shorter cooking grains, cook triticale first and add to other grains the last few minutes of cooking.

Several commercial mixed grain combinations such as Kashi™ and Arrowhead Mills' 7 Grain cereal include triticale.

Triticale flakes can be combined with oatmeal when making granola or combined with barley flakes, oatmeal, or rice flakes for a cooked hot cereal.

WHEAT

Facts and Features

Wheat is one of the oldest cultivated crops and still remains the most commonly used grain throughout the world.

Whole wheat is very nutritious. Out of the 44 known essential nutrients that can be obtained from food, only vitamins A, B12, C, and iodine are completely unavailable. However, much of this nutrition is severely depleted when the wheat's bran and germ are removed during the refining process.

Wheat's versatility is due to the unique properties of its gluten which varies according to the protein-to-starch ratios found in soft, hard, or durum types of wheat. .

Soft wheat is low in gluten and is ground into pastry flour for lighter-textured baked goods that don't rely on baking yeast or sourdough as a leavening. Hard wheat contains more gluten and is used for cooking and ground into bread flour. Durum wheat contains the most gluten. It is ground into flour to make pasta and is used to make couscous.

Varieties and Cooking Guidelines:

Whole-grain wheat, also known as wheat berries, are characterized by short, rounded kernels of varying shades of brown. After cooking, the "berries" can be combined with other grains for texture or used in stuffings, casseroles, salads, or breads. To cook, soak 6-8 hours or overnight. Drain, add to 3 cups water for each 1 cup dry and cook 50-60 minutes until tender. To pressure-cook 1 cup whole wheat, use 21/2 cups water and cook 50 minutes. Wheat berries also make excellent sprouts.

Bulgur is cracked wheat that has been parboiled and cracked into one of three granulations. Use fine granulation for making Lebanese kibbe, bread, and dessert recipes. Medium granulation bulgur, the type most generally available, is considered all-purpose, especially for salads and stuffings. Coarse granulation is more chewy, making it excellent for pilafs, salads, and soups. Since bulgur is partially cooked, it has a more nutty, roasted flavor than cracked wheat. Its cooking time is also dramatically decreased.

Bulgur can be prepared in two ways: For basic stovetop cooking, add 1 cup bulgur to 2 cups boiling water. Return to a boil, reduce to simmer, and cook 25 minutes. Allow to stand, covered, for 10 minutes before serving or using in a recipe.

Another method is to boil 21/2 cups water, add1 cup bulgur, cover, remove from the burner, and allow to steep 1 hour. Drain bulgur in a colander lined with cheesecloth and squeeze out excess moisture. This soaking method will yield a more coarse, chewy texture.

Try adding 1/2-1 cup of bulgar to chili during the last half hour of cooking for a texture remarkably like ground beef. As the bulgur absorbs a lot of liquid, you may need

TRADITIONAL STEAMED COUSC0US

You'll need a couscousiere, the authentic couscous steamer that looks like a double boiler with a narrow, deep bottom half. The top half resembles a colander with very tiny holes. You can also improvise with a colander lined with a double layer of cheesecloth and a large pot.

First, place 1 1/2 cups couscous in a 9" X 13" baking dish and cover with cold water to moisten. Drain through a fine strainer and return the couscous to the baking dish, spreading the grains out evenly. Let sit for 15-20 minutes.

Put water in the lower half of the couscousiere and bring to a moderate boil. When the steam begins to rise through the lined colander, reduce the heat to moderately high and put the couscous in the colander, rubbing the grains to make sure there are no lumps. If the steam seems to be coming out the sides, seal the circumference with a wet dishtowel or aluminum foil. Steam the couscous, uncovered, for 20 minutes.

Return the couscous to the baking dish and add 2/3 cup cold water. Break up any clumping in the couscous and allow the couscous to sit for 20 minutes. Meanwhile, fill the bottom of the couscousiere with the stew and heat until steam begins to rise through the colander. Return the couscous to the colander and steam for 25-30 minutes. Transfer couscous to a bowl, season, and serve.

(Pyramid Servings: 2 1/2 Bread/ Grain Group)

Nutrition Facts

Serving Size 1/3 recipe (179 g)
Servings Per Container 3

Amount Per Serving

Calories 200

	% Daily Value*
Total Fat 0g	0%
Sodium 10mg	0%
Total Carbohydrate 42g	14%
Dietary Fiber 3g	10%
Sugars 1g	
Protein 7g	

Calcium 2%	•	Iron 4%

Not a significant source of Calories from Fat, Saturated Fat, Cholesterol, Vitamin A and Vitamin C.

* Percent Daily Values are based on a 2,000 calorie diet.

---

to add extra water or tomato sauce to get the final consistency you desire.

Don't stop with water and salt when preparing bulgur. Go wild and cook it with fruit juice, vegetable broth, or chicken broth. Close your eyes and reach into your herb and spice cupboard or drawer for one or two seasonings. It's bound to be really good or memorable in one way or another.

Cracked wheat is made by cracking the wheat berries between rollers. Not only does it result in a considerably reduced cooking time, it is more versatile. Use cracked wheat as a cereal, a rice substitute, in casseroles, stuffings, or in making tabouleh, a Lebanese grain-based salad. To cook, combine 2 parts water to 1 part cracked wheat and cook 20 minutes over moderate heat. Allow to stand, covered, for 5 minutes before serving.

Couscous is a bulgur-type grain typically made from semolina, refined durum wheat flour, that has been rolled into thin strands, broken into small pieces, steamed, and dried. In other words, it can be considered as a very finely cracked spaghetti. A whole wheat version made from whole durum wheat is more nutritious and even more flavorful. Refreshing, light, and very quick to prepare, couscous can be cooked as a main or side dish, a breakfast cereal, a salad, or as a dessert.

Couscous is especially good when cooked with fruit juice and pressed into a baking dish. When cool, the couscous can be cut into squares for a sweet snack or dessert. If cooked with vegetable broth, pressed and cooled couscous becomes a wheat-based polenta.

There are two ways to cook couscous. Most people use the quick-cooking method. Bring 11/2 cups water, broth, or fruit juice to a boil and add 1 cup couscous. Reduce the heat to low, cover, and simmer 5 minutes or until all the liquid is absorbed. Stir to fluff and serve.

The more traditional way, cooking couscous over a stew or soup takes considerably more time and yet the results are much more light and fluffy, with each grain soft and separate.

Farina is a refined cereal made from ground and sifted wheat. The bran and most of the germ is removed in the process.

Fu (pronounced "foo") is a wheat gluten product that is toasted, steamed, and dried into doughnut shaped rounds. Unlike seitan, it is not preseasoned. To use, soak in hot water for 10 minutes until softened and squeeze out excess water. (Fu expands considerably when reconstituted.) Add to soups or stews, or boil, saute, steam, or bake. Like seitan, fu absorbs flavors and adds a meaty texture.

Seitan (pronounced say'-tan), also referred as "wheat meat" or "wheat roast" is a concentrated source of protein made by cooking the gluten extracted from wheat flour in a soy sauce and kombu (a sea vegetable) broth. Its chewy texture and full-bodied flavor are remarkably similar to roast beef and it's just as versatile.

Although it has a delicious flavor of its own, seitan readily absorbs the flavors of other vegetables, sauces, or seasonings.

Seitan is at its best cooked in stews, chilis, soups, or lasagna and other casseroles. It can also substitute for corned beef in a veggie reuben sandwich. Ground and seasoned seitan makes a delicious sandwich spread. Or go "all-American" and serve it sliced with gravy and mashed potatoes.

Seitan is high in protein, containing about 15 grams per 31/2 oz. serving but, like any wheat product, it is low in lysine. To enhance seitan's limited protein quality, serve with beans, tofu, sesame or sunflower seeds, cheese, or a soymilk-based sauce. Seitan is low in fat and contains no cholesterol but, because it is cooked and stored in a tamari soy sauce broth, seitan is fairly high in sodium. You may want to forego additional salt in recipes using seitan.

Seitan is generally found in natural food stores refrigerated in small tubs or in shelf-stable jars. For those with extra time on their hands, several cookbooks offer detailed instructions to easily make seitan at home. It involves mixing a high-gluten whole wheat bread flour, unbleached white flour, or extracted gluten flour with water, kneading it into a dough similar to bread dough, allowing it to rest to develop the gluten, and rinsing it under water to separate the starch and bran from the gluten. A 2 hour simmering in a seasoned soy sauce broth completes the process. Reserved "starch water" is an excellent thickener for stews, soups, and sauces.

Stored in its broth, seitan will stay fresh up to one week in the refrigerator. It freezes well, too.

Wheat bran is the outside protective covering of the wheat berry, sometimes called miller's bran or unprocessed bran. Only a small amount of bran should be used per individual serving, ranging from 1/2 teaspoon to 2 tablespoons. Eat with plenty of liquid for digestive ease. More is not always better. Too much bran can have a negative effect of binding up minerals such as copper, iron, and zinc, preventing their absorption.

Wheat flakes are made from whole wheat berries that have been heated and flattened. Cook into a hot cereal, add to granolas, or use in meat or bean loaves for bulk. Wheat flakes require 3 cups water per 1 cup dry flakes. Cook 30 minutes and allow to stand 5 minutes before serving.

Wheat germ, the embryo of the grain, can be sprinkled on foods as a nutritional enhancement or added to baked goods and entrees for its flavor and texture. Because it is so high in natural oils and very prone to rancidity, never buy wheat germ in bulk.

Raw wheat germ is available in shelf-stable nitrogen-packed packages while toasted wheat germ is often sold vacuum-packed. Because the heat treatment inactivates enzymes that can cause rancidity, toasted wheat germ retains its freshness somewhat longer than raw wheat germ.

Once the package has been opened, wheat germ should always be refrigerated or placed in the freezer and used within a week for optimum nutrition. It is better not to eat it at all than to eat rancid wheat germ.

Wheatena or Bear Mush™ is a finely ground hot cereal made from the whole grain. It offers much more flavor than farina. To cook, add 3/4 cup into 3 cups cold water in a medium-sized saucepan. Bring to a boil, stirring constantly. Turn heat to low, cover, and let simmer for 5-10 minutes. Serve with fresh or dried fruit, nuts, milk, or soy milk.

Flavor Enhancers: onion, chives, dill, mushrooms, pepper, garlic, curry, parsley, cilantro, and mint. For a sweet effect, cook with fruit juice instead of water. Dried fruits and sweet spices such as cinnamon, pumpkin pie spices, apple pie spices, ginger, and allspice add variety.

Menu Companions: Add cooked whole wheat berries to rice or barley. Mix equal parts of bulgur and buckwheat or quinoa, add to twice the amount of boiling water, and cook 20 minutes. Substitute 1/2 cup wheat flakes for oatmeal in your favorite granola recipe.

Breakfast Cereals

OVER HALF the adult population in the United States eats cereal for breakfast. Considering that cereal is generally low in fat with its calories primarily from carbohydrates, it's probably one of the best choices anyone could make to start the day.

Since product names and packaging art give few hints about the actual food value of the various cereals, to figure out which ones are worth eating look carefully at the ingredients and the "Nutrition Facts" listed on the label.

Like bread, the best cereals have the simplest list of ingredients: whole grains ground, rolled, flaked, shredded, or puffed processed with or without a sweetener or salt. Reflecting a growing trend for "natural" cereals, old standbys like Grape Nuts™, corn flakes, and shredded wheat are once again getting the good reputation they deserve as simple, wholesome cereals that are high in complex carbohydrates, moderate to high in fiber, and low in simple carbohydrates.

However, the concept of "natural" is often interpreted in several ways. Some brands of cereals rightfully proclaimed as low-fat and high in fiber may still contain artificial flavors, artificial colors, and/or artificial preservatives. While some cereals are technically free of preservatives, they may be sold in preservative-impregnated boxes. Added dried fruit may be treated with sulfur dioxide.

Fortunately, several manufacturers have bucked the trend and offer cereals made from basic ingredients free of questionable additives, confirming that "natural" alternatives can and do exist. New trends include the use of unconventional grains such as kamut, spelt, quinoa, millet, and triticale. Cereals made from organically grown grain are increasingly appearing on grocery shelves, adding another standard of quality.

The subject of sweeteners is another important issue concerning cereals. Avoid any cereal that lists sugar, honey, corn syrup, fructose, molasses, fruit juice sweetener, or malt syrup as the first ingredient. Never assume a "naturally sweetened" cereal will contain less simple sugars than those sweetened with white sugar. Depending on the brand and specific product, some "naturally sweetened" cereals may be equal or even higher in simple sugars.

To evaluate the relative sweetness of a cereal, compare the amount of "Sugars" listed on the "Nutrition Facts" label with "Total Carbohydrate." The total carbohydrate listing will include the sum of both complex and simple carbohydrates. The sugars declaration separates out the amount of simple sugars (glucose, fructose, lactose, and sucrose) present in the cereal.

Included in this figure are added dried fruits and sweeteners such as sugar, corn syrup, maple syrup, honey, fruit juice concentrate, and barley malt. To put the declared figure in more practical terms, consider that 1 teaspoon of sugar weighs 4 grams. So, if a cereal claims that it contains 8 grams of sugars, it would contain the equivalent of 2 teaspoons of sugar added to a plain otherwise unsweetened cereal. Ideally the amount of sugars should be very low, 4 grams or less. The lower this figure, the higher the amount of complex carbohydrates, the preferred type of carbohydrate which digests slowly to provide consistent energy fuel to our bodies.

To determine if the cereal is a good source of dietary fiber, refer again to the "Nutrition Facts" labeling. Choose cereals that contain at least a moderate amount of dietary fiber, about 3-4 grams. Designated high-fiber cereals usually have 5 grams or more per serving. Interestingly enough, ultra-high-fiber cereals usually contain the most sugars, an attempt to make more palatable what could taste like cardboard. When eating any high-fiber cereals be sure to moisten it with plenty of milk or soy milk or drink some sort of beverage with the meal. Since fiber needs to absorb water to be effective as a bulking agent, too little liquid can cause flatulence and constipation.

However, don't expect to get most of your daily fiber needs in one meal. A moderate amount frequently throughout the day is probably easier on your digestive system. Too much fiber can also inhibit trace mineral absorption.

Some cereals are also very high in sodium. Ideally, they should contain less than 140 mg. of sodium, the reference amount indicating "low sodium" content.

Fortification with essential vitamins and minerals may seem like a good idea but, in reality, it creates a false sense of security, making the cereal look much more wholesome that what it has to offer. Cereals based on whole grains naturally provide a wide variety of nutrients, including the B vitamins and some minerals. Not surprisingly, most fortified cereals are made from overly refined grains. Evaluate the nutrition of the cereal on its own merits, not by how many nutrients are artificially added to it.

The new wave of fortification is to provide additional nutrients from natural sources to already nutritious whole grain-based cereals. Beta carotene in the form of alga D. salina, an alga similar to spirulina and chlorellas is added to some cereals to provide a source of antioxidants, a category of nutrients considered beneficial as cancer deterrents. Some companies that prepare their foods according to Ayurvedic health principles add spices such as cinnamon, fennel, fenugreek, and cardamom, to some granolas to improve digestibility and help in the assimilation of nutrients.

VARIETIES AND COOKING GUIDELINES

Hot Cereals

Hot cereal is a centuries-old method of cooking grains quickly. Unlike their whole counterparts, rolled, coarsely cracked, or finely ground grains rarely require more than 20 minutes cooking time.

Rolled grains such as rolled oats, wheat flakes, rye flakes, and barley flakes are processed by briefly heating or steaming the grain, rolling it flat, and drying it before packaging. Although a cooked whole grain provides the most vitamins and minerals, since this process retains the bran and germ, rolled grains are very nutritious.

Grits are grains cracked into small, coarse pieces. For best flavor and nutrition, look for the word "whole" preceding the name of the grain on ingredient labels. Farina is made from refined wheat.

"Cream of" type cereals are made from fine to moderately ground grain. Like grits,

APPLE ALMOND KAMUT

1 1/2 cups kamut flakes
3 cups water
1/4 tsp. salt
1/4 cup dried apples, cut into medium sized pieces
1/2 tsp. vanilla extract
1/4 cup whole almonds

Combine all ingredients except almonds in a saucepan. Bring to a boil, reduce heat to simmer, and cover. Cook about 15 minutes. Add almonds and cook an additional 5 minutes. Serve plain or top with milk or soy milk.

Serves 4
(Pyramid servings: 3 Bread/Grain Group, 1/2 Fruit Group, 5 grams Fat)

Nutrition Facts

Serving Size 1/4 recipe (207 g)
Servings Per Container 4

Amount Per Serving

Calories 120	Calories from Fat 45	

	% Daily Value*
Total Fat 5g	8%
Sodium 180mg	8%
Total Carbohydrate 16g	5%
Dietary Fiber 3g	11%
Sugars 5g	
Protein 3g	

Calcium 2%	•	Iron 6%

Not a significant source of Saturated Fat, Cholesterol, Vitamin A and Vitamin C.

* Percent Daily Values are based on a 2,000 calorie diet.

---

choose the ground whole grain version for taste, texture, and nutrition. Baby cereals usually fit in this category. Choose varieties based on finely ground whole grains free of sugar, salt, and preservatives.

Several premixed single and multiple grain combinations and textures are available. You can also make your own customized blends. See "Whole Grains" chapter to familiarize yourself with the various options. Combine several rolled grains together and cook like oatmeal. Coarsely grind whole grains in a blender or electric nut/seed mill. Roast flour by stirring it constantly in a dry skillet over moderate heat.

Some popular national brands use additives to speed the cooking process of hot cereals. Disodium phosphate, an alkalinizing agent, causes the grains to swell and gelatinize faster. Proteolytic enzymes open up pathways within the grain to facilitate the penetration of water. While these timesavers aren't exactly harmful or even necessarily bad, neither are they necessary. Few "natural" whole-grain hot cereals depend on them.

Cooking hot cereals is somewhat different than simmering whole grains. Pulverization of the grain allows the grain's starch to readily mix with the cooking liquid to create a thick mixture. To prevent lumps in finely ground cereals, bring water to a boil. Combine the cereal with cold water to make a paste and then add to the boiling water, whisking only to mix the grain with the water. An alternative method is to sprinkle the cereal slowly into the boiling water. Minimal stirring when cooking hot cereals will prevent gummy results.

The flavor of cooked cereals is enhanced with longer cooking as the heat converts the starches to dextrins and sugars. Accordingly, opt for low heat, sustained cooking and al-

LOWFAT VANILLA GRANOLA

6 cups rolled oats
1/4 cup sunflower seeds
1/4 cup almonds, chopped
pinch of salt (opt.)
1/2 cup honey, maple
    syrup, or rice syrup
1 tsp vanilla extract

Preheat oven to 325° F. In a large bowl, combine oats, sunflower seeds, almonds, and salt. Warm sweetener in a small saucepan over low heat about 1 minute. Add vanilla extract. Thoroughly mix flavored sweetener in with oat mixture. Spread thinly on 2 cookie sheets. Bake at 325°F about 20 minutes, stirring every 5 minutes to prevent burning. The granola is done when it just begins to turn a golden color. Allow to cool before serving. Store in a tightly sealed container in the refrigerator.

Nutrition Facts

Serving Size 1/2 cup (56 g)
Servings Per Container 13

Amount Per Serving

Calories 210	Calories from Fat 45

	% Daily Value*
Total Fat 5g	8%
Saturated Fat 0.5g	4%
Sodium 25mg	1%
Total Carbohydrate 35g	12%
Dietary Fiber 5g	18%
Sugars 9g	
Protein 7g	

Calcium 4%	•	Iron 10%

Not a significant source of Cholesterol, Vitamin A and Vitamin C.
* Percent Daily Values are based on a 2,000 calorie diet.

Makes 6 1/2 cups.
(Pyramid servings: 1 Bread/Grain Group, 5 grams Fat, 8 grams Sweets)

---

low the cereal to "rest" at least 5 minutes before serving.

Leftover cooked grains can also be made into hot cereals. Heat with milk, water, or juice in a pan. The more liquid, the more creamy the results. Jazz it up with dried fruit, nuts, seeds, or a touch of maple syrup, honey, or your favorite flavoring.

Ready-to-Eat Cereals

Hot cereals are generally more nutritious but ready-to-eat cereals win the prize for convenience. When based on whole grains and free of artificial colors, flavors, and excess sugars, ready-to-eat cereals make a valuable breakfast or late-night snack.

Your best choices are shredded cereals or whole grain flakes unsweetened or lightly sweetened with malt syrup, a more balanced sweetener higher in complex carbohydrates than other sweeteners. Honey- or fruit juice-sweetened cereals generally affect blood sugar levels just as dramatically as comparable amounts of white sugar.

Shredded cereals are most nutritious, simply manufactured by putting the whole grain, including the germ and bran, in a shredding machine followed by baking. Shredded cereals are often sugar-free.

Flakes are manufactured in two basic ways, yielding different textures and nutrition. Roller-flattened toasted flakes are hearty and chewy, providing similar nutrient value as rolled whole grains (see above). Extruded flakes are made from a slurry of ground whole or refined grains and water, flattened by a flaking mill, and toasted. While lighter in texture, undergoing more initial processing, whole- grain versions are slightly less nutritious than roller-flattened toasted flakes. Refined versions offer marginal nutrition, resulting in severely reduced amounts of fiber and several nutrients found originally in their bran and germ.

Puffed cereals are produced by heating moist grains under pressure and suddenly releasing the pressure. This causes steam to expand rapidly, expanding or puffing up the grains, in a similar fashion as popcorn. Because of their high heat processing, they are less nutritious than other cereals. Look for sugar-free brands free of other additives.

Granola is based on rolled grains, nuts, and seeds sweetened and baked with or without oil. High in fiber, granola is also typically high in fat and sugar, depending on the specific ingredients and amounts used. High-quality oiled baked granolas are made with high-oleic expeller-pressed oils. To keep saturated fats to a minimum, avoid granolas made with coconut oil or partially hydrogenated fats. Oil-free granolas can still be high in fat, depending on the amount of nuts and seeds added. Without the luxury of being baked in oil, this type of granola is usually more crisp and chewy than the full-fat version.

Muesli is granola European-style. While the ingredients look very similar to granola, muesli is unbaked and typically sugar-free, relying on dried fruit for sweetness. To prepare, soak overnight in juice, milk, or soy milk. By next morning the flakes will have softened considerably, facilitating their digestion. Top with a grated apple and serve, if desired, with yogurt, milk, or soy milk.

Sprouted baby cereals provide "cream of" texture but require no cooking. Sprouting the grain converts some of the starch into maltose which, besides providing natural sweetness, facilitates digestion of the grain. Sprouting also increases the amount of protein in the grain as well as vitamins A, B, C, and E.

Whole Grain Flour

Renewed interest in grains as well as increasing awareness of sensitivities to gluten and/or wheat has changed the generally accepted definition of "flour." Whereas previously "flour" could be listed as an ingredient in a recipe under the assumption that cooks and bakers would naturally use whole wheat or white flour, now things aren't that simple. A trip to the grocery store will reveal not only the familiar wheat varieties of flour but also exotic options such as amaranth flour, spelt flour, and teff flour.

All whole grains can be ground into flour, but it's not just a matter of substituting them equally with wheat flours. Each contributes its own unique flavors and textures. Some flours are mildly flavored while others are downright assertive. Textures range from silken to sandy. Density and suitability as a primary flour in leavened breads depend on the amount of gluten present in the flour. Recognizing each flour's characteristics can not only make experimentation fun and interesting but yield delicious baked goods as a reward for all your efforts.

BAKING WITH ALTERNATIVE FLOURS

Knowing how to balance textures is most critical when baking with alternative flours. If most of your recipes call for 100% wheat flour, initially it is advisable to start by substituting another flour for only part of the wheat rather than *all* of the wheat flour. A good starting point is to use, for each cup of whole wheat flour, 3/4 cup whole wheat flour and 1/4 cup flour of your choice. Recipes on packages of alternative flours and from many cookbooks prove substitutions of this sort can work, but textures and "crumb" can vary tremendously. Experiment to find as many variations to your basic recipes as you can invent.

Certain recipes for flat breads, muffins, cookies, and pancakes can be made successfully with single nonwheat flours. However, each individual flour's baked textures are accentuated when used alone. For instance, a product made solely with brown rice flour will yield a dry, crisp, grainy texture quite different from the texture and taste of a baked whole wheat product. While cookies or flat bread could be made with 100% brown rice flour with good results, you wouldn't have the same luck with a cake. To remedy the situation without resorting to wheat, the dry, grainy texture of brown rice flour could be balanced with a grain flour that yields a moist texture such as buckwheat, millet, rye, or soy. The converse also applies: when using a flour that yields a product with too moist or gummy a texture, add a dry textured flour.

NONGLUTEN FLOURS ON THE RISE

Gluten is a protein complex that is responsible for the elastic properties in bread doughs and for the appearance and structure of baked goods such as cakes, quick breads, and cookies.

Gluten is comprised of two types of protein, gliadin and glutenin. Gliadins give dough its fluid and sticky characteristics. Glutenins are responsible for the dough's elasticity. The quantity and proportion of these two proteins within a grain will determine the overall density and volume that can be expected in breads and baked goods made with a specific flour. Gluten is developed through gentle stretching and folding of the dough through kneading or, in the case of cake and quick bread batters and cookie doughs, through stirring with a spoon or with an electric mixer or food processor. The gluten then captures the carbon dioxide produced by the yeast, sourdough, baking powder, or baking soda to achieve lighter-textured, higher-volumed results.

Wheat flour contains the best quality and quantity of gluten, but even within the wheat category there are significant variations. The gluten in durum wheat is very strong, good for pasta but too rigid for bread. The gluten in hard wheat is perfect for breads while soft wheats contain just enough to produce quick breads and other baked goods that are light and airy.

Spelt and kamut, ancient ancestors of our modern-day wheat, contain similar gluten properties. Other grains vary from low to no gluten (see chart next page), producing more dense results. Modifications can be made with the inclusion of higher-gluten flours or, to a certain degree, increased amounts of leaveners. Pie crusts made with low-gluten or gluten-free flours need to be pressed into shape instead of rolled.

While gluten produces beneficial baking results, several individuals are sensitive to the gliadin component of gluten, causing major digestive difficulties after eating products made from gluten-containing flours. The gluten in common wheat is most problematic. Although rye contains some gluten, its complex includes only glutenin and not gliadin, the major source of gluten intolerance. For reasons not completely understood, spelt and kamut, two grains with ancestral ties to wheat, appear to be tolerated by many, but not all, people otherwise sensitive to gluten. Barley and oats contain small amounts of gluten.

BUYING AND STORING

Flour can be ground in several ways. Whole-grain flours are usually stone-ground or hammer-milled.

Stone-ground flour is ground between two flat millstones that rub against each other, producing a rather coarse flour somewhat uneven in texture. The stones slowly crush the grain, distributing its bran and nutrient-rich germ throughout the flour. Slow grinding keeps temperatures to a minimum, around 90° F. As the most traditional method of grinding flour, some of its popularity can be attributed to nostalgia. However, its method of grinding and speed may also contribute to increased preservation of nutrients and better flavor. Grinding stones require much maintenance to ensure best results.

Hammer-milled flour is ground in a mill in which bars, swinging on an axle, rotate inside a steel cylinder, crushing the grain against the inner surface. A faster way to grind grains, hammer-milling also controls texture granulation better than stone-grinding.

Refined flours are ground in a **roller mill**, a machine that depends on rollers with smooth to coarse surfaces set various widths

FLOUR AT A GLANCE

Flour	Gluten?	Flavor	Baked Texture
amaranth	no	strong, spicy	smooth, crisp crust moist, fine crumb
arrowroot	no	neutral	lightens wheat-free baked goods
barley	yes	sweet, malty	firm, chewy crust cakelike crumb
buckwheat	no	hearty	moist, fine crumb
carob	no	chocolatey	like cocoa
chickpea	no	sweet, rich	dry, delicate crumb
cornmeal	no	sweet, nutty	grainy, slightly dry
gluten	yes	tangy	fine crumb crisp, thin crust
kamut	yes	rich, buttery	dense, heavy crumb
kuzu	no	neutral	a cooking starch
millet	no	mildly sweet,	dry, delicate crumb buttery smooth, thin crust
oat	yes	sweet, nutty	moist, cakelike crumb, firm crust
potato	no	sweetly pungent	soft, dry crust fine, springy crumb
quinoa	no	nutty	delicate, cakelike crumb
rice	no	nutty	dry, fine crumb
rye	yes	tangy	moist, crumb smooth, hard crust

Flour	Gluten?	Flavor	Baked Texture
soy	no	slightly bitter	moist, fine crumb smooth, hard crust
spelt	yes	sweet, nutty	moderate crumb supple crust
tapioca	no	slightly sweet	lightens wheat-free baked goods
teff	no	sweet, malty	delicate crumb
triticale	yes	nutty, tangy	dense crumb semi-firm crust
wheat	yes	sweet, nutty	coarse, large crumb (whole wheat) fine crumb (pastry flour)

apart. Unlike stone-grinding and hammer-milling, grinding flour in a roller mill makes it possible to quickly separate the bran and germ from the endosperm and completely control the particle size of the flour through continuous grinding and sifting. It also allows for the making of custom flour blends geared for commercial bread bakers, home use, specialty breads, cakes, crackers, and pastries, and pasta production using two or more varieties of wheat. A grain can go through a roller mill up to 26 times to get to the desired results. Temperature goes no higher than 140°F.

Flour can also be ground at home. Several flour grinders are available, some with grinding stones and others with metal burrs, both manual and electric-powered. Some juicers and food processors have special flour grinder attachments.

Some grains such as rice, millet, oats, quinoa can be ground in your blender; however, unless your blender is particularly heavy-duty, too much grinding could burn out the motor. Results are often mixed, as well.

Further Processing of Wheat Flour

Refined wheat flour may also be subjected to further processing including the use of bleaching and maturing agents, dough conditioners, and enrichment.

Artificial bleaching agents were adopted in the early 1900s as a quicker, cheaper way to mature the flour and condition the gluten. Traditionally, flour was stored for several months. During that time, oxygen naturally bleached the flour's yellow tint to an off-white color. It also oxidized the protein, making the gluten stronger and more elastic for better baking results.

Since storage cost money and the flour had to be rotated to make sure all the flour was exposed to oxygen, the discovery of artificial bleaching agents was enthusiastically accepted by many millers. However, while they may save time, space, and money, artificial bleaching and maturing agents adversely affect the flour's nutrients and add additives with questionable long-term safety ramifications.

Benzoyl peroxide is commonly used to bleach the flour white, requiring just a few moments rather than months. Chlorine dioxide and acetone peroxide are used as oxidizing agents to quicken the maturation process of the flour. In the process, vitamin E is completely destroyed. Other oxidizing agents include potassium bromate, azodicarbonamide, and ascorbic acid.

Malted barley flour is added to enhance the flour's natural enzymes when a particular crop of wheat is tested to be deficient. Proper enzyme activity is necessary to enable doughs to rise properly.

How to Store

Whole-grain flour should be stored at cool temperatures below 70°F., preferably in the refrigerator or freezer, to prevent the natural oils found in the bran and germ from going rancid. Keep flour in its original moisture-proof package wrapped in another plastic bag or in airtight plastic containers. Use within 3 months. To ensure better baking, warm the flour to room temperature before using. Proper storage will also deter weevils and mealy moths.

Exploring Your Options

AMARANTH FLOUR

Facts and Features

Amaranth flour adds an unusual nutty/spice flavor and smooth, moist texture to cookies, muffins, pancakes, waffles, and breads. But its real claim to fame is its protein quality which boosts the nutritional content of any recipe.

However, instead of using it as the sole or primary flour in recipes, amaranth flour should be combined in small amounts with other flours to create the right balance in flavor and texture. Too much may result in strong-flavored, overly dense baked goods.

Baking Guidelines

Amaranth flour is gluten-free so it is appropriate only in recipes that don't require baking yeast.

A good rule of thumb is to substitute up to 1/4 of the wheat or other grain flour indicated in a recipe with amaranth flour. Experiment by using 1/4 cup amaranth with 3/4 cup brown rice or oat flour. Or try 3/4 cup amaranth flour with 1/4 cup arrowroot powder, tapioca flour, soy flour, buckwheat flour, potato starch, or ground nuts or seeds in your favorite recipes.

ARROWROOT FLOUR/ STARCH

Facts and Features

Derived from a narrow, 6-inch-long root that hails from the West Indies, arrowroot is true to its name, having the distinction of being used by Indians to draw poison from arrow wounds. Now in its dried and powdered stage, it is used for more peaceful means as an easily digested thickener and flour substitute.

Arrowroot has several things going for it as a thickener. Unlike flour, arrowroot is virtually neutral in taste, so it doesn't need to be precooked to get rid of any raw floury flavor. It also allows the true flavors of the sauce to come through.

While equal in strength to both cornstarch and potato starch, arrowroot has double the thickening power of flour. Because it starts to thicken at lower temperatures, arrowroot thickens quicker than flour, making it perfect for last-minute corrections.

The visual result of sauces thickened with arrowroot is also clear and transparent, presenting an overall beautiful glazed look.

If kept tightly sealed to prevent moisture, arrowroot can keep almost indefinitely.

Baking/Cooking Guidelines

Plan on using about 1 Tbsp. to thicken 1 cup liquid. To prevent clumping, first dissolve arrowroot in cold water. Stir slowly into boiling liquid and continue mixing just until thickened. Then reduce the heat immediately and serve within 15 minutes. With continued cooking, an arrowroot thickened sauce will break down. It doesn't reheat well, either.

Arrowroot is often used as a flour substitute to lighten wheat-free baked goods such as those made with amaranth, brown rice, or millet flours. Experiment using 25-50% in recipes.

BARLEY FLOUR

Facts and Features

Barley flour contributes a sweet, malty flavor, a moist, cake-like crumb and a firm, chewy crust. For optimum flavor and nutrition, look for barley flour ground from hulless barley.

Baking/Cooking Guidelines

Baked goods taste even better if barley flour is lightly toasted in a dry skillet before adding to recipes.

Although it contains some gluten, in yeasted breads or sourdough breads barley flour should be combined with higher-gluten flours such as whole wheat, unbleached white, or spelt in a 1 to 5 ratio.

Cakes, cookies, muffins, pancakes, and quick breads made with 100% barley flour may turn out too moist. You'll have better results balancing barley flour with wheat and/or oat flour. Start with a 50/50 mixture and experiment from there.

And, don't forget barley flour when making flour-thickened gravies and other cooked sauces for an interesting twist in taste.

BUCKWHEAT FLOUR

Facts and Features

Hearty pancakes, paper-thin crêpes, and Japanese soba noodles all develop their distinctive qualities from the robust, somewhat musty flavor of buckwheat flour.

Light buckwheat flour is made from hulled buckwheat while the stronger-flavored dark buckwheat flour includes finely ground parts of the hull. For a drier texture and more mellow flavor, use your blender or electric nut/coffee grinder to grind white unroasted buckwheat into flour.

Baking/Cooking Guidelines

Buckwheat is gluten-free, so its flour needs to be combined with a high-gluten flour such as whole wheat if a yeast-risen bread is in the works. Because its flavor is so hearty and its texture potentially gummy, only small amounts, no more than 1/3 cup per loaf, should be used.

Pancakes, muffins, and crêpes can handle a higher proportion of buckwheat

BUCKWHEAT MAPLE MUFFINS

1/2 cup pecans
3/4 cup buckwheat flour
2 1/4 cup whole wheat
    pastry flour
1 Tbsp. baking powder
1/2 Tbsp. baking soda
1/2 tsp. salt
2/3 cup nonfat yogurt
1/3 cup water
1/3 cup maple syrup
2 eggs or 4 egg whites,
    slightly beaten
3 Tbsp. safflower or
    canola oil
grated peel from 1 large
    orange

Preheat oven to 400°F and oil muffin tins. Chop pecans and combine with other dry ingredients in a large bowl. In a separate bowl, combine remaining ingredients. Form a well in the flour mixture and add liquid ingredients. Mix only until the ingredients are moistened, using no more than 15-20 strokes. Quickly fill muffin cups to the top and place on middle rack of the oven. Bake at 400° for 18-20 minutes. Allow muffins to remain in pans for 1-2 minutes. Remove and allow muffins to cool briefly on a wire rack.

Makes 12 large muffins.
(Pyramid servings: 2 Bread/Grain Group, 1/4 Meat/Protein Group,

Nutrition Facts

Serving Size 1 muffin (69 g)
Servings Per Container 12

Amount Per Serving

Calories 180   Calories from Fat 70

                                          % Daily Value*
Total Fat 8g   12%
    Saturated Fat 1g   4%
Cholesterol 30mg   10%
Sodium 210mg   9%
Total Carbohydrate 25g   8%
    Dietary Fiber 3g   11%
    Sugars 7g
Protein 5g

Vitamin A 2%   •   Calcium 15%
Iron 8%

Not a significant source of Vitamin C
* Percent Daily Values are based on a 2,000 calorie diet.

---

flour. It all depends on just how robust a flavor you want and the types and amount of ingredients, such as eggs or yogurt, that are used for leavening.

Due to its gluey texture when cooked, buckwheat flour is not a good choice when thickening sauces and gravies.

CAROB FLOUR

Facts and Features

Carob is the dried, roasted, and pulverized pod of the honey locust tree that grows primarily in countries surrounding the Mediterranean. With a flavor similar to yet milder than chocolate, carob is generally used as a substitute for cocoa. It is also added as an ingredient in bread doughs to make deep, richly-colored loaves.

Unlike chocolate, carob is naturally sweet, high in fiber, very low in fat, and caffeine-free. It also contains 3 times the amount of calcium (390 mg. of calcium per 1 cup) found in chocolate. Easily digested and rich in pectin, carob is also a traditional remedy to soothe upset stomachs.

Baking/Cooking Guidelines

Substitute carob equally for cocoa in cookies, cakes, candies, and beverages. To replace 1 square of baking chocolate in a recipe, substitute 3 Tbsp. carob plus 1 Tbsp. milk.

For darker-colored bread, add 1-2 Tbsp to 1 loaf bread recipe.

Because of its high fiber content, carob needs to be thoroughly mixed in a blender when making carob drinks to avoid it settling at the bottom of the glass.

CHICKPEA FLOUR (BESAN OR CHANA)

Facts and Features

Like the chickpeas (garbanzo beans) from which it is ground, chickpea flour not only boosts protein, it also adds a sweet, rich flavor. In baked goods it lends a dry, delicate crumb.

Besan, unroasted chickpea flour, is used only for cooking. It is a common ingredient in East Indian fritters called pakoras, and an Indian fried noodle snack called sev.

Roasted chickpea flour makes an interesting addition to baked goods. It also makes quick work of falafel or hummus, substituting for cooked, mashed garbanzo beans.

Both besan and roasted chickpea flour can even be used to thicken soups, stews, sauces, and to bind ingredients together to form bean or grain "burgers."

Baking/Cooking Guidelines

Combine 1 cup roasted chickpea flour with 2/3 cup cold water to equal 1 1/2 cups cooked, mashed garbanzo beans when making dips, spreads, casseroles, or patties.

In muffin and bread recipes, mix small amounts of chickpea flour with other flours. Because it is gluten-free, in yeast or sourdough breads chickpea flour should be combined with wheat or spelt flour in a 1:4 ratio.

As it is more digestible than soy flour, chickpea flour is a good substitute for soy flour in most recipes.

CORN FLOUR

Facts and Features

Mildly sweet and nutty with a grainy, slightly dry texture, even a small amount of cornmeal makes a wonderful contribution of color and crunch to muffins, pancakes, savory crusts, and yeasted or sourdough breads.

Whether you use regular yellow cornmeal, high-lysine cornmeal, or blue cornmeal (see CORN in whole grains chapter for detailed information), the best taste and texture comes from stone-ground corn.

Corn flour is ground to a finer consistency than cornmeal. Use in breads, pancakes, or waffles if a smoother, less grainy texture than found in regular cornmeal is desired. If you have trouble finding it, make your own by grinding regular cornmeal finer in your blender.

Baking/Cooking Guidelines

Great-tasting cornbreads can be made solely from cornmeal. Some people, however, prefer blending in whole wheat or white flour for a lighter, softer texture. Suggested proportions vary but, in general, 3 parts corn to 1 part wheat flour is a good place to start.

Fold in fresh, cooked corn kernels to corn bread batters for added sweetness and texture.

Cornmeal is often used to prevent breads and pizza crusts from sticking to their respective pans. It also adds a delicious flavor and texture to the crust.

CORNSTARCH

Facts and Features

Next to flour, cornstarch holds the honor as the second most commonly used thickener. However, several attributes of cornstarch make it the preferred choice in certain applications. Unlike flour, a cornstarch-thickened sauce has a smooth texture and shiny, transparent appearance. It imparts considerably less flavor to the finished product, although it's still more noticeable than arrowroot. And, cornstarch is also more effective in fruit sauces and pies since it doesn't lose its thickening power as quickly as flour.

To become cornstarch, corn kernels go through rather extensive refining. After the hull and germ are removed, the corn is further processed to separate any remaining protein, resulting in pure starch. It is then washed, dried, and ground into the fine powder so characteristic of cornstarch. Because it is so refined and contributes little nutritive value, many people prefer to use arrowroot powder instead.

Baking/Cooking Guidelines

Use half as much cornstarch as flour and equal amounts as arrowroot and potato starch. Like other thickeners, cornstarch must be dissolved in cold water before adding to the liquid to be thickened. Stir the mixture constantly until thickened, reduce heat, and serve immediately.

GLUTEN FLOUR & VITAL WHEAT GLUTEN

Facts and Features

Gluten flour is a mixture of white flour and concentrated wheat gluten. **Vital wheat gluten** is the undiluted form of dried and ground gluten extracted from wheat flour specially processed to prevent the denaturation of the protein by heat.

Small amounts, about 5-10% of the flour weight for gluten flour and only 2-3% of the flour weight for vital wheat gluten, will help the dough rise higher and more quickly, creating a lightly textured bread that doesn't crumble when sliced. It is especially useful when baking with low gluten flours. Breads leavened with baking powder can also benefit from gluten. It will improve shape and texture, but, unlike yeasted or sourdough breads fortified with gluten, quick breads will not necessarily experience an increase in rising.

The addition of gluten also increases the amount of protein in the bread. However, since it is very deficient in lysine, one of the essential amino acids, the protein quality is affected accordingly.

Similar to the process in making seitan or "wheat meat," gluten is extracted from wheat flour. Formed into a kind of dough, it is kneaded, allowed to rest to develop the gluten, and then rinsed under water to separate the starch and bran from the gluten.

While its benefits sound like a dream come true, the addition of gluten flour or vital wheat gluten has its drawbacks. Because it contributes more gluten than normal, it requires more kneading to allow the gluten to fully develop. Gluten also imparts a distinctive flavor and texture to breads that may or may not be appreciated. On top of that, breads made with extra gluten stale more quickly.

The most important objection to using gluten flour or vital wheat gluten is that, because it is so concentrated, some people who generally have no adverse reaction to wheat-based foods, find breads made with gluten difficult to digest. Obviously, anyone who is allergic to wheat will have a problem if gluten flour is added, which makes its use in low-gluten flour breads which may be otherwise wheat-free incompatible.

Baking/Cooking Guidelines

Use about 2 Tbsp. of gluten flour per cup of flour for whole-grain breads. Since white flour lacks the bran and germ, cup for cup it contains more gluten than whole wheat flour. Therefore, less gluten flour, about 1 Tbsp.+ 1 tsp. per cup white flour, is needed when making white breads.

In whole-grain breads, use 11/2 tsp. vital wheat gluten per cup flour. Cut it down to 1 tsp. per cup flour when making white breads.

Breads that contain bran, nuts, raisins, seeds, and nonwheat flours may need slightly more gluten flour or vital wheat gluten to compensate for the increased bulk.

KAMUT FLOUR

Facts and Features

Ground from the giant, buttery-tasting ancient variety of durum wheat, kamut flour lends a terrific flavor and beautiful amber color to baked goods.

And yet substituting kamut for wheat in any recipe doesn't always work. When working with kamut flour, consider it as an alternative for durum wheat flour, possessing the same high-gluten, hard starch granules that make it such a good flour for pasta. It works well in flat breads, crackers, pizza crusts, and pancakes, but anything that needs to rise higher than these foods, such as yeasted or sourdough bread, will turn out much too dense and heavy.

Much of kamut flour's recent popularity is due to its successful use by many individuals allergic to common modern-day wheat. Anyone severely allergic to wheat should consult with a doctor or health practitioner before experimenting with kamut.

Baking/Cooking Guidelines

When baking or making pancakes with kamut flour, for best results limit kamut flour to 1/4 of the flour required in the recipe. Since it contains a particularly strong gluten, you can also experiment adding small amounts to quick bread recipes using non-gluten flours.

Kamut makes an interesting sourdough culture with a lot of oomph. Just make sure to combine with another flour such as whole wheat or spelt when proceeding with the recipe instead of adding more kamut flour. Sourdough kamut/spelt breadsticks are particularly good.

KUZU

Facts and Features

According to ancient Japanese medicine, kuzu, an easily digested, concentrated root starch, has an alkalinizing effect on the body. Accordingly, it has been used as a rebalancing agent to deal with self-limiting conditions such as intestinal and digestive disorders, headaches, fevers, colds, and hangovers. When cooked with apple juice, sesame tahini, and vanilla as natural health educator and gourmet cook Annemarie Colbin suggests in her landmark book, *Food & Healing* (Ballentine Books, 1986), kuzu helps to reduce body tension when you're feeling overworked or stressed and crave something comforting and creamy.

As much as kuzu is valued for its medicinal qualities, its thickening and "gelling" properties are highly regarded, as well. Like arrowroot and cornstarch, sauces and desserts thickened with kuzu are smooth and transparent. An added plus is that kuzu-thickened pies and puddings remain set after cooling, making dairy-free desserts a delicious possibility.

Kuzu's only drawback is that it is very expensive. Currently it is imported from Japan, an ironic situation since it's a prolific weed growing in the Southern U.S.

ANNEMARIE'S APPLE JUICE PUDDING

Adapted from Annemarie Colbin's Apple Juice-Kuzu recipe found in her book, *Food and Healing* (Ballentine Books, 1986)

3 cups apple juice
1 cup water
2 Tbsp. sesame tahini
1/3-1/2 cup kuzu
2 tsp. vanilla extract

Dissolve kuzu in 1 cup water. Mix with juice and vanilla and cook over medium heat, stirring constantly. When mixture becomes thick and creamy, slowly add tahini and stir 1 minute more. Remove from heat. Serve hot or cold.

Serves 3-4
(Pyramid servings: 1/2 Bread/Grain Group, 1 Fruit Group, 4 1/2 grams Fat)

Nutrition Facts

Serving Size 1/4 recipe (273 g)
Servings Per Container 4

Amount Per Serving

Calories 200   Calories from Fat 40

	% Daily Value*
Total Fat 4.5g	7%
Saturated Fat 0.5g	3%
Sodium 10mg	0%
Total Carbohydrate 38g	13%
Dietary Fiber 1g	4%
Sugars 21g	
Protein 2g	

Vitamin C 2%	Calcium 2%
Iron 6%	

Not a significant source of Cholesterol and Vitamin A.

* Percent Daily Values are based on a 2,000 calorie diet.

Baking/Cooking Guidelines

Kuzu is sold in chunks. Before measuring, crush it with a mortar and pestle or with the back of a spoon. Dissolve it in cold water before adding to the liquid to be thickened and then stir constantly until the desired thickness is achieved. Plan on using about 2 Tbsp. to thicken 1 cup liquid, about the same as when thickening with flour, twice as much as arrowroot and cornstarch.

MILLET FLOUR

Facts and Features

Considering all the flours available, it is particularly important for millet flour to be freshly ground. At its prime, millet flour has an appealing sweet flavor, but when even slightly old, it makes anything baked with it taste bitter. For best results, grind it at home in a small electric nut/spice mill, blender, or flour mill. Store extra flour in the freezer and use as quickly as possible.

Despite these caveats, millet flour is well worth trying. Baked goods made with millet flour have a dry, delicate crumb and a smooth, thin crust.

Baking/Cooking Guidelines

Cookies and muffins can be made with up to 50% millet flour. Combine with whole wheat flour, brown rice flour, or a combination of brown rice flour and tapioca flour to enhance millet's sweet flavor and to balance its texture.

Because millet is gluten-free, yeasted and sourdough breads made with millet flour need a high proportion of wheat or spelt flours. For best flavor and texture results, limit the millet flour to 1/2-3/4 cup per loaf.

OAT FLOUR

Facts and Features

Oat flour-based baked goods turn out especially moist and flavorful with a cake-like crumb, primarily due to its bran which, unlike its coarse wheat counterpart, is high in soluble fibers.

Readily available in natural food stores, it can also be ground fresh at home in the blender, using 11/4 cups rolled oats to make 1 cup oat flour.

An added benefit with oat flour is that baked goods made with it remain fresher longer, thanks to the grain's natural antioxidant. Before chemical preservatives were added to breads and cakes, bakers often added a small amount of oats to their products to prevent them from going stale too quickly.

Baking/Cooking Guidelines

Successful substitution for wheat flour depends on the application. In yeasted breads, use 1/3 oat flour with 2/3 wheat flour. Some muffins and pancakes can be made with up to 100% oat flour while cakes and cookies need at least a 50/50 balance of oat flour with another flour. In wheat-free recipes, oat flour can be combined with brown rice flour, arrowroot, tapioca flour, or homeground white buckwheat flour.

Oat flour also works as a good thickener in sauces, soups, and stews.

OAT/RICE PANCAKES

1 1/2 cups oat flour
1 1/2 cups brown rice flour
1/2 tsp. salt
2 tsp. baking powder
2 eggs
1 cup soy milk or milk
1 cup water
1/2 tsp. almond extract
2 Tbsp. oil or prune puree or apple butter

Preheat pancake griddle over medium heat. Stir together all the dry ingredients. Beat the eggs lightly and combine with the milk, water, extract, and oil. Add mixture to the dry ingredients and stir briefly. Ladle batter onto a lightly oiled griddle. Cook over medium heat, turning once when bubbles come to the surface and the edges are slightly dry.

Makes 18 average or 8 large pancakes
(Pyramid servings: 1 Bread/Grain Group, 3 grams Fat)

Nutrition Facts

Serving Size 1 pancake (55 g)
Servings Per Container 18

Amount Per Serving

Calories 110   Calories from Fat 30

	% Daily Value*
Total Fat 3g	5%
Cholesterol 20mg	7%
Sodium 120mg	5%
Total Carbohydrate 16g	5%
Dietary Fiber 2g	6%
Sugars 1g	
Protein 3g	

Vitamin A 2% • Calcium 6%

Iron 4%

Not a significant source of Saturated Fat and Vitamin C.

* Percent Daily Values are based on a 2,000 calorie diet.

POTATO FLOUR

Facts and Features

Potato flour is a mild-tasting flour made from cooked potatoes that have been dried and ground. Used primarily as a thickener and binder, like arrowroot and cornstarch, potato flour-thickened sauces are translucent and glossy. It can also be used as a substitute for flour in cakes and cookies.

Baking/Cooking Guidelines

Use in equal proportions to arrowroot and cornstarch but only half as much as suggested in flour-thickened sauce recipes.

When combined with other non-gluten flours, potato flour can also be used in wheat-free cakes and cookies. Experiment with the following proportions: 1/4 cup potato flour + 1 cup soy, 1/3 cup potato flour + 1/3 cup rye, and 1/4 cup potato flour + 3/4 cup rice flour.

QUINOA FLOUR

Facts and Features

Baked goods made with quinoa flour have a delicate crumb and delicious flavor. Leavened breads made with quinoa flour are lighter in texture. Like its whole-grain counterpart, quinoa flour is also an effective protein booster.

Quinoa flour may be difficult to locate. Fortunately, it can easily be ground in your blender at home.

Baking/Cooking Guidelines

To make 1 cup quinoa flour, grind 3/4 cup whole quinoa in a blender. Its texture will be similar to a finely ground cornmeal. Dry-roasting the flour will enhance its flavor.

Quinoa flour is gluten-free so it should be combined with wheat flour in yeasted or sourdough breads at a ratio of approximately 1 part quinoa flour to 4 parts wheat.

Biscuits, pasta, and tortillas will also turn out better if a small amount of wheat flour is added to balance quinoa's delicate qualities. Experiment using up to 50% in cakes, cookies, pancakes, and waffles.

Try using quinoa flour as a substitute for wheat flour to thicken sauces and gravies, too.

RICE FLOUR

Facts and Features

Rice flour has a delicious nutty flavor and a very grainy, somewhat gritty texture. While it adds variety when used in small amounts to replace wheat flour, developing recipes based primarily on rice flour can be challenging. However, once you get familiar with its ideosyncracies, the results will be worth the experimentation.

No matter what you intend to bake, some type of binder is required to balance rice flour's texture. Excellent flat breads, cookies, and cakes can be made if "gummy" flours such as rye, oat, or potato flour are added to the recipe.

Satisfactory, sliceable breads made from 100% rice flour are possible with the addition of vegetable gums such as methylcellulose and guar gum. Methylcellulose can be purchased from Ener-G Foods, Inc., a company specializing in hypoallergenic foods and mixes. Ask your local store to order it for you or order it direct from Ener-G Foods, P.O. Box 84487, Seattle, WA 98124-5787.

The company also manufactures a product called "Brown Rice Baking Mix™" that includes methylcellulose along with brown rice flour, tapioca flour, almond meal, safflower or sunflower oil, pear juice, plain gelatin, rice bran, calcium propionate (Note: this is a preservative), vinegar, and calcium chloride as ingredients. Several recipes are printed on the package for brown rice-based

PECAN CRISPIES

1½ cups brown rice flour
2 cups oat flour
1/2 tsp. salt
1½ cups chopped pecans
1/4 cup canola oil
1/2 cup rice syrup or
    maple syrup
1/3 cup apple juice
1 tsp. vanilla extract (omit
    if using maple syrup)

Mix dry and liquid ingredients separately and then combine them to form a very thick dough. Divide the dough into 4 balls and chill 2 hours.

Preheat oven to 350°. Form the chilled dough into flat, 3" cookies, smoothing out edges. Place on an oiled cookie sheet. Bake 25 minutes until firm but not browned. Cool to crisp.

Variation: Make a small indentation in the center of each cookie and fill with an unsweetened jam or jelly. Bake as usual.

Makes 36 cookies
(Pyramid servings: 1/2 Bread/ Grain Group, 5 grams Fat, 2 grams Sweets)

Nutrition Facts

Serving Size 1 cookie (25 g)
Servings Per Container 36

Amount Per Serving

Calories 100   Calories from Fat 50

% Daily Value*

Total Fat 5g	**8%**
Sodium 35mg	**1%**
Total Carbohydrate 13g	**4%**
Dietary Fiber 1g	**5%**
Sugars 3g	
Protein 2g	
Iron 4%	

Not a significant source of Saturated Fat, Cholesterol, Vitamin A, Vitamin C and Calcium.
* Percent Daily Values are based on a 2,000 calorie diet.

---

yeasted bread, buns, bagels, pizza crusts, and pasta. The mix is also available in a refined rice flour version.

Another manufacturer, Fearn Natural Foods, sells their own version of Brown Rice Baking Mix for quick breads, muffins, pancakes, waffles, and a yeasted pizza crust. Instead of methylcellulose, Fearn uses guar gum to help bind the rice flour. Other ingredients include soy powder, nonaluminum baking powder, and salt.

Because its natural oils can turn rancid in long-term storage, for best flavor brown rice flour should be purchased as fresh as possible. Readily available in most stores, brown rice flour can also be successfully ground at home. Use short-grain or medium-grain rice for a less sandy texture.

Baking/Cooking Guidelines

To make wheat-free cookies, flat breads, and muffins based on rice flour, use approximately equal amounts oat flour to brown rice flour. Other successful combinations include 2/3 cup rice flour with 1/3 cup rye flour or 3/4 cup rice flour with 1/4 cup potato flour.

Smoother-textured, all-rice flat breads can be made by toasting brown rice flour in a skillet and then combining it with enough hot water to make a very stiff dough. After patting it into an oiled baking pan, it should be baked for about 30 minutes at 350°. While not exactly light, delicate fare, it is deliciously nutty in flavor, making a tasty breakfast bread that is especially good topped with almond butter or sesame tahini and applesauce. To save some time, substitute preroasted dry cream of rice-type cereals for the rice flour.

RYE FLOUR

Facts and Features

Rye flour has interesting, sometimes irritating characteristics. Thanks to its low gluten content and high levels of cereal gums called pentosans, breads or other baked goods made with 100% rye flour are very moist, compact, and heavy.

Occasionally you'll find a 100% rye bread that "eats well." More than likely it will be made with white rye flour, an off-white, grayish-colored flour that has had most of the bran and germ removed. It will also be leavened with a sourdough culture with or without the addition of baking yeast. Since too alkaline a dough makes for a gummy bread, the sourdough is an effective acidifier to moderate rye's otherwise goopy potential. Most 100% rye breads are sliced very thin to counter its heavy texture.

Pumpernickel rye flour or medium rye contains more of the bran than white rye and is less finely ground.

Whole-grain rye flour is the darkest rye flour and most nutritious, retaining most of the bran and germ. Baked goods made with whole-grain rye flour will also be the most heavy.

Baking/Cooking Guidelines

For best results with homemade rye breads, combine rye flour with wheat flour at an approximate ratio of 1 part rye to 3 parts wheat.

Cookies, pancakes, and waffles can also be made with rye. Try balancing its texture by combining 1/3 cup rye with 2/3 cup rice flour or 2/3 cup rye with 1/3 cup potato flour. The flavor and texture of cornmeal also complements rye flour.

SOY FLOUR

Facts and Features

Like amaranth and chickpea flours, soy flour is used primarily as a protein-booster. It also makes baked goods more moist. However, due to its strong flavor, only small amounts should be added to recipes.

Since low fat and defatted soy flours are the by-product of soy oil production, generally involving the use of a chemical solvent, look for full-fat soy flour, lightly toasted for better flavor and digestibility.

Baking/Cooking Guidelines

Use no more than 25% soy flour in quick breads, cookies, or cakes. It should be used even more sparingly in yeasted breads. Too much can over-condition the dough, making the bread rise too soon.

When improvising with soy flour in favorite recipes, reduce baking temperature to compensate for soy flour's tendency to brown prematurely.

Save your taste buds and don't even bother trying to use it as a thickener for sauces and gravies.

SPELT FLOUR

Facts and Features

Similar in gluten and starch properties to high-protein wheat, spelt flour, an ancient strain of wheat, makes excellent breads, baked goods, and pasta.

Spelt is especially popular as a wheat alternative for those who are typically sensitive to gluten. Still, anyone with a serious wheat allergy should check with a health professional before experimenting with spelt.

Baking/Cooking Guidelines

Since spelt absorbs water more readily than wheat, the liquid to flour ratio needs modification when substituting spelt for wheat in familiar recipes. Start by reducing the recipe's liquid component by 25%. Add more water only if more seems to be needed to obtain the optimum consistency of batter or dough as needed for a particular recipe.

Spelt's gluten is also very fragile. Make sure not to knead it too much. One rising might be plenty.

TAPIOCA FLOUR

Facts and Features

Tapioca flour is a gluten-free, grain-free, slightly sweet powdered starch made from the root of the cassava plant cultivated in South America and in Florida. Not to be confused with its pearl or quick-cooking form, tapioca flour's thickening and baking properties are very similar to arrowroot.

Baking/Cooking Guidelines

Like arrowroot, tapioca flour can be used as a flour substitute to lighten wheat-free baked goods such as those made with amaranth, brown rice, or millet flours. Experiment using 25-50% in recipes.

However, it's possible to make muffins and cakes with 100% tapioca flour if baking powder and plenty of beaten egg yolks and egg whites are also included. Refer to wheat-free cookbooks or recipes listed on tapioca flour packages for details.

TEFF FLOUR

Facts and Features

Introduced to the United States in the 1980s, teff flour's sweet, malty flavor and light, delicate crumb have proved it to be an exciting alternative for baking and cooking. Its high calcium, iron, copper, and zinc content makes it particularly appealing, too.

Brown and white teff flour are ground from two different varieties of teff, each with distinctive flavors. Brown (or red) teff flour gives baked goods a rich, molasses-like flavor while results with white teff flour are more subtle.

Baking/Cooking Guidelines

Teff flour is gluten-free so when baking yeasted or sourdough breads, it must be combined with wheat flour for yeast-risen breads. Substitute up to 20% teff flour in your favorite recipe to take advantage of teff's unique flavor and nutrition.

Teff also makes a terrific thickener for gravy, sauces, soups, and stews.

When roasted a couple of minutes in a pan over medium heat, teff flour can be used to make a cream of teff breakfast cereal.

TRITICALE FLOUR

Facts and Features

Triticale flour, ground from the grain developed from a cross between wheat and rye, is slightly higher in protein than wheat and has a better amino acid balance than many other grains. Baked goods made with triticale flour have a delicious nutty/rye-like flavor.

Baking/Cooking Guidelines

In yeasted breads, triticale flour should be combined at least 50/50 with wheat flour. Since its gluten is very delicate, kneading should be done with a gentle hand. To pre-

PEANUTTY TEFF COOKIES

1/2 cup roasted peanut
    splits
1/4 tsp. baking soda
1/4 tsp. salt
1 1/4 cups teff flour
1/2 cup barley flour or
    whole wheat pastry
    flour
1/4 cup canola oil
1/3-1/2 cup rice syrup or
    honey
1 egg, slightly beaten
1/2 tsp. vanilla

Preheat oven to 350°F. Combine peanuts, soda, salt, and flour. In a separate bowl, beat oil and sweetener together. Add egg and vanilla and beat well. Fold into flour mixture. The dough should be very stiff; add extra flour if necessary. Drop dough by rounded teaspoonfuls onto oiled cookie sheets. Using a fork, press cookies to about 1/2 inch thickness. Bake for 12-15 minutes or until bottoms are golden. Remove and cool on a wire rack.

Makes 24 cookies
(Pyramid servings: 1/2 Bread/ Grain Group, 4 grams Fat, 1 gram Sweets)

Nutrition Facts
Serving Size 1 cookie (21 g)
Servings Per Container 24

Amount Per Serving

Calories 90   Calories from Fat 40

                               % Daily Value*

Total Fat 4g   6%
Cholesterol 10mg   3%
Sodium 40mg   2%
Total Carbohydrate 11g   4%
    Dietary Fiber 1g   6%
Protein 2g

Iron 4%

Not a significant source of Saturated Fat, Sugars, Vitamin A, Vitamin C and Calcium.
* Percent Daily Values are based on a 2,000 calorie diet.

---

vent overly dense loaves, bread dough should be allowed only one rising.

Proportions of triticale flour to wheat and baking techniques are not as critical in quick breads, drop biscuits, cookies, and pancakes.

WHEAT FLOUR

Facts and Features

Wheat flour's distinction of being the most widely used flour is due to its unique type of protein. When mixed with water it forms gluten which can respond to various types of leavening: yeast, sourdough, baking powder, baking soda, as well as natural yeasts in the air, to make light baked goods, hearty breads, and textures in between.

Accordingly, the different varieties of wheat are classified according to the protein-to-starch ratio found in the endosperm, an indication of how much gluten is present and the best application for the flour.

Very Hard Wheat

Durum wheat, referred to as very hard wheat, contains the most protein and the least starch. It is the wheat of choice for making pasta as its high levels of protein make a tough dough that allows it to stretch and expand without disintegrating during cooking. (Think of the word "durable.")

Whole wheat pastas are made from unrefined durum wheat.

Semolina is durum flour with the bran and germ removed. High-quality "white" pasta is made from semolina flour. Unlike most refined wheat flours, semolina flour is never bleached since its buttery yellow color is generally valued in pasta. Semolina flour is also used in some breads to add extra flavor and texture.

Hard Wheat

Bread flour ground from hard spring or winter wheat is high in protein with a strong gluten that makes for light, airy loaves. It is available in both whole wheat and refined white versions.

Graham flour is hard whole wheat ground so that the outer bran layer is left coarse and flaky while the endosperm and germ are ground fine. Although most famous for its use in graham crackers, it adds a pleasant texture and chewiness to all baked goods.

White flour is made from wheat that has had both the bran layer and the wheat germ removed, severely depleting several nutrients in the process. White flour contains only 7% of the fiber found in whole wheat flour. Fifty percent of linoleic acid, an essential fatty acid, is lost. Twenty-two vitamins and minerals are reduced by 70-80%. And, much of the vitamin E is gone, too.

In an attempt to make white flour look like it has at least some food value, each pound of flour is often enriched with four nutrients: 2.9 mg. thiamine (B_1), 1.8 mg. riboflavin (B_2), 24 mg. niacin (B_3), and between 13-16.5 mg. iron. Only a fraction of the nutrients found naturally in whole wheat flour are replaced.

White flour is the only flour to which the terms "bleached" and "unbleached" have any application. Unlike whole wheat flour, white flour needs to be aged to strengthen its gluten, making higher-volumed breads and cakes. Unbleached white flour is aged naturally for a couple of months in a warehouse. During the interim, white flour's natural light yellow color turns off-white from the effect of oxygen in the air.

Storing flour in a warehouse costs both money and time, so most flour producers use chlorine dioxide to make the flour look whiter and bake better in just a few minutes instead of waiting for weeks. Despite the fact this bleaching and aging chemical is a suspected carcinogen, it is allowed to be used since the residue that remains in the finished flour is below the FDA levels set as "safe." If potential carcinogens aren't bad enough, the bleaching further depletes naturally occurring vitamin E and essential fatty acid.

Insist on using only unbleached white flour in your baking and cooking. Your health is worth the manufacturer's time and money.

White Whole Wheat Flour is a light golden-colored, mild-flavored flour ground from the entire kernel of a special variety of hard wheat. Three genes control the color of bran. Regular hard wheat has a reddish-colored bran while, as its name suggests, the genes present in white whole wheat produce yellowish/white colored bran. Flavor varies, too, depending on the color of bran. White whole wheat's whitish-colored bran contributes a more subdued flavor than wheat surrounded with red bran. When baking for someone who objects to regular whole wheat's nutty flavor and brownish hue, white wheat flour will satisfy picky criteria without sacrificing nutrition.

Whole wheat flour is made by grinding the entire wheat berry to include the outside bran layer, the starchy endosperm, and the

WHOLE WHEAT PASTRY CRUST

1 1/2 cups whole wheat
    pastry flour
1 1/2 cups unbleached
    white flour
1/4 tsp. salt
1/2 cup canola oil
1/2 cup cold water

Mix flours and salt. Cut in oil with a fork until mixture has a pebble-like consistency. Gradually add water until dough forms into a damp but smooth ball. Handle the dough as little as possible to avoid a tough crust. Cover dough and refrigerate for 30 minutes. Roll out on a floured pastry cloth or on waxed paper to desired size. Transfer crust to an oiled pie plate. Proceed with pie recipe, prebaking as required or baking after the crust is filled.

Makes one 9" double crust or two single crusts
(Pyramid servings: 2 Bread/Grain Group, 14 grams Fat)

Nutrition Facts

Serving Size 1/8 recipe (69 g)
Servings Per Container 8

Amount Per Serving

Calories 260   Calories from Fat 130

	% Daily Value*
Total Fat 14g	22%
Saturated Fat 1g	5%
Sodium 75mg	3%
Total Carbohydrate 30g	10%
Dietary Fiber 2g	10%
Protein 5g	

Calcium 2%	•	Iron 4%

Not a significant source of Cholesterol, Sugars, Vitamin A and Vitamin C.
* Percent Daily Values are based on a 2,000 calorie diet.

germ of the kernel. Consequently, whole wheat flour is the most nutritious. Because the bran cuts into the gluten strands, breads made with whole wheat flour won't rise as much as ones made with white flour. However, the difference isn't so appreciable that it should stop you from making 100% whole wheat breads. Besides, its more full-bodied flavor and coarser texture makes a better-eating loaf.

Although the results can be somewhat dense and heavy, whole wheat flour can also be used in unyeasted baked goods. While these qualities are enjoyed by many, others prefer to combine whole wheat flour with white flour or substitute with whole wheat pastry flour for a lighter texture.

When substituting whole wheat flour for 1 cup white flour, start with 3/4 cup. The bran in whole wheat flour absorbs liquid more readily than white. The other alternative is to increase the liquid in the recipe.

Soft Wheat

Soft wheat is higher in starch and lower in gluten than both durum and hard wheats, making it most appropriate for light-textured

CURRIED SPINACH SAMOSAS

The crust:
1/2 cup water
1/3 cup organic safflower oil
pinch of salt (optional)
3 cups organic whole wheat flour

The filling:
1 Tbsp. sesame oil
1 bunch green onion, finely chopped
1/2 small onion, finely chopped
3 medium carrots, diced
pinch of salt
1/4 tsp. curry powder
3/4 -1 lb. fresh spinach, thoroughly washed, dried, and chopped
1 Tbsp. tamari (wheat-free soy sauce)
1/4 cup water
1 Tbsp. kuzu (Japanese arrowroot)

Combine water, oil, and salt in a small saucepan and bring to a boil. Remove from heat and beat the mixture with a whisk until it has a milky appearance. Add to flour in a large bowl. Gently knead the dough just until mixed well. Form into a ball and let sit for 30 minutes (or cover and place in a refrigerator until needed and then bring to room temperature.)

Meanwhile start to prepare filling.

Heat oil in a skillet. Sauté onions and carrots for 1 minute. Sprinkle with salt and curry powder and add chopped spinach. Cover and steam over medium heat until spinach wilts and the carrots are tender, about 4 minutes. Season with tamari. Dissolve kuzu in 1/4 cup water, add to spinach mixture, and cook for about 1 minute, stirring constantly, to thicken and glaze.

Preheat the oven to 375°F. Divide the dough in half and roll out until about 1/8 inch thick. Using a saucer or a small plate as a guide cut the dough into 4-inch-diameter circles. Place 2 tablespoons of filling in the middle of each circle. Fold over and pinch edge shut. Using a fork, poke a few holes in each samosa. Place on an oiled cookie sheet and bake for 30 minutes. Delicious hot or cold.

Makes 16
(Pyramid servings: 1 Bread/Grain Group, 1 Veg. Group, 6 grams Fat)

Nutrition Facts

Serving Size 1 samosa (82 g)
Servings Per Container 16

Amount Per Serving

Calories 140 · Calories from Fat 50

	% Daily Value*
Total Fat 6g	9%
Saturated Fat 0.5g	3%
Sodium 115mg	5%
Total Carbohydrate 20g	7%
Dietary Fiber 4g	16%
Sugars 2g	
Protein 4g	

Vitamin A 100%	•	Vitamin C 15%	
Calcium 4%	•	Iron 8%	

Not a significant source of Cholesterol
* Percent Daily Values are based on a 2,000 calorie diet.

unyeasted cakes, cookies, pie crusts, and quick breads. It is available in both whole wheat and refined flour versions.

Cake flour is "white" pastry flour ground from soft wheat with its bran and germ removed. It is ground finer than whole wheat pastry flour and chemically bleached. Some cake recipes specify it for an increased light, delicate texture as it allows for a higher ratio of sugar to fat to be absorbed. In the interest of nutrition, whole wheat pastry flour is a better bet. If you need lighter results, use a combination of whole wheat pastry flour with unbleached white flour.

Whole wheat pastry flour is ground from the whole soft wheat kernel, retaining its bran, germ, and endosperm. Like regular whole wheat flour, it is significantly more nutritious than refined pastry flours.

Because it absorbs less liquid than white flour, pie crusts made with whole wheat pastry flour tend to be more crumbly and harder to manage. Try using a combination of whole wheat pastry flour and unbleached white flour for smoother, more tender results. Other baking projects can use 100% whole wheat pastry flour with excellent results. This flour can also be used to thicken sauces and gravies.

Miscellaneous Wheat Flours

Several other wheat-based flours are available, variations of the basics already mentioned above.

All-purpose flour is a blend of hard and soft wheats, a middle-of-the-road flour yielding average results in breads and pastries. Breads made with all-purpose flour don't rise as much as breads made with hard wheat. Cookies, cakes, and pies are heavier in texture than those baked with soft pastry flours. However, if no particular flour is suggested in a recipe, all-purpose flour is a safe bet. It is available in both whole wheat and refined white as well as bleached and unbleached. Look first for whole wheat all-purpose flour. If you have to resort to white, make sure it is unbleached.

Self-rising flour is all-purpose flour that includes salt and leavenings such as baking powder and/or baking soda. To substitute for 1 cup self-rising flour as called for in some recipes, add 11/2 tsp. baking powder and 1/2 tsp. salt to 1 cup all-purpose flour.

For a discussion about gluten flour and vital wheat gluten, see "Gluten Flour.".

Breads

FEW FOODS are as satisfying and centering as chewy crusted whole-grain bread. Unlike its refined, additive-laden counterparts, high-quality traditionally-made bread presents a blend of subtle and complex flavors that is nothing short of wonderful.

Not only do they naturally contain at least three times more fiber than breads made with refined flour, whole grain breads supply more vitamin E, B6, pantothenic acid, and folic acid, as well as the minerals zinc, copper, iron, chromium, magnesium, and manganese.

Clever marketing, however, has made it more difficult to separate the chaff from the "wheat." Names like "old-fashioned," "multi-grain," and "country" sound a lot better than what the bread actually has to offer. "Wheat" bread is just another name for refined white bread. And, although definitely preferable to breads made with chemically bleached flour, those based on unbleached white flour are still lacking fiber and nutrients.

You can't even judge a bread by its color. Several breads are tinted brown with a substance called caramel color. Despite the fact that caramel color is nothing more than burnt sugar and, therefore, fairly benign as far as additives go, it serves only to pretend to be something it is not.

Fortunately, increased interest in fiber, flavor, and nutrition has made whole-grain breads easier to find. In order to discover them, it's important to know which ingredients to look for and which to avoid.

BIOLOGICAL LEAVENING AGENTS

Breads depend on leavening to rise. Through its interaction with the simple and complex sugars in the dough, the leavener helps produce carbon dioxide. The gluten present in the dough captures the carbon dioxide and, during its rising time, stretches to make the bread rise.

Both sourdough culture and baking yeast are considered biological leavening agents since the carbon dioxide they provide is the result of yeasts and bacteria that feed on the carbohydrates in flour and sugars.

The required rising time for yeasted and sourdough breads allows for the development of flavor, texture, and digestibility. It also triggers an enzyme to break down phytic acid, a nonnutritive component found in the bran layers of whole grains that binds iron, calcium, zinc, magnesium, and copper. As the bread dough ferments, these minerals are liberated and, consequently, made more bioavailable to the body.

Sourdough

Sourdough-leavened breads can be traced back to the Egyptians around the year 2300

B.C. The leavening power of the sourdough culture results from the interaction of bacteria and wild yeasts found naturally in the air with the thick mixture of flour and water. To make bread, the prepared starter culture is combined with fresh dough and allowed to rise and ferment a couple of hours before baking.

The predominant type of yeast found in sourdough is called Saccharomyces exiguus, meaning small or scanty. Because these microorganisms vary according to the environment in which the breads are made, each bakery and household will make uniquely-flavored sourdough bread.

Sourdough breads are renowned for their superior flavor, moist texture, improved digestibility, and long shelflife. As a pre-fermented base added to the bread dough, sourdough culture facilitates the breakdown of complex carbohydrates into simple more easily digested sugars. Constant careful maintenance of the culture and the proper balance of time, temperature, and dough consistency are required to yield finely grained, not-too-sour breads.

Homemade starters take about 1 week of daily flour and water feedings to the base batter for a viable culture to develop. Commercial sourdough starter kits usually include baking yeast in their mix to ensure more foolproof results.

Once developed, the starter must be stored in the refrigerator and fed with more flour and water at least once per week. Best baking results occur when the sourdough culture is fed the day before or at least twelve hours before using it to leaven.

There are two basic categories of sourdough, distinguished by the kind of flour used to make it.

Rye- based Northern European sourdough primarily produces lactic acid bacteria, making it milder in flavor than wheat-based sourdough. The leavener of choice in areas that depend heavily on rye breads, it provides enzymes that break down pentosans, the heavy cereal gums found in rye flour, to produce lighter, less dense loaves than would be possible if leavened with baking yeast.

Wheat-based sourdough is pungent with a vinegar-like flavor, a result of the significant amount of acetic acid bacteria produced in the fermentation of wheat flour. Despite the fact it has been used for centuries throughout the world, in the United States wheat-based sourdough is often referred to as "San Francisco-style sourdough," no doubt because wheat-based sourdough was the saving grace of breads and pancakes that fueled California's Gold Rush miners.

A modern-day twist on sourdough culture is the development of pure monocultures featuring only one type of bacteria chosen specifically for its bread-making ability. Less critical control of the baking process is needed; once the sourdough reaches a certain pH level during rising, the fermentation stops. Breads made with isolated monocultures will have consistent results day after day. On the other hand, as the monoculture doesn't require the presence of wild yeasts, the bread may lack the unique regional differences that would normally occur in typical sourdough breads found throughout the country.

Sourdough breads can even be made by simply mixing together a dough of flour, water, and fresh or leftover whole grains and allowing it to ferment up to a day or two to take advantage of the natural yeasts and bacteria found in the air. Although these natural-rise breads can be made without developing or maintaining a prepared culture, they tend to be more heavy and pungent.

Wheat-based **desem** (Flemish for starter) "sourdough" is related to typical sourdough except that it relies on the organisms and enzymes that naturally occur in organically grown wheat instead of airborne yeasts and bacteria. Breads made with desem culture are particularly light and flavorful. A few natural bakeries specialize in desem breads. They can also be made at home.

It takes about 2 weeks, steady temperatures of 50° to 65°, and ten pounds of flour to make a desem starter. Instead of developing into a batter like typical sourdough culture, a desem starter looks like a ball of dough. For detailed instructions, refer to *The Laurel's Kitchen Bread Book* by Laurel Robertson with Carol Flinders and Bronwen Godfrey (Random House, 1984).

Baking Yeast

Modern yeast-leavened bread also has its roots in antiquity. Bakers living in Egypt around 300 B.C. made bread by combining the yeasty froth from beer with flour and water and allowing the dough to ferment. Even through the 1800s, distilleries were the source for packaged yeast cakes made from starch, water, and the yeast skimmed off the top of their beer-brewing vats. Accordingly, this particular strain of yeast is called Saccharomyces cerevisiae, meaning "brewer's sugar fungus."

Bakers find this type of yeast more convenient, quicker, and more predictable than sourdough. However, since baking yeast consists of a single isolated strain of yeast, breads made with it lack the richness, complexity, and digestibility found in traditional sourdough breads. Some breads are made with both sourdough culture and baker's yeast to try to capture the best traits each has to offer.

Instead of being a by-product of the brewing industry, modern-day yeast is now grown in a solution of molasses, mineral salts, and ammonia. Commercial bakers typically rely on **compressed yeast**, a mixture of yeast and starch that is relatively inexpensive and ready to use without having to rehydrate it as with active dry yeast. Compressed yeast must be kept refrigerated and used within 2 weeks. It can also be frozen up to 2 months.

Active dry yeast was developed during World War II to provide a low-moisture product with a longer shelf life. Although it can be stored without refrigeration, it lasts even longer when kept cool. To give active dry yeast a proper jump-start, it must be dissolved in water ranging in temperature from 105° to 115° F. One packet of active dry yeast is equivalent to 2 teaspoons or 1/4 oz. It can substitute for 1 square of compressed yeast.

A more recent innovation, instant or **rapid-rise yeast** has been dried at high temperatures in a special process that allows it to rehydrate easily and leaven more quickly. However, since longer proofing times allow for more development of flavor and aroma, time-saving is the only real advantage to using rapid-rise yeast.

ADDITIVES IN BREAD

The best breads are a simple mix of flour, leavener, and water as basic ingredients. However, a glance at some labels illustrates that it's hard for some bakeries to leave well enough alone. Like all additives, some are useful as well as nutritious and can even be added when making your own bread at home. Others benefit only the manufacturer, adding nothing to the wholesomeness or inherent quality of the bread.

In general, additives used to aid production or modify the appearance and texture of the final baked product are called dough conditioners. There are six basic categories of dough conditioners: acidulants and buffers, fermentation accelerators, emulsifiers, enzymes, oxidizing agents, and reducing agents. Preservatives used to extend the shelflife of the bread include antioxidants and antimicrobials.

Acidulants and Buffers

Acidulants and buffers affect flavor and pH of the dough. **Lactic acid** and **sodium diacetate** impart a sour flavor. Pseudo-sourdough breads that contain no real sourdough but imitate its flavor rely heavily on these acidulants. Acidulants also retard staling and mold growth.

Calcium salts and other minerals make the dough more alkaline to strengthen the gluten. These appear harmless but unnecessary in high-quality breads.

Fermentation Accelerators

Fermentation accelerators act as fuel for yeast. **Ammonium sulfate** or **ammonium chloride** provide nitrogen, an element considered beneficial for optimum development of the yeast. Sweeteners, sprouts, or malted barley flour induce yeast activity through a different route, by furnishing the yeast simple sugars.

Emulsifiers

In deference to the old saying, "Oil and water don't mix," emulsifying agents attract both, keeping them in suspension. In breads, emulsifiers retard spoilage and distribute the fat throughout the dough for a softer texture.

Common emulsifiers are **mono- and diglycerides**, isolated from vegetable oils, and soybean **lecithin**. Of the two, lecithin is more familiar and available to the home baker. Both are acceptable additives. However, less processed and more nutritious ingredients such as milk, eggs, butter, or vegetable oils could be added instead to enhance texture. As for spoilage potential, bread should be expected to spoil but it should be eaten or frozen before it does.

Even more potent emulsifiers are **calcium stearyol-2-lactylate** and **sodium stearyol lactylate**. In addition to performing basic emulsifying work, they improve volume and strengthen the dough by interacting with proteins and carbohydrates.

The use of these emulsifiers is even harder to justify than mono- and diglycerides or lecithin. Mass-produced bread is generally made according to the time-saving continuous production method in which the ingredients are mixed and extruded directly into loaf pans, bypassing the fermentation period of the dough. Quick techniques such as these often need all the help they can get to "improve" volume and texture, hence the reason emulsifiers such as calcium stearyol-2-lactylate and sodium stearyol lactylate are often added.

Some may argue that the addition of calcium compounds makes the bread nutritious. However, if obtaining calcium from bread is one's aim, the addition of real dairy products in the dough or consumed with the bread is a better option, supplying a wider spectrum of nutrients than the dough conditioner could ever contribute.

Enzymes

Enzymes are catalysts that increase the rate of chemical reactions. When flour is combined with water to make a dough, starch enzymes (amylase) naturally present in the flour are responsible for breaking down the complex starches into simple sugars to fuel the yeast.

From year to year, enzyme values in wheat can vary. When flour tests out to be deficient in these starch enzymes, malted barley flour made from sprouted whole barley is commonly added to ensure proper baking results.

Malted barley flour is made by sprouting whole barley. During the sprouting process, some of barley's stored-up starch is converted by amylase into maltose, a sweet simple sugar. Once sprouted to its peak enzyme activity, it is ground and dried into malted barley flour. So reactive is malted barley flour that only a small amount is generally added at the flour mill. In fact, when adding it to homemade bread dough, more than 1/4 teaspoon per loaf would provide too much enzyme activity, resulting in a gooey loaf that won't bake properly.

Malted barley flour does more than help provide more food for yeast. It also naturally sweetens the bread and makes the crust more dark and crispy. Malted barley flour can be found in natural food stores, sometimes referred to as dimalt or diastatic malt.

Malted barley flour can be made at home. Sprout whole hulless barley, dry sprouts in a food dehydrator or in an oven heated to about (but no more than) 120° F. until brittle, and grind them in a grain grinder, nut/seed mill, or blender. One cup of hulless barley, sprouted and dried, will make about 2-3 cups of malted barley flour.

Malt syrup is not a suitable replacement. While it will make bread sweet and flavorful, malt syrup has been heated to stop enzyme activity, so it won't help bread rise.

Fungal alpha-amylase or fungal proteases may also be used as enzyme enhancers. Manufactured much like digestive enzymes sold as food supplements, these are harmless ingredients listed on the labels of some breads.

Alpha-amylase acts similarly to malted barley flour, supplementing the amylase enzymes naturally present in flour that degrade the flour into dextrins and maltose sugars. The addition of alpha-amylase provides more fuel for yeasts and improves flavor.

Protease enzymes enhance the natural enzymes in flour that break down some of the flour's protein into amino acids and peptides. The addition of fungal proteases increases extensibility of the dough, thus making it easier to handle during manufacture.

Raw soy flour is also high in enzymatic activity, making breads rise higher more quickly. Only small amounts are recommended, no more than 3 tablespoons per loaf, to prevent the dough from ripening too fast. In addition to conditioning the dough, soy flour also makes a higher-protein bread.

Oxidizing Agents

Oxidizing agents are added to flour at the mill to make breads made with it more springy, softer in texture, finer-grained, and more voluminous. They also make the dough tougher and drier so it won't stick in the kneading and baking machines. Common oxidizing agents are potassium bromate, azodicarbonamide (ADA), and ascorbic acid. Good, soft-textured, well-formed loaves can be made without these additives. Ascorbic acid contributes nutrients in addition to conditioning the dough. However, it is hard to accept or condone the use of other oxidizing agents that may not only be unnecessary but potentially harmful as well.

Potassium bromate-treated flour is often listed as bromated flour on labels. In Germany potassium bromate is banned as a potential carcinogen. It has also been declared a carcinogen in California under Proposition 65, thus requiring bakeries who use it in their breads to caution consumers of its health hazard via labels or signs. Retailers in California decided they'd rather not sell a bread with such alarming information, so bakers were forced to use other oxidizing agents or eliminate them altogether. A national ban on potassium bromate by the FDA is expected in the future but, in the meantime, it remains permissible.

Azodicarbonamide (ADA) was approved by the FDA in 1962. It appears to have no carcinogenic potential; however, ADA is often used in tandem with the more potentially harmful potassium bromate to modify the protein in bread flour to promote loaf volume and shape.

Ascorbic acid is the only oxidizing agent permitted in Germany and France. It is about 2/3 as effective as potassium bromate. Since ascorbic acid is a safe, nutritious additive that works nearly as well as the other oxidizing agents, more bakers in the United States will likely switch to it in the future.

Reducing Agents

Reducing agents do the opposite of oxidizers. Rather than strengthening the protein chains, reducing agents break them to soften the dough so that it requires less mixing of ingredients. The most common reducing agent is **L-cysteine**, an amino acid. Reducing agents are used when dough is developed chemically rather than allowed to naturally ferment, so while L-cysteine on its own may be harmless, its inclusion in bread doughs indicates a shortcut manufacturing method, likely producing a mediocre bread.

Preservatives

Preservatives include antioxidants and antimicrobials. Antioxidants such as **ascorbic acid (vitamin C)**, and **D-alpha tocopherol (vitamin E)**, **BHA**, and **BHT** work by retarding the oxidation of fats to decrease the odds of rancidity. The addition of vitamins C and/ or E adds valuable nutrients while preserving naturally. BHA (butylated hydroxyanisole) and BHT (butylated hydroxytoluene) have been linked as possible carcinogens.

Antimicrobials inhibit the growth of mold and bacteria, often added since the internal temperature of the bread may not get high enough to kill all bacterial spores. Both **calcium propionate** and **potassium sorbate** are considered the least problematic of food additives and yet they should still be considered unnecessary additives. High-

quality breads which are sold quickly and stored at home appropriately have no need for added synthetic preservatives.

Good alternatives to synthetic antimicrobials include **vinegar, raisin juice, honey,** and **other sugars.** Not only do they naturally inhibit bacteria by creating an acidic environment unfavorable to many microorganisms they flavor breads, as well.

Salt inhibits the growth of molds and bacteria by causing their cells to dehydrate. It also controls the action of the yeast. Breads made without salt may rise too quickly, affecting the overall flavor and integrity of the bread. Sometimes potassium chloride is added to salt-free breads to boost flavor.

VARIETIES OF LEAVENED BREADS

Beyond the "sandwich" variety, bread comes in all shapes and sizes including English muffins, bagels, dinner rolls, burger and hot dog buns, pizza crusts, focaccia, baguettes, and pita bread. Not all breads are wheat-based, either. Familiar to most, only a few may need some explanation.

Armenian Soft Cracker Bread is a traditional thin, large, round, pliable bread that is filled, tightly rolled, and sliced in 1-3 inch pieces. It can also be torn into smaller pieces and topped with spreads or used like a huge pizza crust when feeding a crowd.

Bagels are doughnut-shaped breads that are cooked in boiling water a minute before being baked. Bagels are also very low in fat— when eaten without cream cheese or butter, that is. They make a good substitute for doughnuts and other sweet breads at breakfast and are a good choice for a high-complex carbohydrate pre- or post-workout snack.

Baguettes, a.k.a "French bread," taste best the day they are purchased, due to their high ratio of crust to crumb. Authentic versions are crisp crusted and contain no fat or sugar.

Focaccia is a leavened Italian flat bread, similar to a thick pizza crust. It is often baked with herbs such as rosemary and basil, onions, garlic, and sometimes cheese. Serve it warm, plain, spread with olive oil, or with simple toppings.

High-fiber breads are white, whole wheat, or rye breads made with extra fiber in the form of wheat bran, oat bran, flaxseeds, sesame seeds, sunflower seeds, pea fiber, or soy fiber. Since phytic acid is concentrated in the husks of grains, legumes, and seeds, the consumption of high-fiber breads may inhibit bioavailability of trace minerals. A good, balanced diet eaten in conjunction with high-fiber breads should minimize mineral deficiency. As with all high-fiber foods, plenty of water should be ingested to compensate for the extra liquid absorbed by the fiber.

Kamut breads supply another alternative to modern wheat. Kamut flour is most suited for making pasta; accordingly, breads made with it may be somewhat dense. Some kamut breads are made with a combination of kamut and spelt to create a lighter loaf. Like spelt, its gluten is often tolerated by those sensitive to wheat gluten. Individuals with severe wheat allergies should consult a health professional before experimenting.

Pita bread, sometimes called pocket bread or Bible bread, is a round, flat bread usually made from whole wheat flour. A traditional bread originating in the Middle East, small pieces were torn off and used in place of utensils when eating meals. When pita is cut horizontally, a handy pocket is revealed, ready to be stuffed with a sandwich filling or salad. The pocket is formed from the rapid conversion of water into steam, a result of baking the bread at 500°.

Rice breads made with 100% rice flour depend on vegetable gums such as methyl-cellulose or guar gum as binders to compensate for rice's gritty texture. As a specialty item, rice breads are often located in the frozen food area of stores.

Rye breads are often made with the addition of wheat flour to create a milder-flavored, less compact-textured bread. Breads made with 100% rye flour are leavened solely with sourdough or with a combination of sourdough and baking yeast to modify rye flour's usual sticky, moist texture.

Special rye breads imported from Germany are sold in oblong, thinly sliced loaves. Most of these breads are very high in fiber, using coarsely ground whole rye flour sometimes supplemented with whole grains, sunflower seeds, or flax seeds (linseeds). Since the breads are pasteurized before packaging to eliminate the bacteria that can cause breads to mold, they remain fresh at room temperature before opening for up to 6 months without preservatives. Once opened, the bread will remain moist for at least another 4 days at room temperature.

Spelt breads offer an alternative for individuals who are allergic to wheat or like to vary their diet. As an ancient bread wheat, spelt breads have a similar look and texture to typical wheat breads. While its gluten is often tolerated by those sensitive to wheat gluten, individuals with severe wheat allergies should consult a health professional before experimenting.

Yeasted sprouted-grain breads are made by adding yeast, salt, and honey with freshly ground wheat sprouts (or a combination with other sprouted grains) instead of flour to form the dough. These breads are exceptionally good and nutritious, thanks to the increased protein and vitamin content and transformation of complex starches into maltose that occur during sprouting. Some people find them easier to digest than flour-based breads.

PUMPERNICKEL BREAD BOWL

Here's a great way to serve your favorite dip at special occasions. Preheat oven to 350° F. Cut a slice from the top of a round loaf of pumpernickel rye bread. Remove bread from the center, leaving a 1-inch shell. (Removed bread can be reserved for bread crumbs or cut into bite-sized pieces and toasted in an oven to make croutons.) Brush inside of bread shell with 3 tablespoons of sesame oil. Place on a cookie sheet with the reserved bread. Bake for 20 minutes. Let shell cool and then fill with dip.

Variations: Any type and shape of bread can be used instead of pumpernickel rye.

QUICK BREADS

Quick breads are descendants of the most ancient forms of bread when flour and water were simply mixed together, formed into flat cakes, and baked over an open fire. Today most use baking soda, baking powder, or eggs to replace yeast or sourdough culture for leavening.

Tortillas, chapatis, muffins, pancakes, waffles, and crackers made in this manner lack the fermentation time required to deactivate the mineral-binding phytic acid present in grains. However, this usually won't present a problem if the rest of the diet contains good food sources of the minerals iron, calcium, zinc, magnesium, and copper.

Chemical Leaveners

Baking soda and baking powder are considered chemical leavening agents since the carbon dioxide responsible for the rising action is a result of their respective reactions with another alkaline or acidic substance. Although the word "chemical" may sound disconcerting, it merely describes the process. Both baking soda and baking powder should be considered safe.

Baking soda (bicarbonate of soda) is used as a chemical leavening agent when acidic ingredients such as sour milk, yogurt, vinegar, honey, barley malt, rice syrup, lemon juice, or fruit juice are found in the recipe.

Ammonium bicarbonate is used in the cookie and cracker industry for lighter results. Like baking soda, it creates carbon dioxide when moistened and subjected to heat. Since cookie and cracker doughs are porous, the odorous ammonia gas is allowed to escape instead of permeating the dough and affecting flavor.

Baking powder is a combination of baking soda and acids, with an inert filler such as cornstarch or calcium carbonate to act as a buffer between the two. Varieties of baking powders vary according to the type of acid they contain.

The original baking powders were **single acting**, a combination of baking soda and cream of tartar. Rarely will you see it available commercially since it reacts quickly as soon as it is moistened, usually before you have the chance to get the pan into the oven.

Double-acting baking powders react twice to give off carbon dioxide, once when moistened and next when heated, giving a second chance for better results. The two varieties most used by home bakers differ according to whether they contain aluminum compounds or not.

The presence of **sodium aluminum sulfate (SAS)** gives an extra boost to the second carbon dioxide release, thus giving somewhat better results. On the negative side, if too much is used, it can impart a bitter aftertaste in baked goods. More significant, the presence of aluminum has caused some people concern due to its questionable link to Alzheimer's Disease.

Even though the issue remains controversial, to be on the safe side you can use **nonaluminum baking powders** in your own baking and choose products that specify their use. They work almost as well, especially if you are quick to get foods into the oven.

Low-sodium baking powders are made with potassium bicarbonate instead of sodium bicarbonate (baking soda) to reduce the amount of sodium in baked goods made with regular baking powder. For best results, you should use 1 1/2 to 2 times more of the low-sodium variety than called for in your recipe. Another approach to reduce sodium is to continue using your regular baking powder and cut back on the amount of salt specified in the recipe.

Commercial bakers often use sodium acid pyrophosphate baking powder, also known as **SAPP baking powder.** It offers the advantage of slower reaction time, allowing more flexibility when getting pans or trays into the oven.

VARIETIES OF QUICK BREADS

Several quick breads still popular today are based on traditional breads from around the world.

Chapatis are round flat breads made from a kneaded dough containing wheat flour, water, oil, and salt and cooked on a griddle. They are traditionally served with curries and other vegetable dishes all over India. Because they are made without baking powder, chapatis are thinner and flatter than tortillas.

Essene bread is made solely from sprouted wheat or rye sprouts ground, formed into a loaf, and baked at a very low temperature. Chewy, dense, and naturally sweet, Essene bread can be eaten alone, spread with butter, nut butter, or any sandwich filling. Besides plain wheat and plain rye, Essene bread is available in other varieties: wheat with raisin, rye or wheat with seeds (sunflower, sesame, flax), wheat fruitcake (dried fruits and nuts added), multigrain, and wheat with dates and cinnamon.

Naan is another round East Indian flatbread traditionally baked in a hot clay oven called a tandoor in which temperatures exceed 700° F. These chewy, blistered breads are made from white or whole wheat flour, water, oil, and salt. While the dough is traditionally leavened using milk curds and a fermentation process, baking powder is usually the contemporary leavener of choice.

Tortillas made from corn or wheat are the most familiar flatbreads. **Corn tortillas** are made from water and ground masa harina, yellow or blue corn treated with slaked lime (calcium hydroxide). The mixture is rolled into a ball and flattened into a circle either by hand or with a special tortilla press. Both sides are briefly cooked on a hot griddle. Corn tortillas can also be deep-fried to make them crisp and retain certain shapes. Both tostada and chalupa shells are flat while taco shells are made into a U-shaped form.

Simple corn tortillas free of additives are generally easy to find. Avoid those made with artificial colors or preserved with calcium propionate or potassium sorbate. Although safe, the addition of gum arabic, a plant exudate from the Anogeissus latifolia tree, is unnecessary. While it helps keep the

RASPBERRY GEMS

1 1/2 cups unbleached white flour
1 1/2 cups whole wheat pastry flour
3 tsp. baking powder
1/2 tsp. baking soda
3/4 tsp. sea salt
4 Tbsp. canola oil
2 eggs or 4 egg whites
1/2 cup brown rice syrup or honey
1 tsp. almond extract
1/4 cup water
1/2 cup nonfat yogurt
1/4 cup raspberry jam

Preheat oven to 400°F. and oil muffin tins. Combine dry ingredients. In a separate bowl, blend oil, eggs, sweetener, almond extract, water, and yogurt until smooth. Form a "well" in the dry ingredients and pour in the yogurt mixture. Mix only until the ingredients are moistened, using no more than 15-20 strokes. Fill muffin cups half full and top each with 1 teaspoon jam. Top the jam with the remaining batter, filling each cup to the top. Quickly transfer the muffin tins to the middle shelf of your preheated 400° F. oven. Bake 20 minutes. Allow muffins to remain in tins for 1-2 minutes before removing. Cool muffins briefly on a wire rack and serve.

Makes 12 large muffins
(Pyramid servings: 2 Bread/Grain Group, 6 grams Fat, 2 grams Sweets)

Nutrition Facts

Serving Size 1 muffin (73 g)
Servings Per Container 12

Amount Per Serving	
Calories 190	Calories from Fat 50

	% Daily Value*
Total Fat 6g	9%
Saturated Fat 0.5g	3%
Cholesterol 35mg	12%
Sodium 310mg	13%
Total Carbohydrate 30g	10%
Dietary Fiber 2g	7%
Sugars 3g	
Protein 6g	

Vitamin A 2%	•	Calcium 10%
Iron 4%		

Not a significant source of Vitamin C
* Percent Daily Values are based on a 2,000 calorie diet.

---

tortillas from falling apart, fresh tortillas that are stored properly should have no need for this additive.

Wheat tortillas are typically made from white or whole wheat flour, water, salt, a source of fat, and baking powder. The dough is kneaded, allowed to rest, and then rolled out into a circle. Both sides are then briefly cooked on a hot griddle.

To avoid the high amounts of saturated fats and cholesterol found in lard or hydrogenated vegetable shortening, choose tortillas made with vegetable oil. The best-quality tortillas will list the specific type of oil instead of the generic term "vegetable oil" whose quality and source are undetermined.

Avoid varieties that are made with dough conditioners, artificial color and artificial flavor, or preservatives. Tortillas that are purchased fresh, used quickly, and stored properly have no need for these unnecessary additives.

CRISP BREADS

Crackers, both leavened and unleavened, are commonly made with wheat, rye, or rice flour. Depending on thickness and flavor, crackers can be topped with spreads, nut butters, or cheese or served as a crisp accompaniment to the meal. While some crackers are very simple and subtle in flavor, others are quite rich and reminiscent of cookies.

Crackers made with water such as matzoh crackers, water biscuits, and rye crisp breads will be crisper and harder than those made with milk or yogurt.

Savory crackers depend on some type of fat to produce their characteristic rich flavors. To keep saturated fat intake to a minimum, avoid those made with lard, vegetable shortening, palm kernel oil, coconut oil, margarine, or butter.

Given crackers' long shelf life, it's hard to imagine why some brands contain preservatives. It's just as perplexing why artificial colors and artificial flavors are often used as ingredients. High quality crackers have no place for either in their ingredient listings.

Pretzels are experiencing a resurgence in popularity as a high-carbohydrate, low fat snack. In the United States, the most highly regarded pretzels are made in Pennsylvania where the area's highly alkaline water used in pretzel dough enhances both flavor and texture.

Like good bread, high-quality pretzels are made with simple ingredients: whole wheat or wheat flour, water, yeast and/or sourdough culture, and salt. The dough is twisted by hand or by machine and baked in a stone hearth oven to create hard, crisp results.

Unfortunately, to save time and labor, most pretzels are now extruded from a machine with a pretzel-shaped die, rendering uniform, smooth, flat, boring pretzels instead of the uniquely fashioned, "knot in the middle," traditionally made variety. Other modern aberrations include vegetable shortening and corn syrup.

Pretzels' brown glazed appearance and unique flavor can be attributed to the use of sodium hydroxide (caustic soda) as a processing aid. Before baking, the pretzels are sprayed with a very dilute (1%) solution of sodium hydroxide that has been heated to 200° F. The heat and moisture combine to form a starchy gel on the outside of the pretzels. The dough is then salted and baked in a very hot oven for about 5 minutes. As a result of the alkaline reaction contributed by the sodium hydroxide, the starchy gel hardens to a brown, shiny finish. The final step is a long, slow bake to yield a dry, crisp pretzel.

During the baking process the sodium hydroxide reacts with the carbon dioxide derived from the yeast or sourdough to form sodium bicarbonate, commonly known as baking soda. Laboratory analysis reveals the pH (acid/alkalinity) of baked pretzels to fall between 6.3-6.7, indicating that no residual lye (sodium hydroxide), whose pH would be 9.0 or higher, remains.

Pretzels made without sodium hydroxide are tasty but resemble pretzel-shaped hard crackers rather than the appearance, texture, and flavor you would normally expect in a pretzel.

Rice cakes are a special kind of fat-free cracker that makes a great snack or light meal when topped with a sweet or savory spread.

Good-quality rice cakes are thick, sturdy, and flavorful. If your experience with rice cakes in the past has been less than memorable, try switching to another brand. Quality of ingredients and manufacturing expertise make a world of difference.

Rice cakes are made by placing 1-2 Tbsp. whole grain brown rice in a vacuum-sealed cooking mold. When the mixture has cooked for the proper amount of time, the cover is opened, thus releasing the vacuum. With the decrease in pressure, the grains "explode," pressing into each other within the mold to form the rice cake.

Tortilla chips are running a close second to potato chips in terms of popularity as an American snack food. Made from yellow, white, or blue corn, tortilla chips are basically tortillas cut in wedges and fried. High-oleic safflower oil is the best frying oil for tortilla chips since, unlike commonly used partially hydrogenated oils, it contains 75% monounsaturated fat, the type of fat that helps reduce the amount of low-density lipoproteins that can lead to cholesterol buildup.

Even better, however, are the new oil-free baked tortilla chips. With only 1.5 grams of fat per ounce instead of the 8 grams found in typical fried chips, baked tortilla chips are a great choice for snacks, especially if eaten with an equally low fat dip or salsa.

Read the ingredient label carefully to avoid any preservatives, artificial coloring, and monosodium glutamate (MSG) that may appear in some brands.

HOW TO STORE BREADS

Cold refrigerated air makes bread stale much faster than when stored at room temperature. Storing bread in plastic bags inside the refrigerator or at room temperature is even worse. Moisture becomes trapped, encouraging mold growth and making the crust soggy. A bread box, paper sack, perforated cellophane bread bag, or a clean towel are your best bets. Each allows the bread to breathe, helping maintain good texture, crisp crust, and maximum flavor. The crust may become more chewy as the days progress but inside the bread will remain moist.

The only exception to this rule are quick breads such as tortillas, chapatis, and Essene bread. When unrefrigerated they begin to mold within a day or two.

Breads such as French breads dry out within a day but, like all breads, can be re-vived by cutting into pieces and steaming in a vegetable steamer for 3 minutes. To reheat bread in the oven, wrap bread in foil, sprinkle with water, and bake 10-15 minutes at 350°. Tortilla warmers give even better results.

If you can't finish the loaf within three days, slice the rest, double-wrap it in a plastic or foil, and pop it in the freezer. Freezing slows the staling process, trapping water inside the bread's cells. For best flavor, use within 3 months. Individual slices will thaw in about 10 minutes. Frozen bread can also be thawed in the oven in about 20 minutes at 350° F.

Crisp breads such as crackers, pretzels, rice cakes, and tortilla chips shouuld be stored tightly sealed in a dry environment. To rejuvenate crispness, put in a 300° F. oven for about 5 minutes and allow to cool.

Pasta

NO OTHER food is as versatile, economical, and easy to prepare as pasta. And now, after enduring years of mislabeling as a high-fat, high-calorie fast food, pasta is finally getting the kudos it deserves.

High in complex carbohydrates, moderate in protein, and nearly fat-free, pasta is one of the best examples to show that you don't have to give up the foods you like to eat a healthy diet. A typical 2-cup cooked serving (4 oz. dry) contains 420 calories, 84 grams of carbohydrates, 16 grams of protein, and only 2 grams of fat. It's only when you smother pasta with oil, butter, cream sauces, and too much cheese that it becomes a nutritionist's nightmare.

As one of the most easily digested complex carbohydrate-rich foods, pasta is also a favorite fuel for athletes to boost muscle and liver glycogen stores for readily available energy. After hard workouts or events, a meal of pasta is one of the most nutritious ways to help restore depleted glycogen to previous levels.

Every culture and cuisine—be it Italy, France, the former Soviet Union, Israel, Egypt, Thailand, Japan, China, India, or Jamaica—features pasta in one form or another. While the tastes, textures, and appearances may vary, the common link to all kinds of pasta world-wide is its basic ingredients: flour and water.

Exploring Your Options

DURUM WHEAT-BASED PASTA

The best European and North American wheat-based pasta is made from durum wheat. High in gluten, durum flour makes a tough dough that allows pasta to stretch and expand without disintegrating during cooking. In contrast, a pasta made with regular wheat flour is lackluster in flavor and quickly turns soggy on the plate. White, starchy cooking water is a sure sign that your pasta wasn't made with 100% durum flour.

Brightly colored pastas are made by adding at least 3% vegetable solids from dried powders or purées. Even though wholesome vegetables such as spinach, carrots, tomato, and beets may be used, consider it more for fun and eye appeal than nutrition. When it comes to flavor, spinach pasta is the most obvious—you'll either love it or hate it. The other vegetables contribute only a slightly sweet taste.

Manufacturing of Durum Pasta

Using a good-quality flour is not enough to make a high-quality pasta. It also takes a great deal of skill and the right type of equipment.

Because semolina is so difficult to knead into a smooth, elastic dough that sticks together, whole durum or semolina pastas are best made by machine. Spaghetti, elbow macaroni, fusilli, and all other shaped pasta are *extruded:* created by forcing the mixture through a specific die. The speed at which the dough is squeezed through the die is very important. If processed too fast as commonly occurs in many pasta factories geared towards ultraefficiency, the excess stress and heat affecting the wheat reduces the nutrient level, cooking quality, and flavor of the pasta.

Even the composition of the die makes a difference. The best quality shaped pasta is extruded through bronze dies that produce a rough, porous surface, the kind that is more absorbent of sauces. If your pasta has a smooth, polished look, you can bet it was extruded through a Teflon™ die. Unfortunately, Teflon™'s effect on pans is comparable when it comes to pasta: sauces don't like to stick.

Flat ribbon pasta such as fettucini, linguine, lasagna, and egg noodles is best when rolled and cut instead of extruded. After the dough is mixed and kneaded, it goes through a series of rollers until it has the appropriate thickness. The long, continous sheets are then cut as they pass through a series of knives. Although it is more time-consuming and intricate, the extra effort with the roll and cut method makes for firmer-cooking pasta with better texture and flavor than is possible with extruded flat pasta.

Drying time and temperature are the final determinants of flavor. Pasta dries from the inside out. If dried too fast, it will become brittle; if dried too slow, it could sour. Low temperatures using circulating air for 48 hours or more make a better-tasting, high-quality pasta than the conventional quick drying method using hot drying rooms.

Fresh Pasta

Not all pasta is subjected to the drying process. "Nests" of golden yellow semolina and vibrant vegetable-colored plain and herbed fresh pastas grace grocery stores and specialty markets throughout the country. Much like the warm, homey feeling one gets from the aroma of freshly-made bread, fresh pasta is a comfort food, hailing back to simpler, less harried times when noodles or spaghetti came not from a box or a cellophane package but were made from "scratch" in one's own kitchen.

And yet, fresh isn't necessarily better. Although top-notch fresh pasta may be more porous and delicately textured, when both are wellmade, there is little appreciable flavor and textural difference between a good-quality fresh or dried pasta. In contrast, poor-quality fresh pasta is thick, heavy, and rubbery, an unpleasant experience that no affiliation with the concept of fresh can mollify.

Neither is fresh pasta any more nutritious than dried pasta. When it comes down to it, much of fresh pasta's appeal can be attributed to its brief preparation. Once a pot of water has come to a boil, all it takes is one to three minutes' cooking time. With pesto, olive tapenade, or your favorite sauce, a meal of fresh pasta is about as quick as it gets.

Tightly wrapped in the refrigerator, fresh pasta is best cooked as soon as possible after manufacture with a maximum refrigerator life of up to 3 days.

To extend shelf-life up to 120 days, some large manufacturers are now using modified atmosphere packaging, a technique that dramatically alters the definition of "fresh pasta". Before packaging, the pasta dough is conditioned, heated to dry the outside surface, and then cut into the specific shape. The pasta is then steam pasteurized, cooled, and packed in a thermoformed polyvinylchloride rigid-base tray sealed with a ethylene vinyl oxide barrier lid. Normal air is displaced with a high concentration of carbon dioxide and an oxygen-absorbant desiccant packet is added to each package to control microbial growth.

Modified atmosphere packaging seems to be an interesting process, but what's the point? If you're concerned about keeping fresh pasta for long periods of time, just buy a good quality dry pasta and store it on a shelf until you're ready to use it.

Since fresh pasta still contains the moisture that is removed from dried pasta, you'll get fewer servings per pound. Plan on cooking about 6 oz. of fresh pasta per person.

Whole Wheat Pasta

For optimum nutrition, look for whole wheat pasta made from whole-grain durum flour. Since it contains all the nutrients found naturally in the whole grain, pasta made from whole durum flour never needs to be "enriched" as is most "white" pasta sold in the United States. Similar to the nutritional differences between whole wheat bread and white bread, whole grain pasta contains more calcium, copper, magnesium, manganese, pantothenic acid, phosphorus, potassium, protein, B6, and zinc. It also contains three times more fiber, making it more filling yet equal in calories to its refined counterpart.

After tasting a good quality whole wheat pasta, you'll find most pastas made from refined flour bland in comparison. The rich, nutty flavor of whole wheat pasta makes it the focal point of the meal, needing only the simplest sauce or a light dressing of oil for enhancement. Hearty toppings such as pesto, Italian-style sauces, beans including tofu and tempeh, and nut butter-based dressings also blend well with the robust flavor of whole wheat.

Unfortunately, not all whole wheat pastas are created equal. If in the past you've considered it to be heavy, gummy, and slightly rancid-tasting, try a couple of other brands before condemning the entire category. Better-quality flour and more attention to production details separate the mediocre from the memorable.

"White" Pasta

Although it lacks the nutrients found in whole grain pasta, there's nothing wrong with occasionally opting for a more subdued, lighter-texture pasta, especially when the sauce or other components of the meal are the featured elements. The finest "white" pasta is actually amber-colored, a result of being manufactured from semolina. Refined of its bran and germ, semolina is the golden endosperm of durum flour ground to the consistency of fine sand. Its coarse texture makes pasta more resistant to overcooking, very receptive to sauces, and more flavorful than pastas made from common flour.

Occasionally you may see the term "fancy patent durum flour" listed on pasta labels. This finely ground version of semolina has some of the outside endosperm layer replaced that had originally been removed during refining. The smoother texture of fancy patent durum flour facilitates the traditional roll and cut manufacturing method for making ribbon- type pastas. Nutritionally speaking, it is marginally higher in fiber and protein than pure semolina.

Pastas that list plain durum flour on their labels often use a high percentage of the less desirable by-products of semolina milling. For the best tasting white or amber-colored pasta, stick with pasta made with durum semolina.

Egg Noodles

Technically, flour and water pastas are called macaroni and egg-enriched pastas are called noodles. Egg noodles are slightly higher in protein, fat, iron, and vitamin A than eggless pastas. However, they also contribute an additional 50 calories and 50 mg. of cholesterol per cup cooked.

More delicate in texture, egg noodles absorb sauces better than macaroni. Unless you have a hankering for a plate of gummy glop, avoid using heavy or oily sauces with egg noodles. Instead, dress them with something mildly flavored and light.

The amount and source of eggs are key facts to know when buying a high-quality egg noodle. Sometimes egg yolks are used instead of the whole egg to achieve a darker yellow, more rich-looking pasta. Egg whites are rarely used alone since they would dilute the color that is expected in an egg noodle.

Italian producers are required to make egg noodles with 20% egg solids from fresh eggs. In the United States, however, only 5.5% egg solids are mandatory and the use of frozen or powdered eggs, pasteurized to eliminate the possibility of salmonella, is the norm.

Precooked Pastas

New on the pasta scene is precooked lasagna that allows the cook to eliminate boiling the pasta before making lasagna or other casseroles. Instead of the preferred roll and cut method, a pasta sheet is extruded into the characteristic shape of lasagna noodles. It then goes into a near-boiling water bath, after which air and water sprays wash away surface starches. Twenty minutes in a special dryer reduces the after-cooking moisture content from 75% to 12.5%, making it ready for packaging. When used to make lasagna, the noodles are layered directly with the sauce, cheese, and other ingredients. Baking time is reduced by about a third since only rehydrating and heating of the dish are required.

This same process is already used for pastas combined with dehydrated vegetables and seasonings in "meal-in-a-cups." Pre-cooking of the pasta allows for its rapid rehydration within 5 minutes after boiling water is added to the cup's contents.

Convenience, not quality, remains the rationale behind pre-cooked pasta.

Specialty Wheat Pastas

Addition of other flours to durum wheat contributes both flavor and nutrition.

Jerusalem artichoke pasta is a blend of durum and the flour made from the dried Jerusalem artichoke (sunchoke), an unusual root vegetable that contains no starch. Compared to other pastas it has a particularly mild, pleasant flavor and a slightly lower carbohydrate content.

Kamut pasta is made from an ancient form of durum wheat. With the same high-gluten properties of modern-day durum wheat and a rich, buttery flour, kamut flour makes an excellent whole wheat pasta. It also freezes well, retaining its cooked texture. Some individuals normally sensitive or allergic to wheat are able to tolerate it with little problem.

(Note: anyone severely allergic to wheat should consult with a health practitioner before experimenting with kamut pasta.)

Lupini pasta is made from durum flour and sweet lupin flour, a legume similar in protein content and quality to soybeans. The lupin/semolina blend contains over twice the amount of protein and four times the fiber as 100% semolina pastas. A darker-colored version includes triticale flour, contributing even more protein, fiber, and flavor. An added benefit of lupini pasta is that it keeps naturally loose and separate after cooking without requiring the addition of oil.

Sesame-rice pasta is made from 80% durum wheat, 10% brown rice flour, and 10% sesame flour (the by-product of making sesame oil) for a very flavorful pasta that is slightly higher in protein.

Spelt pasta is made from another ancient variety of wheat that makes a very tasty, whole-grain pasta, available in various shapes and sizes. As spelt seems to digest quite easily, choosing pasta made from it may be a particularly good choice for athletes. Like kamut, spelt is well tolerated by many individuals normally sensitive to wheat.

ORIENTAL PASTAS

Oriental pastas are traditionally served with thin broths or dipping sauces. Although you'll find them softer and more porous than European/North American durum wheat pastas, there's no reason to use them only when serving Japanese, Chinese, or other Oriental-ethnic cuisine. Udon and soba are equally delicious with fish, beans, tofu, tempeh—served plain, topped with salad dressing, gomasio (sesame salt), tamari shoyu, or with just a sprinkling of rice vinegar.

Bifun noodles are clear, "cellophane-type" noodles made from rice flour and potato starch. **Saifun** are transparent noodles made from mung bean starch. Both varieties are sold folded in skeins and are well suited for salads, clear soups, sukiyaki, and fried noodle dishes. Boil 5-6 minutes or soak in hot water 10-20 minutes. To stop cooking and to remove excess starch, rinse cooked bifun or saifun noodles under cold water until thoroughly cool.

Kuzu kiri are light-colored noodles made from kuzu powder and potato starch that are traditionally used in sukiyaki, salads, or served in a light broth. Unlike bifun and saifun, kuzu kiri require 20 minutes' cooking.

Ramen are extruded thin wheat noodles that are precooked and dried in blocks. Here's where the phrase, "you get what you pay for," couldn't be more true. Cheap "5 for a dollar" ramen features a label that looks like chemical soup. Its noodles are generally made with white flour, monosodium glutamate (MSG), and vegetable oil. The accompanying seasoning packet usually contains more MSG, synthetic soy sauce, corn syrup, sugar, and even more artificial flavor enhancers (disodium inosinate and disodium guanylate). Before drying into ramen's characteristic blocks, it is precooked in oil.

A high-quality ramen is priced a bit more than a dollar per package. Its noodles are nutritious and simply based on whole wheat flour combined with either a small amount of white flour, buckwheat flour, or brown rice flour. Its seasoning packet is derived from a combination of naturally aged soy sauce, miso, natural seasonings, and a variety of sea and land vegetables. Before drying, it is pre-cooked with steam. Considering nutrition and flavor, the natural version is clearly the better value.

Always keep a couple of packages of ramen on hand. It's invaluable for quick meals ready in less than 10 minutes or for a stress-free way to feed unexpected or extra-hungry dinner guests.

Rice sticks, mai fun, sen mee, bun, or banh pho noodles are brittle and off-white

THE SHAPE OF THINGS

Ever wonder why the shapes of European and North American pastas are so varied? Aesthetics have something to do with it, but the primary reason is that the different shapes were developed according to their ability to retain heat, absorb liquids, and hold sauces.

There are six basic categories of shapes:

1. Long rods without a hollow center: spaghetti, vermicelli, and capelli d'angelo (angel's hair) call for smooth tomato and olive oil sauces that are intended to coat the pasta.

2. Flat ribbons: fettucini, tagliatelle, and linguine absorb and attract rich butter and cream sauces.

3. Hollow shapes: elbow macaroni, ziti, penne, and rigatone are perfect for meat or vegetable sauces as they cling to the bends and crevices in the pasta.

4. Fun shapes: farfalle (bow ties), shells, radiatori, and rotelle trap chunky sauces and dressings in cooked dishes and cold pasta salads.

5. Tiny shapes: orzo (rice-shaped pasta), alphabets, and stars are used sparingly in soups to contribute substance.

6. Stuffed and layering pastas: tortellini, lasagne, and cappelletti depend on vegetable, seafood, or meat fillings to complement their shape.

in color. A familiar entree in Thai restaurants, Pad Thai is made with rice sticks that look like vermicelli. Depending on their thickness, rice sticks should be cooked 1-5 minutes or soaked in hot water for 15 minutes followed by stir-frying. Use the narrow ones for soups and cold noodle accompaniments and the wide noodles for stir-fries.

Soba are dark brown, thin buckwheat flour-based noodles traditionally eaten cold in summer and hot in winter. Like udon, soba is available in different flour combinations. One hundred percent buckwheat soba is a gluten-free alternative for those allergic to wheat. Although delicious, it has a very strong buckwheat flavor and hearty texture. Lighter versions made from 40-60% buckwheat flour mixed with unbleached white flour are more popular and more versatile.

Mugwort soba is made with dried mugwort, a plant rich in iron. Like spinach pasta, mugwort soba is green in color and very flavorful. Although not a traditional way to serve soba, it is terrific mixed with sauteed onions, cubed yellow finn potatoes, and red bell peppers.

Jinenjo soba is made with dried Japanese wild mountain yam, a vegetable traditionally used to promote strength and vitality. When used to make pasta, it adds a terrific nutty flavor and soft texture.

Somen is a thinner, more delicate wheat noodle traditionally served cold during the summer months. Generally made from unbleached white flour, occasionally you may find it in its whole wheat version.

Udon noodles look like cream-colored fettucini. Instead of using hard durum flour, udon, like all wheat-based Oriental pastas, is made from a lower-gluten wheat to create a more tender texture. Salt is added to strengthen the gluten and help bind the dough. After kneading, the dough is allowed to rest for several hours to develop the gluten before being rolled into a long continu-

USE YOUR NOODLE WHEN COOKING PASTA

You need to know more than how to boil water to make perfect pasta. It's also essential to know how much water to use, when the pasta is done, and how to treat it immediately after it is cooked.

Pasta should be cooked in plenty of water to allow it to move freely during cooking. For 1/2 lb. pasta, bring 3 quarts of water to a boil. For 1 lb., 4 quarts is the minimum. Once it reaches a rolling boil, add salt to taste, about 1 teaspoon per 1/2 lb. pasta. Obviously, don't go overboard, but if you use too little, you'll probably end up using more sauce (read calories) or salty condiments to make up for the lack of proper seasoning.

Add the pasta at once and stir it to prevent sticking. Bring the water back to a boil, covering the pot briefly if necessary. Fresh pasta should be checked after 1/2-1 minute. If using dried pasta, start testing for doneness with thin varieties such as capelli d'angelo (angel's hair) and cappellini after about 2 minutes and thicker types after 4 minutes.

Depending on its thickness, fresh pasta requires only 1/2 to 3 minutes total cooking time. The pasta is ready to remove from the pot when it is firm, yet tender with a very minute chalky white center remaining visible. Plan on about 4 minutes total cooking time for thin dried pasta and 8-10 minutes for thicker strands, ribbons, and special shapes. Since the pasta continues to cook after it leaves the pot, it will be perfectly done by the time it is drained and ready to serve.

Removing pasta is also an art. Instead of draining it in a colander, try lifting it out of the pot. A small amount of water will cling to the pasta, just enough for it to absorb so the pasta will stay soft. Instead of dumping the pasta cooking water down the drain, save some of it for making sauces. Not only is it flavorful, the starch that remains in the water helps with thickening. If not too salty, it can also be used as a flavorful way to moisten your dog's dry kibble.

Never rinse pasta or you'll remove the starchy coating that helps sauces cling to the strands. Instead, transfer the cooked pasta to a bowl and add the sauce. If you're not planning on adding the sauce right away or not using one at all, toss the pasta with a tablespoon or two of oil. The oil will bind with the starchy coating and lower the odds of it sticking to its neighbor noodles. This is especially important if you are planning to serve the noodles cold.

Oriental udon and soba noodles need special cooking treatment. Since udon and soba noodle dough is already made with salt, never add extra to its cooking water for further seasoning.

While they can be cooked in the same fashion as Western wheat pasta, the "shock method" is more traditional. For every 1/2 lb. of udon or soba, bring about 21/2 quarts of water to a boil. Drop in the noodles and stir just to separate them as they start to cook. When the water returns to a boil, add 1 cup of cold water to the pot. When the water returns again to a boil, add another cup of cold water. After another round of boiling, add the final cup of cold water. The noodles should be perfectly done—just tender and tasty with a uniform color when broken in half.

Unlike durum wheat-based and other "Western" pastas, udon and soba should

(Continued)

be rinsed after cooking to stop the cooking and to remove the excess starch on the noodles that results from their use of softer gluten flour. Udon cooking water is especially good to save for flavoring and thickening sauces or soups. Excess pasta water also makes a great moistening agent for your dog's dry kibble.

If the noodles need to be reheated, submerge them in a pot of boiling water for a few seconds.

ous sheet and cut. It is then naturally dried for over 30 hours, similar to the methods used for producing high-quality flat western pastas.

Udon made with 100% whole wheat is the most nutritious and flavorful. For lighter, smoother-textured noodles, several brands use "sifted wheat flour." Because both the bran and wheat germ found in whole wheat flour tend to cut through the gluten "glue strands" during the kneading process, small portions of each are removed. Other varieties are made from combinations of whole wheat and unbleached white flours. Tsuru udon is made from a blend of 60% whole wheat and 40% white flour. Genmai udon contains 30% brown rice flour and 70% wheat flour (whole wheat in some brands).

WHEAT-FREE PASTAS

While some individuals must avoid wheat altogether because of food sensitivities or allergies, switching to a wheat-free pasta for a change of pace can be a treat for anyone.

In addition to 100% buckwheat noodles, bifun, saifun, kuzu kiri, and rice sticks, a few other types of wheat-free pastas are available.

Brown rice pasta made with 100% brown rice flour makes a more nutritious alternative than bifun noodles and rice sticks made with refined flour. Available in familiar pasta shapes, it can be substituted for wheat pasta in several recipes. Like corn, brown rice pasta also lacks gluten and must, therefore, be cooked until done and no longer. Since it has the tendency to be very starchy, be sure to use plenty of water to cook brown rice pasta.

Corn pasta made from a blend of refined corn flours is available in several forms and shapes, including spaghetti, rotini, and elbows. Its rich, natural corn flavor is especially good served with black, pinto, or kidney beans and cheese. Since it lacks gluten, it is especially critical not to overcook corn pasta to avoid ending up with a soft and pasty mass. In addition to plain corn pasta, look for colorful vegetable corn pasta made with natural dried vegetable powders.

Nutritionally, plain and vegetable corn pasta contains about half the amount of protein and less vitamins and minerals as found in durum wheat pasta.

Quinoa/corn pasta is made by combining quinoa flour with corn flour for a higher-protein, more nutritious pasta. Quinoa's unique nutty flavor also comes through, making a particularly delicious alternative to 100% wheat pasta.

Sev are noodles made from unroasted chickpea flour (besan). A familiar snack in India, sev is fried instead of boiled. Often spicy, it is eaten alone or mixed with other ingredients—a savory Indian trail mix. Although it will probably be hard to find in most food stores in the United States, check ethnic groceries or try making them on your own.

PASTA PRIMAVERA

8 oz. whole wheat udon or ribbons
2 Tbsp. olive oil
2 cloves garlic, finely minced
1 yellow squash, sliced in rounds
1/2 lb. snow peas
3 green onions, cut diagonally into 1/2" pieces
1 red bell pepper, stemmed, cored, and cut into fine julienne strips
1/4 cup fresh basil, finely chopped
2 Tbsp. freshly grated Parmesan cheese (optional)
freshly ground black pepper

Cook pasta al dente. Lift pasta from water and drain. Immediately toss with olive oil and garlic. Lightly steam yellow squash and snow peas. Add to pasta with the remaining ingredients. Season with freshly ground pepper and serve.

Serves 3.
(Pyramid servings: 3 Bread/Grain Group, 2 Vegetable Group, 13 grams Fat)

Nutrition Facts

Serving Size 1/3 recipe (246 g)
Servings Per Container 3

Amount Per Serving

Calories 420   Calories from Fat 110

	% Daily Value*
Total Fat 13g	**19%**
Saturated Fat 2g	**10%**
Cholesterol 5mg	**1%**
Sodium 310mg	**13%**
Total Carbohydrate 64g	**21%**
Dietary Fiber 7g	**30%**
Sugars 12g	
Protein 15g	

Vitamin A 35%	•	Vitamin C 160%
Calcium 10%	•	Iron 10%

* Percent Daily Values are based on a 2,000 calorie diet.

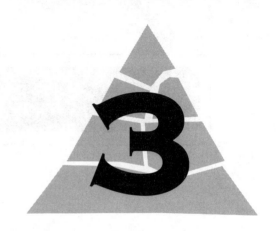

VEGETABLE GROUP

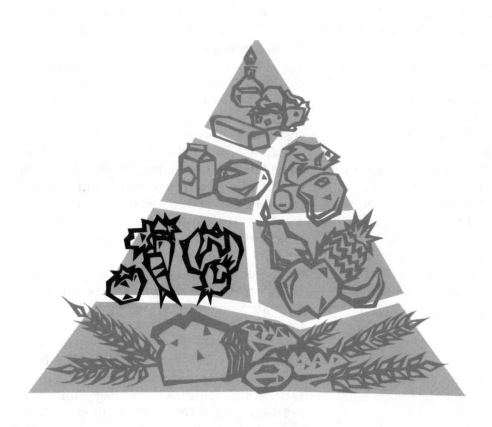

Vegetables

RESULTS FROM the Continuing Survey of Food Intakes by Individuals conducted by the U.S. Department of Agriculture during 1989-1991 revealed that about 80% of Americans eat at least one vegetable each day. While potatoes appeared to be the popular choice, most other vegetables didn't fare so well. About 25% of consumers had at least one serving of lettuce on any given day. Only 10% claimed they ate a dark green or yellow vegetable.

It's a far cry from the daily 3-5 servings the Food Guide Pyramid suggests to get all the nutrients we need to develop and maintain strong, healthy bodies, but with more awareness, it's a goal that is definitely within reach of anyone.

A serving is only 1 cup of raw leafy vegetables, 1/2 cup of other vegetables (both cooked or raw), or 3/4 cup of vegetable juice. These servings should be low in fat, too, with only minimal amounts of spreads, toppings, sauces, and salad dressings. Since different types of vegetables provide different nutrients, variety is another key component when choosing which vegetables to include in your diet.

NUTRITION

Orange and yellow vegetables, dark leafy greens, and cruciferous vegetables are highest in nutrition.

Carrots, winter squash, pumpkins, sweet potatoes, and dark leafy greens such as kale, mustard greens, arugula, collard greens, chard, escarole, and chicory are high in beta-carotene. In addition to naturally converting in our bodies into vitamin A, beta-carotene and other carotenoids have high antioxidant activity, rendering potentially destructive oxygen free radicals harmless. It's these free radicals that are suspected of causing cellular damage leading to cancer, heart disease, and premature aging.

Greens' high folic acid content is of particular interest. Studies have shown that women whose diets provide at least 400 micrograms (mcg.) of folic acid each day have significantly lower odds of giving birth to children with neural tube defects, including spina bifida or the related abnormality, anencephaly. If taken from the very early days of pregnancy, it is estimated that 50-70% of the 1500-3000 cases of neural tubal defects that affect children in the United States each year could be prevented.

Some studies also suggest that folic acid may decrease the risk of a child being born with abnormalities of the heart, limbs, and urinary tract.

Many of the dark leafy greens are also considered cruciferous vegetables. This family of vegetables that includes broccoli, Brussels sprouts, cauliflower, cabbage, bok choy, radishes, and turnips, in addition to kale, collards, arugula, and mustard greens, is called "cruciferous" since the flowers that bloom from the plants have four petals that form the shape of a cross.

Cruciferous vegetables are highly regarded due to the presence of certain compounds which help stimulate the production of protective enzymes that detoxify potential carcinogens.

Label Claims

So universally accepted are the beliefs that a diet high in vegetables can reduce the risks of coronary heart disease and cancer that three health claims are allowed to be used in connection with vegetable products that specifically link vegetables with reduced health risks:

•fiber-containing grain products, fruits, and vegetables and a reduced risk of cancer

•fruits, vegetables, and grain products that contain fiber and a reduced risk of coronary heart disease

•fruits and vegetables and a reduced risk of cancer.

Designer Vegetables

With the discoveries of an increasing amount of potentially beneficial nutrients and compounds comes the emergence of "designer vegetables" bred to emphasize or eliminate particular components within the food. The trend has already begun. Carrots have been developed that are much higher in beta-carotene, beets are being bred for increased levels of folic acid, and new varieties of garlic contain more of a protein that makes blood less likely to clot.

Some, but not all, of these new breeds are being developed through biotechnology, a process in which new varieties of food are produced by removing the specific genes or group of genes responsible for a certain trait and splicing in genes viewed as more desir-

VEGETABLES HIGH IN FOLIC ACID	
The Daily Value for folic acid is 400 mcg.	
1/2 cup cooked spinach	110 mcg.
1/2 cup cooked asparagus	88 mcg.
1 cup romaine lettuce, chopped	76 mcg.
1 cup loose leaf lettuce, chopped	60 mcg.
1/2 cup cooked broccoli	53 mcg.
1/2 cup cooked beets	49 mcg.
1/2 cup cooked dandelion greens	41 mcg.
1/2 cup cooked cauliflower	32 mcg.
1/2 cup cooked winter squash	30 mcg.
1/2 cup cooked collard greens	28 mcg.
1/2 cup raw parsley	27 mcg.

able. The source of the desirable gene could be from bacteria, plants, insects, fish, or animals.

But the production of vegetables higher in nutrients isn't all that is being explored in biotechnology. Besides genetically altering a vegetable for nutritional reasons, changes are being made to enhance flavor, appearance, texture, and "freshness."

The "Flavr Savr™" tomato broke the ground for the emergence of the new biotechnology-derived breed of vegetables. In order to offer a new tomato that could be picked ripe but still withstand the rigors and time associated with sending it to market, scientists for Calgene, the company that developed the special tomato, inserted a gene to block the production of an enzyme within the tomato that would otherwise break down the pectins and other compounds in the tomato that make it ripen quickly. As a result, the Flavr Savr™ tomato can be picked later at a more flavorful stage of ripening and still look and taste good after its trip to market.

To try to allay consumer fears, the Calgene company submitted their tomato to extensive FDA testing. In May 1994, the government approved the sale of the Flavr Savr™ tomato, claiming it as safe as any tomato bred by conventional means.

Still, several consumer groups object to the use of foods created in this manner, particularly because no labeling is required to differentiate them from those that are conventionally bred. Other concerns have been raised as well. (For more information, see "Biotechnology" in the Additives and Alternatives chapter.)

Many more new genetically altered products are expected for the future, including potatoes that absorb less fat when fried and crops that require fewer pesticides and herbicides. Consumer acceptance and the safety results after long-term use remain to be seen.

BUYING ORGANIC

High-quality produce departments will offer a variety of organically grown vegetables. With the emphasis on maximum yields, produce tends to be more heavily treated with synthetic fertilizers and pesticides than most foods. High yields are worthy goals, but the use of synthetic chemicals ignores and disrupts our complex ecologic system. Soil vitality and fertility is depleted and chemical residues enter the food chain and, ultimately, end up in our bodies. (For more information on pesticide use in the United States, refer to "Organically Grown" in the Additives and Alternatives section.

If consumers begin to demand safer food, farmers will be forced to reduce their use of pesticides and make changes that will significantly benefit our health and protect the environment.

Buy certified organically grown vegetables and fruit whenever possible. Avoid imported produce from nations with weak pesticide regulatory programs. Patronize stores that allow consumers to make informed choices by providing "country of origin" tags on every product within the department.

Also note how much locally grown produce is offered. Locally grown produce has the potential to be much fresher and, therefore, more nutritious, especially considering that other vegetables may already be a couple of days old when the long journey from field to market is factored in. Even better is to buy produce straight from the farm or at a farmer's market. Several small producers are using little or no farm chemicals so it shouldn't be too hard to find local organically grown produce.

Exploring Your Options

While basic vegetables such as carrots, green beans, peas, and potatoes are very nutritious, it's important to eat a wide variety of vegetables throughout the day, not only to make meals more interesting but also to provide different proportions of nutrients to your diet.

No doubt, you've seen some of the following greens, roots, squashes, and mushrooms at your favorite store or farmer's market. Make it a habit to buy at least one unfamiliar vegetable each time you shop.

CABBAGE FAMILY

Facts and Features

The cabbage family, also known as cruciferous vegetables, include a wide variety of vegetables. Arugula, collard greens, kale, and mustard greens have dual citizenship in the leafy greens category. Daikon, radishes, rutabagas, and turnips are cruciferous vegetables that are generally classified as roots. What's left are "flowers" and round vegetables, including broccoli, Brussels sprouts, cauliflower, green and red cabbages, and the few mentioned below that you may not be as familiar with.

All cruciferous vegetables are very nutritious, rich in beta-carotene, vitamin C, calcium, carbohydrates, fiber, and unique compounds that can enhance the deployment of potential carcinogens.

Varieties and Cooking Guidelines

Broccoflower is a cross between broccoli and cauliflower, easily identified by its light green color and cauliflower-like shape.

Flavorwise, broccoflower is also a cross between its parental roots, sweeter than cauliflower but milder than broccoli. It can be eaten raw, steamed, or sautéed.

Chinese cabbage, also known as napa cabbage, is a tall, elongated cabbage with pale green, crinkled leaves and broad-ribbed stalks. A favorite for stir-fries, its mild, delicate flavor and crisp texture is also good in salads and soups. When steamed whole, it can be used as a wrap to encase savory fillings.

Radicchio looks like a small, ruby-red cabbage with thick, white-veined leaves. Slightly bitter, radicchio provides an interesting flavor contrast in salads. It can also be used like other cabbages—steamed, braised, or stir-fried.

CHILE PEPPERS, FRESH AND DRIED

Facts and Features

Hot chiles provide flavor, character, and spirit to foods that may otherwise border on bland. Their popularity has also risen today partially in response to interest in reducing fat and sodium in our diets. Let's face it, some chiles are so hot that you'll likely be preoccupied with surviving the flames and forget about whether a dish is salty enough or not.

While just as many people say they feel even better eating on the mild side, others report that eating foods highly seasoned with hot chiles provides them with a sense of well-being as the brain releases natural pain killers called endorphins to ease the burning sensation on the tongue and throat.

Many cultures also include hot chiles in their cuisine because in the hot climates in which they are typically consumed, the inevitable sweating that occurs from eating spicy food appears to have a cooling effect on the skin.

Chiles are available both fresh and dried. They are also classified according to how much capsaicin, the fiery compound responsible for their heat, they contain. A scale to measure the varying levels of heat found in chiles was devised in 1912 by a pharmacologist named Wilbur Scoville, based on the number of grams of water it would take to cancel the heat of a single gram of chile. Ranging from 0 for green and red bell peppers as well as sweet banana peppers, the Scoville rating goes as high as 300,000 heat units for habeñero peppers. In general, the smaller the chile, the higher on the Scoville scale.

How do you cool the heat? Some people suggest yogurt, sour cream, rice, bread, or something sweet seems to provide some balance. Interestingly enough, the various cuisines that include liberal use of hot chiles include one or more of these buffers in the menu.

Nutritionally, fresh chiles are rich in vitamin C and beta-carotene. Ripe, red varieties are higher in these nutrients than when consumed in their green stages of maturity. Dried chiles are much lower in vitamin C, due to the dehydration process.

Varieties and Cooking Guidelines

Always use caution when working with hot chiles. To avoid potential burning, wear rubber gloves or cover your hands with plastic bags. Wash your hands thoroughly when done.

Roasting fresh peppers makes for a richer flavor. Broil them in the oven or directly over a gas flame until the skin turns black. Place them in a covered pot to steam and cool. Then peel, remove the stems and seeds, and proceed with your recipe.

Chiles are appropriate not only in Mexican, Thai, or Indian dishes, but also in many of your old favorite family recipes. Experiment, treading lightly at first.

Anaheim or **New Mexico** chiles are green or red, long-shaped and mild, similar in taste to bell peppers but hotter. They are used fresh, roasted, or dried. Leave whole and stuff with cheese or chop and add to cornbread batter, omelets, and salad dressings. The Scoville rating for Anaheim (New Mexico) chiles is 1000-1500 heat units.

Ancho chiles, large, flat, and reddish black in appearance with a flavor faintly reminiscent of raisins, are the dried form of poblano peppers. They are widely used in many Mexican sauces, including adobo, a marinade of chiles, vinegar, garlic, and oregano. Quite often you'll find them sold as ristras, with several anchos strung together. Hang them in your kitchen, removing only what you need for the meal at hand. The Scoville rating for anchos is 2500-3000 heat units.

Cayenne peppers are long, very thin, crinkled chiles sometimes found fresh, but more commonly dried. Used in both African and Cajun cooking, cayenne provides plenty of fuel for the fire. Their heat is a close match to that of piquin chiles, 35,000-40,000 Scoville units.

Chipotles are smoked and dried ripe jalapeño peppers that have a rich, slightly chocolate-like flavor. They are used extensively in sauces. Like jalapeños, chipotles have a Scoville rating of 3500-4500 heat units.

Habañeros, also known as "Scotch Bonnet," should undoubtedly be sold with warning labels since it ranks as the hottest chile in the world. While its name means "from Havana," it is actually grown in the Caribbean. A habañero looks like a small, short and squatty orange pepper and has a unique apricot-like flavor and aroma. Its Scoville rating is 200,000 to 300,000 heat units. The red habañero is even hotter, ranging from 300,000-400,000 Scoville units.

Jalapeños are small, 2-3 inch long, medium-hot chiles that, when dark green, are slightly bitter, changing to sweet if left to ripen until red. Their Scoville rating is 3500-4500 heat units.

Pasilla are thin, dark green chiles about 5-6 inches long. Its name means "little raisin," suggesting that its flavor is similar to its namesake. They are moderately hot.

Piquin chiles are very small in size, little more than 1/4 inch in width and 3/4 inch across. They are very hot, similar to cayenne pepper, with a Scoville rating ranging from 30,000-40,000 heat units.

Poblano chiles are dark green, about 3 1/2-4 inches long whose width tapers down to a point. They are a favorite chile pepper for chiles relleños, mildly hot with a Scoville rating of 2500-3000 heat units.

Serranos are a favorite chile for making salsa and fresh pico de gallo. They are about 2-3 inches long and very hot, with a Scoville rating of 10,000-23,000 heat units.

Thai bird chiles are short, tapered, very hot red or green chilis used in Thai cooking and sauces. They have a Scoville rating of 50,000-100,000 heat units. Green Thai chiles are hotter than the red.

Yellow Wax Hot chiles, also known as **Hungarian Wax**, were developed from the milder banana pepper and introduced into the United States from Hungary in 1932. They are yellow and shiny in appearance and have a subtle, slightly lemony flavor. Their Scoville rating is 5,000-10,000 heat units.

LEAFY GREENS

Facts and Features

The greens category encompasses a wide variety of leafy vegetables, including the more familiar lettuces such as iceberg, Romaine, red leaf, green leaf, and Bibb to the more bitter and hardy greens that are typically steamed, braised, or sautéed rather than eaten raw.

While all leafy greens provide potassium, the darker, hardier types are also good sources of vitamin C, beta-carotene, calcium, iron, and fiber. Many are also considered cruciferous vegetables, members of the cabbage family that contain unique enzymes that protect against cancer.

Varieties and Cooking Guidelines

Arugula is a cruciferous vegetable with dark green jagged leaves and a pungent hot flavor. Use raw in salads and sandwiches or cook briefly with other vegetables.

Belgian endive looks like a cigar made from pale yellow leaves. Its bitter flavor is a good contrast to milder flavored lettuce in a salad. Braise in vegetable or chicken broth for 5-10 minutes for a delicious hot vegetable.

Bok choy has soft, dark green leaves and long, thick white stalks and a sweet milk flavor. Best known for its use in stir-fries, bok choy remains crisp, even when cooked to a tender stage. Because the stalks require a longer cooking time, cut the leaves from the stalks and add during the last few minutes of preparation to prevent overcooking. Bok choy can also be added to salads and soups or simply steamed.

Collard greens are a cruciferous vegetable with leathery, gray-green leaves. For best flavor, buy during fall and winter months, choosing small/medium leaves for

EXPLORING VINEGARS

A splash of a flavorful vinegar over salad greens can easily take the place of high-fat salad dressings. Vinegars can also perk up steamed veggies, cooked grains, and even fruit salads.

Used since 5000 B.C. as a flavor enhancer, preservative, and folk remedy, vinegar was often traditionally served at high-protein meals to aid digestion. Unlike distilled or overly-filtered vinegars, the most nutritious varieties will be slightly cloudy, still containing the "mother," a strand-like mixture of active enzymes and beneficial bacteria.

Several different types of vinegar are available, with acidity and flavor dependent on the carbohydrate source that has been fermented to produce ethyl alcohol from which the vinegar is produced, as well as the particular production method utilized.

Apple cider vinegar is an all-purpose vinegar whose tart, apple-like flavor and golden color is good when used as an ingredient in salad dressings and as a condiment. The best varieties will be based on hard apple cider made from organically grown apples.

Balsamic vinegar is a dark, dense, syrupy vinegar that is both sweet and slightly tart. It is aged at least 3 years in wooden barrels but is at its best when older than 10 years. The complex production process for making balsamic vinegar involves transferring the vinegar each year into increasingly smaller barrels. The evaporation of the vinegar in the various exotic woods gives the vinegar its noted bouquet and flavor. Use balsamic vinegar in salad dressings, marinades, and as a condiment for fruit, vegetables, and grains.

Brown rice vinegar or rice wine vinegar has a slightly sweet, smooth, mellow flavor with about half the sharpness of cider vinegar. It is delicious in salad dressings, sauces, and as a condiment on fish, vegetables, and grain dishes.

Distilled vinegar, also known as grain vinegar, is made from distilling alcohol from corn, rye, or barley. It is the least nutritious and flavorful of all the vinegars. The strong, acidic flavor of distilled vinegar is too potent for salad dressings or as a condiment,

best flavor. Steam, braise, or sauté.

Dandelion greens are a pungent-flavored, cruciferous vegetable that is characterized by its deeply notched leaves. Young leaves can be used in salads. Older ones are best for stews.

Endive (also called chicory) has curly, frilly, coarse leaves with dark green edges and pale yellow stems. It is very high in fiber. Use raw in salads for a bitter accent or cook briefly for a more mild flavor.

Escarole has broad, coarse, flat leaves that are slightly bitter. Use raw in salads or cook briefly to mellow the bitter flavor.

Kale is a cruciferous green with dark bluish/green, finely curled, plume-like leaves and a subtle cabbage-like flavor. Steam, braise, or sauté.

Mizuna is a leafy cruciferous vegetable with a pungent, exotic flavor that's exceptional mixed with other greens in a salad.

Mustard greens are a cruciferous vegetables with curly edges and a spicy, peppery flavor. Steam, braise, or sauté.

but excellent for pickling and as a cleaning agent.

Fruit vinegars, most notably raspberry, strawberry, and blueberry vinegars, are made by infusing the flavor of the fruit into white wine vinegar. They have a light, fresh flavor that is delicious as a condiment with vegetables, fruit salads, and grains or as a tart addition to salad dressings and marinades.

Herb vinegars are cider, red wine, or white wine vinegars steeped with herbs, such as rosemary, basil, oregano, thyme, and tarragon. They are particularly good with salads.

Malt vinegar is made by fermenting the liquid extract of sprouted barley. It adds a distinctive flavor to hot and cold vegetable dishes, sautéed potatoes, and, of course, fish and chips.

Red wine vinegar is made from various types of red wine. Its robust flavor is excel-

lent with pungent greens, meats, and cheese dishes and salads.

Sherry vinegar has a mellow, full-bodied flavor with a sweet aftertaste. It is excellent in dressings for fruit salads and vegetable salads featuring cheeses.

Umeboshi vinegar is not a true vinegar, but the liquid drawn off from pickled umeboshi plums and shiso leaves. Its salty, tart flavor is delicious in salad dressings, dips, and marinades. Try substituting umeboshi vinegar for salt and lemon in chickpea-based Middle Eastern hummus. A 11/2-teaspoon serving of umeboshi vinegar equals the flavor and saltiness of 1 umeboshi pickled plum.

White wine vinegar is made from various types of white wine, from Chardonnay to Sauvignon Blanc. Its delicate flavor blends well with most dishes but is best with salads featuring mild-tasting varieties of greens.

Sorrel has a sour lemony flavor and bright green color, resembling young spinach leaves in appearance. Use sparingly in salads and cooked vegetable medleys and soups.

EDIBLE FLOWERS

Facts and Features

Although eating a salad that contains flowers we normally admire in gardens or arrange in vases may seem a bit odd, when you think about it, it's no more strange than eating the greens or lettuce, or any plant we grow specifically for food. Edible flowers provide flavor, color, and drama to salads, soups, entrees, and desserts.

However, it is very important to eat only those flowers that have been sanctioned as non-toxic. Never experiment unless you are positive of the flower's identification as one that is safe to eat.

You should also buy edible flowers only from produce departments or farmer's markets where they are grown specifically to be consumed. Even better, you can grow your own organically.

Avoid flowers from florists and, in many cases, even wildflowers. They may be treated with pesticides, herbicides, or fungicides.

Varieties and Cooking Guidelines

You'll need only a few petals per individual salad. Since they are very delicate, add immediately before serving. Although only the petals should be eaten on some flowers, others, such as violets, nasturtiums, and Johnny-jump-ups can be eaten in their entirety, including the stems and leaves.

Common, edible flowers and their respective flavors include:

Begonias: sweet, lemony
Borage: cucumber-like
Chive blossoms: onion-like
Chrysanthemums: slightly bitter
Geraniums: lemony
Hollyhocks: mild
Johnny-Jump-Ups: mild, lettuce-like
Lavender flowers: strong, lemony
Marigolds: lemony
Pansies: mild, lettuce-like
Nasturtiums: peppery, watercress-like
Rose petals: strong, fragrant
Tulip petals: sweet, pea-like
Violets: sweet

FRESH HERBS

Facts and Features

Fresh herbs are most valued for their flavor-boosting characteristics, making the simplest salad or sandwich a masterpiece. They also provide a small amount of nutrients, including vitamin C, beta-carotene, and potassium.

Varieties and Cooking Guidelines

Herbs (and spices) can be classified according to their overall predominance of flavor.

Strong, dominantly-flavored herbs and spices include: bay leaf, rosemary, sage, cardamom, curry, ginger, mustard, black pepper, and hot peppers.

Mild-flavored herbs and spices include: basil, celery seeds and leaves, dill, fennel, tarragon, garlic, marjoram, mint, oregano, savory, thyme, and turmeric.

Delicately-flavored herbs include: burnet, chervil, chives, and parsley.

While there are no hard and fast rules, you may want to create a balance between strong and mildly flavored herbs instead of mixing two very strong herbs and spices together. Strong, dominantly-flavored herbs should be used sparingly in recipes. Delicately-flavored herbs mix well with most other herbs and spices and can be used quite liberally.

As a general rule, you can use three times as much fresh herb as dried. Except for rosemary, thyme, and winter savory, fresh herbs should be placed in sauces and soups only during the last 10-15 minutes of cooking—just long enough to lose their volatile oils without losing flavor or becoming bitter.

Fresh herbs in dips, salads, herb butters, and cheese spreads should be added several hours before serving to allow the full development of flavor.

MUSHROOMS

Facts and Features

Throughout the centuries in China and Japan, mushrooms have been valued not only for their flavor, but for their medicinal qualities, as well. Although there has never been a question about mushrooms' culinary contributions, Western scientists are now discovering that the traditional use of mushrooms to enhance better health is, likewise, supported in fact. Some mushrooms, including the common button mushroom, shiitake, enoki, and oyster mushrooms are beneficial for the immune system. Wood ears have been found to inhibit blood clots.

Mushrooms also provide fiber, B vitamins, and potassium. The vegetable highest in protein next to beans and peas, mushroom's protein quality is enhanced when served with whole grains, bread, and pasta which complement the otherwise limited amino acids.

Ounce for ounce, dried mushrooms are more concentrated nutrients than their fresh counterparts. While fresh mushrooms are best for texture in quick sautés and stir-fries, dried mushrooms provide more depth of flavor.

Varieties and Cooking Guidelines

When buying fresh mushrooms, allow for the fact that during the cooking process the volume of mushrooms is reduced by 1/3 due to water shrinkage. Therefore, each pound of fresh mushrooms will yield 6 cups chopped mushrooms or 2 cups cooked.

Store fresh mushrooms in a paper bag and refrigerate; a plastic bag will make them deteriorate prematurely. Fresh button mushrooms will last up to a week, but exotic varieties should be used within 2-4 days. To clean fresh mushrooms, wipe them with a damp cloth or soft vegetable brush, using minimal water to prevent loss of nutrients and a change in texture. Some mushrooms, such as chanterelles and morels, may need to be briefly rinsed with running water to remove dirt embedded within crevices.

Except for button mushrooms, criminis, and enokis, most other varieties should always be cooked, both for health consider-ations and to intensify the flavors.

Dried mushrooms should be reconstituted by bringing them to a rapid boil in a moderate amount of water and then simmered for about 30 minutes. The liquid can then be used as the base for a soup or sauce. Although most of the flavor will be in the cooking liquid, chop or slice the reconstituted mushroom to provide a chewy texture to the entrée.

Mushrooms that are commonly used in cooking can be simply divided into two main categories, those of European descent and Oriental-based varieties.

European Mushrooms

Button mushrooms are the white, button-shaped, mild-flavored mushrooms commonly sold in supermarkets. Although this type of mushroom, the agaricus bisporus, has been commercially cultivated since 1650 in France, the white variety to which we are so accustomed was discovered by a Pennsylvania farmer in 1926. Button mushrooms are harvested when the gills underneath the cap are tightly enclosed; however, they are most flavorful when they are allowed to "ripen" in the refrigerator after purchase until the gills are exposed. To enhance the flavor of the mushrooms, sauté, steam, bake, or marinate.

Cèpes are woodland forest mushrooms gathered during late summer to late fall. Light brown in color, they have flat, very large caps, chunky stems, and a rich, meaty, nutty flavor. In Italy they are called porcini mushrooms which is translated to mean "little pigs." Instead of gills underneath its cap as found in many other mushrooms, this variety of mushroom has a spongy layer consisting of pores and tube-like crevices. Grill the caps, braise, or sauté and add to sauces or pasta and grain dishes. Dried cèpes are also available.

Chanterelles are a beautiful trumpet-shaped, forest mushroom now widely grown throughout the Pacific Northwest. Golden-colored chanterelles have a light, delicate, almost fruity flavor and aroma and a slightly chewy texture. Dramatic black varieties have a more earthy flavor. Use chanterelles quickly after purchase. While admittedly expensive, you owe it to yourself to experience, at least once, their incredible flavor in pasta, sauces, or soups. Dried chanterelles are also available.

Crimini mushrooms, also known as Italian Brown mushrooms, are a brown variety of the agaricus family which also includes the common button mushroom. Criminis are much richer in flavor and more meaty in texture, primarily due to their lower moisture content. Use as you would button mushrooms.

Morels look like elongated sponges or honeycombs with stems. They can be yellow, brown, or black in color. Gathered from woodland areas during the spring, morels have a deep, earthy flavor that is terrific with pasta and rice dishes, fish, or poultry. Because the whole mushoom is hollow inside, they are also perfect for stuffing. Use quickly after purchase. Dried morels are also available.

Pom-pom mushrooms, also called bear's head or lion's mane, look like small heads of cauliflower with a slightly furry texture. Their delicate flavor is enhanced when sliced and sautéed or baked whole.

Portabello mushrooms are very flavorful, meaty-textured, dark brown mushrooms whose caps range from 3-8 inches in diameter. Unlike its button and crimini cousins in the Agaricus family of mushrooms that are picked while the gills are still enclosed, portabellos are picked when their gills are fully exposed. Sometimes referred to as "vegetarian steak," portabellos are exceptional when marinated and grilled. They can also be sliced and sautéed with seasonings such as tamari soy sauce, olive oil or butter, and rosemary to be served with a thick piece of crusty bread or as a side dish to accompany the rest of the meal.

Oriental Mushrooms

Enoki mushrooms are mild-flavored, creamy white mushrooms with long slender stems and very small round caps. Originally grown on stumps of the enoki tree in the mountain ranges of Japan, enoki mushrooms are commercially produced on a growing medium of moist sawdust and rice bran that is packed in plastic bottles to yield a more "leggy" appearance. Their crisp, tender texture makes them a good raw addition to salads or briefly added to stir-fries just before serving.

Shiitake mushrooms are large mushrooms whose woodsy, almost smoky, flavor and meat-like texture make them a favorite in both Oriental and Western dishes. Grown in Japan on the wood of the shii tree, an evergreen oak tree, in the United States they are grown on oak tree logs. Only one or two are needed to impart a delicious flavor to soups, stews, stir-fries, and pasta dishes. Dried shiitakes are also available.

Straw mushrooms are typically sold dried, rarely fresh. Their interesting name relates not so much to their appearance but because they are produced on a soaked-rice growing medium. Use in stir-fries and soups.

Tree oysters are fan-shaped mushrooms that grow on one another on the trunks and limbs of trees. True to their name, they not only look like oyster shells, they even have a similar taste to oysters. Lightly sauté and add to sauces, soups, pasta, and rice.

Wood ear mushrooms are grown on logs, looking very much like the shape of an ear when fresh. Firm, yet gelatinous, wood ear mushrooms add an interesting texture to stir-fries, pasta, and rice dishes. Dried wood ear mushrooms are also available.

RICH AND ZESTY CREAM OF SHIITAKE SOUP

1 Tbsp. sesame oil
1 clove elephant garlic, diced
1/4 cup millet
1 stalk celery, cut on diagonal 1/2 inch thick
4 green onions, thinly sliced (reserve one for garnish)
4 small or 2 large shiitake mushrooms, thinly sliced
2 carrots, cut in 1-inch chunks
1/2 tsp. coriander
1 Tbsp. tamari soy sauce
6 cups water
1/4 tsp. orange zest (grated organic orange rind)

Heat oil in a soup pot. Sauté garlic for 3 minutes. Add millet, green onions, celery, mushrooms, carrots, coriander, tamari, and water. Bring to a boil, cover, and reduce heat. Simmer 45 minutes. Remove soup from heat. Stir in orange zest, allowing its flavor to permeate the soup for 5 minutes before serving. Taste and adjust seasonings. Garnish with reserved green onion slices.

Serves 4.
(Pyramid servings: 1/2 Bread/ Grain Group, 1 Veg. Group, 4 grams Fat)

Nutrition Facts

Serving Size 1/4 recipe (443 g)
Servings Per Container 4

Amount Per Serving	
Calories 110	Calories from Fat 35

	% Daily Value*
Total Fat 4g	6%
Saturated Fat 0.5g	3%
Sodium 270mg	11%
Total Carbohydrate 16g	5%
Dietary Fiber 3g	11%
Sugars 3g	
Protein 3g	

Vitamin A 200%	•	Vitamin C 10%
Calcium 4%	•	Iron 4%

Not a significant source of Cholesterol
* Percent Daily Values are based on a 2,000 calorie diet.

ROOTS AND TUBERS

Facts and Features

Roots and tubers grow underground, substantial vegetables that, indeed, provide a kind of grounding energy to our diet. Potatoes, carrots, and beets are most familiar, but many other roots and tubers of all shapes, sizes, and colors are also available.

Yellow and orange root vegetables are excellent sources of beta-carotene. All are high in fiber and mineral, particularly potassium. Some, such as potatoes and sweet potatoes, are also fair sources of vitamin C. Because of their high complex carbohydrate content, roots and tubers (potatoes are the exception) taste sweet, a property that intensifies with longer cooking. When eaten raw, flavors within this family of vegetables may range from bland to biting.

Varieties and Cooking Guidelines

Burdock is a long slender root vegetable with an earthy flavor. Scrub but do not peel. It is somewhat tough and often is boiled 10 minutes before adding other vegetables. Plan on twice as much cooking time as carrots. To keep firm during long storage, wrap the burdock in a damp cloth before refrigerating.

Celery root or celeriac is a tough knobby root that comes from a different variety of celery than the one raised for its stalks. Since it is difficult to clean due to its tough skin, it is often peeled before use.

ROASTED ROOT SOUP

1 carrot
1 rutabaga
4 jerusalem artichokes
3 parsnips
1/4 cup water
1 Tbsp. fresh rosemary or
    1/2 tsp. dried
1 tsp. sesame oil
2 tsp. tamari soy sauce
2 tsp. sesame oil
1 cup mushrooms,
chopped
1/2 cup onions, chopped
1 stalk celery, chopped
3 Tbsp. pearled barley
6 cups water

Preheat oven to 400° F. Cut all root vegetables into small chunks and combine in a baking dish with water. Top with rosemary and drizzle with oil and tamari. Cover with foil and roast in the oven for 35-40 minutes or until tender.

Meanwhile, sauté mushrooms, onions, and celery in sesame oil for 5 minutes. Add barley and water, bring to a boil, and simmer for 1 hour. Add roasted root vegetables and any accumulated cooking liquid to the barley base. Simmer 20 minutes and adjust seasoning before serving.

Nutrition Facts

Serving Size 1/4 recipe (577 g)
Servings Per Container 4

Amount Per Serving

Calories 170   Calories from Fat 35

	% Daily Value*
Total Fat 4g	6%
Saturated Fat 0.5g	3%
Sodium 200mg	8%
Total Carbohydrate 31g	10%
Dietary Fiber 6g	26%
Sugars 8g	
Protein 4g	

Vitamin A 110%	•	Vitamin C 35%
Calcium 8%	•	Iron 20%

Not a significant source of Cholesterol
* Percent Daily Values are based on a 2,000 calorie diet.

Serves 4.
(Pyramid servings: 1/2 Bread/Grain Group, 2 Veg. Group, 4 grams Fat)

Celery root has a subtle celery flavor. It can be cooked like carrots or turnips or used in its raw state. It is especially good when grated and combined with a mustard salad dressing. To soften the root when used raw, it is advisable to add 11/2 teaspoons of salt per 1 pound of celery root with 11/2 teaspoons lemon juice or vinegar. Refrigerate for 30 minutes, rinse thoroughly, and use a towel or paper towel to squeeze out moisture. Then add a salad dressing and marinate for 2 hours.

Daikon is a white radish that is similar to an icicle radish but much larger in size. It has a hot taste that is good raw in salads. When cooked in soups, stews, or alone as the feature vegetable, daikon becomes surprisingly sweet.

Elephant garlic looks, not surprisingly, like a giant bulb of garlic. Although it is much more mild in flavor than regular garlic, it can be used in any recipe that calls for garlic. Elephant garlic is especially good drizzled with oil while still in its papery wrapper and baked at 350° F. for 30-45 minutes. When soft, the insides of the elephant garlic can be squeezed out and spread on bread, baked potatoes, or whatever.

Fennel/Anise—Fennel is a compact greenish-white bulb with a licorice flavor that can be used raw or cooked in casserole salads, soups, stews, stuffings, or by itself.

Anise is the feathery top which can be used as an herb for seasoning.

Jerusalem artichokes have no resemblance to an artichoke. They are a brown-skinned root which can be cooked like potatoes— either sautéed, boiled, baked, simmered in soups, eaten raw in salads, or used as a substitute for water chestnuts.

Jicama (pronounced: he' cah mah) is a light brown-colored root grown in Mexico that can be sautéed, boiled, or used raw in salads or for dips. Peel the tough skin before use. When raw, it has a texture similar to an apple with a somewhat sweet, refreshing flavor. It stays crisp when cooked.

Parsnips look like white carrots and are, indeed, related to carrots but are unique in flavor. Their sweet, nutty flavor complements bean dishes, soups, stews, and curries.

Rutabagas are roundish in shape with a yellow-brown skin and yellow flesh. Its nutty, sweet flavor becomes even more sweet the longer it is cooked. Raw grated rutabagas add an interesting flavor and texture to salads.

Taro root is a vegetable most familiar to people living in Japan, Egypt, Syria, New Zealand, Hawaii, and other islands in the Pacific Ocean. It looks like a hairy potato and can, indeed, be cooked like a potato— baked, steamed, boiled, or used in soup. Remove skins after cooking.

SQUASHES

Facts and Features

Squashes can be divided into two categories, summer and winter. Summer squash includes zucchini, straight or crookneck yellow squash, and pattypan or scallop squashes, which look like flattened versions of the previous two.

Winter squash, more correctly stated as fall and early winter squash, have hard rinds and are sweeter in flavor. Acorn squash is most familiar, but it's only a hint at the other terrific varieties that are also available.

Spaghetti squash and chayote fit somewhere in between summer and winter squashes—sweeter than typical summer squashes but with thinner rinds and higher water content than winter squashes.

Squashes are high in potassium, fiber, and folic acid, and contain good amounts of vitamin C and several B vitamins, including thiamine, niacin, and riboflavin. Winter squashes are also excellent sources of beta-carotene. All types can be steamed, braised, or baked.

Varieties and Cooking Guidelines

Banana squash is a very large, yellow-brown banana-shaped, sweet-flavored squash that is often precut into smaller more reasonably sized pieces.

Blue hubbard squash is a sweet-flavored, blue-grey, thick skinned squash that can also be quite large. It is often stuffed and baked as you would a turkey.

Buttercup squash looks like a dark green globe with a light green crown. Its flavor is very sweet.

Butternut squash is a light yellow, bottle-shaped squash with a sweet, nutty flavor.

Chayote is a squash with a soft pale green rind that has a flavor somewhat similar to zucchini but with the fibrous texture similar to a winter squash. It can be baked, steamed or sautéed.

Delicata squash is an elongated yellow vegetable with green stripes with a delicate(!) sweet flavor.

Golden nugget squash is a small round squash with a very thick inedible orange skin. It has a sweet nutty flavor.

Hokkaido squash (also known as Kabocha), with its blue-green skin and

GOLDEN POPPYSEED SOUP

1 tsp. safflower or canola oil
1 onion, diced
1 medium-sized butternut squash, seeded and cut into 1-inch chunks
1 stalk celery, diced
1 carrot, diced
4 cups water
1 Tbsp. hulled white sesame seeds or 2 tsp. sesame tahini
2 Tbsp. white miso
1 Tbsp. poppy seeds
2 squares mochi, cut into 1/2-inch squares

Heat oil in a soup pot and sauté onion for 5 minutes. Add squash, celery, carrot, and water. Bring to a boil and reduce heat. Simmer for 30 minutes. In a food processor or blender, purée soup with the sesame seeds or tahini until smooth and return to the soup pot. Dilute miso in 1/2 cup of the soup. Blend in the poppy seeds and return mixture to the soup. Add mochi squares and simmer soup for another 5 minutes to cook the mochi into "dumplings." Serve immediately.

Serves 6.
(Pyramid servings: 2 Veg. Group, 3 grams Fat)

Nutrition Facts

Serving Size 1/6 recipe (287 g)
Servings Per Container 6

Amount Per Serving

Calories 130   Calories from Fat 25

	% Daily Value*
Total Fat 3g	4%
Sodium 220mg	9%
Total Carbohydrate 23g	8%
Dietary Fiber 4g	14%
Sugars 3g	
Protein 3g	

Vitamin A 180% • Vitamin C 30%
Calcium 8% • Iron 6%

Not a significant source of Saturated Fat and Cholesterol.

* Percent Daily Values are based on a 2,000 calorie diet.

---

pumpkin shape, is the sweetest of all the squashes.

Pumpkins are available in two basic types, the less flavorful jack-o'-lantern and the sugar pumpkin which is used for cooking and baking. Pumpkins are not as sweet as other winter squash and often need additional sweetening.

Spaghetti squash, as the name implies, can be a vegetable substitute for spaghetti. Bake or steam this yellow-skinned, oblong-shaped squash until tender and then use a fork to separate the fibers to produce the mildly sweet-flavored "noodles."

TOMATILLOS

Facts and Features

Tomatillos, also known as the Mexican tomato, look like green cherry tomatoes that are wrapped in a thin, parchment-like husk. Grown in Mexico and central California on weedy plants that grow up to 4 ft. high, tomatillos are not actually tomatoes, although they do belong to the nightshade family which includes tomatoes as well as potatoes, eggplants, and peppers.

Tomatillos are a good source of vitamin C.

Varieties and Cooking Guidelines

Tomatillos have a tart, slightly sweet apple or plum flavor that is delicious raw in salads, as a filling in tacos, and in fresh salsas and dressings. Even so, its flavor is enhanced with cooking, making tomatillos a common ingredient in Mexican cuisine for cooked green salsas, stews, and casseroles, an especially good complement to seafood, cheese, and chicken dishes.

Store tomatillos with husks on in a paper bag in the fridge for up to 3 weeks. When ready to use, discard the husk and wash the tomatillo well to remove its sticky residue.

VEGETABLE JUICES

A serving of vegetables can also be fulfilled with 3/4 cup vegetable juice. Vegetable juice is lower in calories than fruit juice. Like its fruit counterpart, vegetable juice is a good source of potassium, vitamins, and minerals. Water-soluble vitamins are at their highest potency level immediately after juicing. Each subsequent hour after juicing, the nutrient levels continue to decrease. For best results, buy your juice at a juice bar, make it from your own juicer, or buy a fresh frozen vegetable juice and thaw it in the refrigerator.

Carrot juice is the most popular vegetable juice. It takes about 1 pound of carrots to make 1 cup of carrot juice.

Wheatgrass juice is very high in chlorophyll. Devotees claim that it is energizing, helps improve blood sugar, and "purifies" the blood.

PEAK SEASONS FOR VEGETABLES

JANUARY, FEBRUARY

broccoli	leeks
cabbage	mushrooms
carrots	mustard greens
celery	rutabaga
collard greens	spinach
fennel	winter squash
kale	

MARCH, APRIL, MAY

artichokes	leeks
asparagus	mustard greens
broccoli	peas
cabbage	new potatoes
carrots	sorrel
collard greens	spinach
dandelion greens	watercress

JUNE, JULY, AUGUST

arugula	fava beans
asparagus (June)	kohlrabi
beets	lima beans
cabbage	okra
carrots	pattypan squashes
chard	peppers
corn	radishes
cucumbers	sorrel
eggplant	spaghetti squash
garlic	yellow squash
green beans	zucchini

SEPTEMBER, OCTOBER, NOVEMBER, DECEMBER

arugula	leeks
beets	mushrooms
Belgian endive	mustard greens
broccoli	parsley
Brussels sprouts	peppers
cabbage	snow peas
carrots	potatoes
cauliflower	pumpkin
celery root	rutabaga
chard	sweet potatoes
fennel	yams
garlic	winter squash
kale	

Sprouts

SHORT OF harvesting vegetables from your own garden immediately before preparation, sprouts are often the freshest vegetable available. Some stores grow their own while others are supplied by local vendors on a frequent basis. Sprouts labeled as certified organically grown must be grown from organic seeds.

Sprouts also are very easy to grow yourself. No special equipment is needed, no large growing area is needed, and no large amounts of money need be invested.

NUTRITION

Sprouts are the very young shoots from the germinated seeds of vegetables, beans, or grain. Not only do the sprouts contain the concentrated amounts of protein, vitamins, and minerals found in the seed, during the process of sprouting the nutrient level increases dramatically. For instance, vitamin C and the B complex can increase up to 600% and Vitamin E can triple. Their protein may also be more easily digested.

Still, however, their nutrient content remains about comparable to lettuce—slightly higher in some values but lower in others. Sprouts' real claims to fame are that they are grown without pesticides and herbicides, and that they have a higher likelihood to be fresher, therefore, potentially more viable in nutrients. Like other vegetables, each day after harvest brings reduc-

tions in nutrient levels, so use them as quickly as possible. Maximum refrigerator life is 1 week.

Research has shown that it is important to keep your consumption of raw alfalfa sprouts to a moderate amount. What with all the high esteem people generally have about sprouts, relating information such as this may seem akin to saying something nasty about Santa Claus. However, it's simply a reminder that no food is so perfect that it warrants going overboard.

In the case of alfalfa sprouts, small amounts of a natural toxin, called *saponins*, are found. Consistent consumption of very large amounts could lead to red blood cell damage. Another natural toxin is canavanine which, again, if consumed in abnormally large quantities, could lead to weakening of the immune system. Although you don't need to avoid them, alfalfa sprouts are generally considered harmless if consumed in normal amounts within a diet that contains plenty of variety from other vegetables. Other leafy green types of sprouts don't seem to be connected with these concerns.

While occasional small amounts of raw sprouted legumes is considered acceptable, all sprouted legumes should be cooked to inactivate a toxin that can also affect the immune system.

HOW TO SPROUT

Almost any seed, bean, or grain will sprout. Red clover, alfalfa, cabbage, zippy radish sprouts, sunflower, and buckwheat will sprout into leafy greens. Starchy beans and grains grow shoots and roots.

Basic equipment includes a wide-mouthed quart-sized jar, a rubber band, and cheesecloth or clean nylon stockings. Special equipment can be bought ranging from sprouting jars with lids of plastic or stainless steel grids to 3-tiered or dome-shaped mini sprouting greenhouses. The amount of seed needed depends on the size of the seed. Seeds as small as alfalfa seeds require 1 Tbsp. to fill a quart jar while seeds as large as beans or grains require 4 Tbsp.

Place the seeds in the jar, add water to cover the seeds plus 1" depth. Cut a piece of clean cheesecloth or nylon stocking 2" larger than the diameter of the mouth of the jar, and fasten it tightly with the rubber band. Let the seeds soak overnight or 8 hours. Then invert the jar to drain the soaking water. (Instead of pouring it down the drain, use it to water your plants. The nutrients in the water will make your plants thrive.)

Fill half the jar with water through the cheesecloth covered opening, shake it to moisten the seeds, and drain again. Water should remain in the jar only the first night. Place the jar on its side or in a dish drainer upside down with the mouth pointed toward the sink. Cover with a towel to provide a dark environment. Most seeds require this rinsing technique twice per day. Some of the beans, such as garbanzo beans and soybeans, need 5-6 rinsings per day to prevent spoilage.

Sprouts are ready within 2-5 days depending on the seed, bean, or grain used. In general, seeds need 3-5 days to grow 1-2 inches, beans need 3-5 days to grow 1 inch, and grains need 2-3 days to grow the original length of the grain used.

Store in the sprouting jar or a plastic container and use quickly.

COOKING GUIDELINES

Use delicate sprouts like alfalfa or red clover raw. Grain sprouts can be used raw or cooked. Sprouted beans are best cooked. (Note: potato sprouts are toxic. Never eat them!)

Sprouts are good in sandwiches, soups, salads, stir-fries, and omelettes.

You can make your own natural malt sweetener from grain sprouts by drying wheat or barley sprouts in an oven at the lowest temperature possible for about 2 hours. When dry, grind in a seed mill or blender. Use with cereals, breads, and cookies.

Sea Vegetables

NUTRITION

Sea vegetable or seaweed? If sea vegetables mean no more to you than slimy underbrush that entangles your feet while swimming in lakes and bays, think again. Many cultures, Japanese, Irish, Scottish, English, Welsh, Russian, French, Canadian, Scandinavian, and even our own colonial ancestors in New England have enjoyed sea vegetables as a delicious addition to soups, breads, and meat and seafood dishes.

Whether you know it or not, the typical American diet still contains a significant amount of sea vegetables. More recently it's been in the form of stabilizers, thickeners, emulsifiers, and suspending agents found in baked goods, ice cream, puddings, cheeses, and as a fat replacement in ground beef and hot dogs. However, recognition of its superior nutritional content and remarkable textures and flavors has led to the "rediscovery" of an ancient food source.

Nutritionally, sea vegetables are a rich source of iodine, iron, magnesium, calcium, sodium, phosphorus, and other nutrients in a well-balanced form.

They also contain sodium alginate, a hydrophilic colloidal substance that reacts with various radioactive substances in the body produced from nuclear reactions, their fallout, and X-rays, as well as with heavy metals, including lead, cadmium, barium, strontium, excess iron, plutonium, and ce-sium. Once chelated with these harmful pollutants, the sodium alginate neutralizes them into harmless salts that are then safely eliminated from the body. The addition of moderate amounts of sea vegetables in the diet, then, can be both preventative and therapeutic in its effects.

The concept of moderation must be emphasized. Eating too large a quantity of sea vegetables puts you at risk of assimilating too much iodine. We need iodine for the healthy functioning of the thyroid, the gland that regulates body temperature, the metabolic rate, growth, reproduction, the making of cells, and nerve and muscle function. However, too much can contribute to hyper-activity, mental and emotional imbalances, rough skin, acne, and excessive weight loss.

Much of the excessive iodine found in some people's diets comes from the liberal use of iodized salt in fast foods and from dough conditioners used in the baking industry. Since they also contain a wide array of nutrients, sea vegetables provide a superior source of iodine in the diet.

For adults and children aged 4 or older, the Daily Value for iodine is 150 micrograms (mcg.). A little seaweed goes a long way.

Cooking Guidelines

Adding small amounts of sea vegetables to soups, stews or beans is a good way to experience the unique flavors, textures, and colors. The mild flavors of arame, dulse, and nori make them good sea vegetables to use initially.

Since rehydrating sea vegetables can expand their volume up to sevenfold, only a small amount is required in recipes. Most sea vegetables should be quickly rinsed with water to remove any lingering dust, sand, or excess naturally-occurring sea salt. Depending on the variety, they should then be briefly soaked before cooking with other quickly prepared vegetables, grains, beans, or seafood dishes. No soaking is needed when used in long-simmered soups and stews.

Dried sea vegetables will keep indefinitely if stored in a tightly sealed container in a cool, dark place such as a cupboard or pantry away from the stove. Cooked sea vegetables will keep 4-5 days refrigerated.

Exploring Your Options

AGAR-AGAR

Facts and Features

Agar-agar is made from several varieties of red seaweed processed into lightweight translucent bars called kanten that may also be further processed into flakes or powder. Its primary use is as a gelling agent to make a vegetarian fruit "gelatin" dessert, vegetable aspics, puddings, and pie fillings. Quicker to use, the flakes and powder are also less expensive and yield a harder gel than the more traditional agar bars.

Cooking Guidelines

To gel 2 cups of liquid, plan on 3-4 tablespoons agar flakes, 2 teaspoons agar powder, or 1 kanten bar. Agar flakes and powder do not have to be soaked prior to use.

If using a kanten bar, first break it into pieces and place them in water to soak for 30 minutes or until spongy. Squeeze out excess water and add kanten to 2 cups juice, broth, or water. Bring to a boil, lower to simmer, and cook for 10 minutes, stirring to thoroughly dissolve the kanten. Transfer to a heatproof mold or glass baking dish and allow to set.

Agar will set at room temperature, but the gelling process is much quicker in the refrigerator (about 45-60 minutes).

ALARIA

Facts and Features

Alaria is dried from its fresh golden-brown leaves that grow off the coast of Maine. With a taste similar to but more pronounced than wakame, it is delicious in salads, miso soups, stews, and cooked with grains.

Cooking Guidelines

Alaria needs at least 20 minutes to bring out its sweet, mild taste and soft, chewy texture. For use in salads, first soak alaria in water or marinate in vinegar or lemon juice.

ARAME

Facts and Features

Arame is a brown alga whose large tough leaves are parboiled for about seven hours to make them tender before they are dried and shredded into long black strands. It has a rich flavor similar to but much more mild than hijiki. Use in vegetable sautées, salads,

AGAR "GELATIN"

3 cups juice
1 cup water
1/3 cup agar flakes or 2
    bars agar
pinch of salt
1 Tbsp. kuzu (Japanese
    thickening agent—
    optional)
1 cup sliced fresh fruit
    (optional)

Add agar flakes to juice, water, and salt, bring to a boil. (NOTE: If using agar bars, first break bars into small pieces, soak in water for 30 minutes, and wring out excess water before adding to juice and water.) If a creamier texture is desired, dilute the kuzu in a small amount of water and add to the boiling mixture. Reduce heat and simmer 10 minutes. Add fresh fruit and simmer an additional 3 minutes. Pour into heat-proof mold or glass dish and let cool to room temperature. Refrigerate 2 hours or until firm.

Nutrition Facts

Serving Size 1/4 recipe (292 g)
Servings Per Container 4

Amount Per Serving

Calories 120

	% Daily Value*
Total Fat 0g	0%
Sodium 80mg	3%
Total Carbohydrate 30g	10%
Dietary Fiber 1g	5%
Sugars 25g	
Protein 0g	

Vitamin A 4%	•	Vitamin C 8%
Calcium 2%	•	Iron 6%

Not a significant source of Calories from Fat, Saturated Fat and Cholesterol.
* Percent Daily Values are based on a 2,000 calorie diet.

(Pyramid servings:)

---

and casseroles. Once soaked and cooked, arame doubles in volume.

Cooking Guidelines

Before cooking, rinse arame and briefly soak for 5 minutes. An excellent introduction to arame is to add it to onions and carrots that have been sautéed in sesame oil. Add a small amount of water, a dash of tamari soy sauce, and simmer over low heat for 30 minutes. For extra richness, during the last 3 minutes of cooking, dilute a dab of sesame tahini in a small amount of water or mirin and mix in to coat the vegetable/arame mixture.

This recipe can also be the filling for a terrific vegetable struedel.

CARRAGEENAN (IRISH MOSS)

Facts and Features

Carrageenan is the gelatinous substance found in Irish moss that is extracted and dried into a powder. It is used in commercial food production as a stabilizer, emulsifier, thickener, gelling agent, and suspending agent in ice creams, salad dressings, cheese spreads, puddings, and to replace the fat in ground beef, hot dogs, and processed poultry products.

Cooking Guidelines

Carrageenan is used in commercial food production. Irish moss, its parent plant, is rarely sold for home use.

DULSE

Facts and Features

Dulse is a reddish-purple sea vegetable harvested commercially in eastern Canada. A traditional staple in Ireland, Scotland, Wales, and parts of New England, it can be eaten raw as a salty snack or rinsed and cooked with chowders, stews, salads, grains, or sandwiches (hint: try it with peanut butter).

Dulse is also sometimes available in its powdered form as a condiment. It has the highest concentration of iron of all the sea vegetables.

Cooking Guidelines

Unlike other sea vegetables, dulse can be eaten right out of the bag. However, to reduce its saltiness, it's probably best to first give it a light rinse or very brief soaking. Watch out for seashells!

When cooking add dulse during the last 5 minutes of cooking.

HIJIKI (HIZIKI)

Facts and Features

Hijiki looks like a chubby version of arame but has a more pronounced, although delicious, flavor. To soften its naturally tough strands, it is first dried, steamed for 4 hours, and dried again.

The traditional use for hijiki was to help maintain hair and skin. In fact, its name is translated from Japanese as "bearer of wealth and beauty." Hijiki is also a good addition to casseroles, salads, noodle dishes, cooked rice, soups, and stews.

Hijiki expands fivefold after soaking and cooking.

Cooking Guidelines

Hijiki should be rinsed 3-4 times and then soaked for 5-10 minutes before cooking. Allow a simmering time of 30 minutes to one hour.

KELP

Facts and Features

Kelp is most often found in powder and tablet form. Like all sea vegetables, it is a good source of trace minerals, most notably iodine. Use as a salt substitute or condiment.

Domestically harvested kelp is also called Atlantic kombu. Like Japanese kombu, it is naturally high in glutamic acid, making it a natural tenderizing, flavor-enhancing agent for soups, beans, and stews. Atlantic kelp is also rich in mannitol, a natural sugar similar to sorbitol, that gives the sea vegetable a slightly sweet taste.

Cooking Guidelines

Atlantic kelp cooks quickly. Unlike Japanese kombu which remains fairly tough even after long cooking, Atlantic kelp will dissolve if allowed to cook for more than 20 minutes in a soup, stew, or with beans.

Besides boiling, it can also be marinated, pickled, or pan-fried.

KOMBU

Facts and Features

Kombu is the backbone of Japanese cooking. These stiff, broad flat dried leaves harvested off the coast of Japan are used to make dashi, the all-important broth that is used as a stock for noodles and soups. What makes kombu so unique and invaluable is its ability to enhance the flavors of foods, due to its naturally-occurring unbound glutamic acid content. Unlike monosodium glutamate (MSG), it is a safe, more nutritious, more balanced type of flavor enhancer.

Use kombu to make soup stocks, broths, and vegetable stews. Beans cook faster and digest and taste better when a small piece of kombu is added. It can also be made into side dishes, condiments, and candies.

Kombu doubles or triples in size after soaking or cooking.

Cooking Guidelines

Rinse quickly under cold water to remove excess salt. When preparing side dishes and condiments, kombu is best soaked in cold water for 3-5 minutes prior to cooking. However, be careful not to oversoak. It makes kombu very slippery and hard to cut.

Cook kombu at least 30 minutes.

NORI

Facts and Features

Nori, the familiar "wrapping" used in making sushi, is a cultivated sea vegetable grown on bamboo-supported nets. It is then washed, chopped into small pieces, ladled onto bamboo mats, pressed into sheets and dried.

Most nori sheets are a dark, iridescent green. Flavor and digestibility are improved when the raw purple nori sheets are toasted. Sushi nori are large pretoasted sheets made specifically for preparing sushi.

Besides sushi, nori can be used to wrap rice balls or cut into thin strips and used as a garnish for soups, salads, grain dishes, noodles, casseroles, and even popcorn. A rich-tasting condiment for grains and beans is made by cooking nori with a small amount of water and tamari soy sauce until the water evaporates and the nori becomes a thick paste.

Cooking Guidelines

To toast green-tinged nori, simply hold it a couple of inches above a flame or heating element on a stove. Within seconds it will turn green, ready to crumble or cut into

strips as a garnish and condiment or to use to make rice balls or sushi.

SEA PALM

Facts and Features

Sea palm is a sea vegetable unique to the Pacific Northwest. Its delicious, subtly sweet flavor makes sea palm a favorite even with those who are preconvinced that they will not like sea vegetables.

Use sea palm in soup, salads, and sautés.

Cooking Guidelines

For use in salads, sea palm should be soaked in water for 1 hour prior to use.

Soak it for 20 minutes in water before adding it to soup or sautés.

WAKAME

Facts and Features

Wakame is a long dark green leaf that grows along the coasts of Korea and China. Traditionally, it is known as an effective detoxifier and strengthening agent for the body.

It is also acclaimed as one of the most tender sea vegetables. Wakame is a common ingredient in miso soup and is a tasty addition to vegetable dishes and salads.

Wakame expands up to 7 times its original volume.

Cooking Guidelines

Rinse to remove surface dirt, soak 3-5 minutes, and then cook 5-10 minutes in soups, stews, or with veggies. The same soaking time is appropriate for wakame intended for use in a salad. Longer soaking time would make it too slippery.

SPLIT PEA WAKAME SOUP

1 cup split peas
    wakame, 4-inch piece
4 cups water
2 ribs celery, cut in 1-inch
    diagonals
3 carrots, cut in 1-inch
    chunks
1 onion, chopped
1 bay leaf
1/4 tsp dried marjoram
1/2 tsp. salt or 1 Tbsp
    tamari shoyu or miso

Rinse split peas to remove any dirt. Quickly rinse wakame in water to remove excess salt. Cut wakame into 1-inch pieces. Add split peas and wakame tot he rest of the ingredients. Bring to a boil, lower flame and simmer 2 hours or until done. Add salt, tamari shoyu, or diluted miso 15 minutes before serving. Garnish with croutons, chopped parsley or scallions.

Serves 4.
(Pyramid servings: 2 Meat/Protein Group, 1 Veg. Group, 1/2 gram Fat*)

Nutrition Facts

Serving Size 1/4 recipe (363 g)
Servings Per Container 4

Amount Per Serving

Calories 200	Calories from Fat 5

	% Daily Value*
Total Fat 0.5g	**1%**
Sodium 75mg	**3%**
Total Carbohydrate 36g	**12%**
Dietary Fiber 15g	**58%**
Sugars 8g	
Protein 13g	

Vitamin A 310%	•	Vitamin C 10%
Calcium 6%	•	Iron 15%

Not a significant source of Saturated Fat and Cholesterol.

* Percent Daily Values are based on a 2,000 calorie diet.

FRUIT GROUP

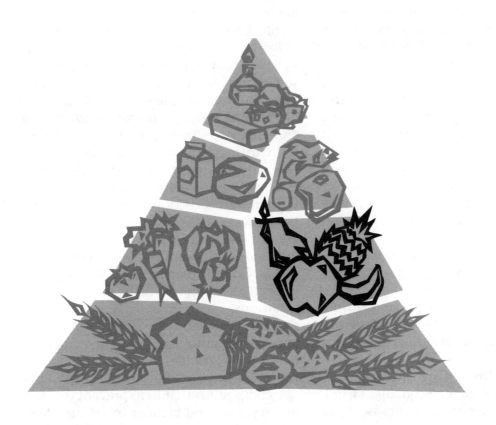

Fresh and Processed Fruit

NUTRITION

All fruits contain some of the nutrients for which they, as a class, are most noted: beta-carotene, vitamin C, and potassium, but some fruits offer significantly more than others.

Fruits that supply high amounts of beta-carotene and vitamin C help neutralize the free radicals that damage cells and contribute to cancer. Fruits high in beta-carotene can be distinguished by their deep yellow or green coloring: apricots, peaches, avocados, mangos, papaya, cantaloupe, and watermelon. Citrus fruits score high in vitamin C content, but so do papaya, cantaloupe, strawberries, mangoes, watermelon, kiwis, pomegranates, raspberries, and blackberries.

Fruits particularly high in potassium, the mineral that helps protect against strokes and muscle weakness, include cantaloupe, watermelon, bananas, apricots, oranges, peaches, and apples.

An important B vitamin not usually linked with fruits, folic acid, is found in both citrus, especially oranges and orange juice, and avocados. A moderate amount of folic acid, 400 mcg. per day, has been shown to help prevent neural tubal defects in newborn infants.

Fruit contains both soluble and insoluble fiber. The high fiber content of whole fruits helps balance their naturally occurring simple sugars: glucose, fructose, and sucrose which otherwise could be absorbed much too quickly, giving the pancreas a workout to stabilize blood sugar levels. The insoluble fiber found in berries and the skins of fruits helps increase transit time through the colon.

Pectin, most familiar for its role in gelling jams, is a soluble fiber especially rich in apples, the white layer of citrus rinds, and in blackberries. Like its action in jams and jellies, pectin forms a gel in our digestive systems, slowing down the absorption of sugars into the bloodstream, thus stabilizing blood sugar levels. It also helps lower blood cholesterol by binding with fats and cholesterol to eliminate them from the body.

Cutting, cooking, and other types of food processing can dramatically deplete water-soluble vitamins in fruit. A sure sign that vitamin C is slowly being destroyed is the dark color that accompanies fruits that are bruised, peeled, cooked, or cut and left exposed to air. Canning also destroys vitamin C. On the other hand, beta-carotene and potassium are more stable nutrients in all situations.

Fruit also contains several compounds beyond vitamins, minerals, and fiber that help keep us healthy. For instance, blueberries and cranberries both contain antibiotic-like compounds that help prevent recurring urinary tract and bladder infections. Many other fruits also contain antibacterial and antiviral agents. All in all, considering fruit's package deal of vitamins and minerals plus fiber, you've got as near perfect a food to satisfy sweet cravings as could possibly be imagined. Even so, fruits still need to be eaten in moderation, especially tropical fruits, which tend to be high in sucrose.

How Much Do We Need?

The Food Guide Pyramid suggests 2-4 servings of fruit each day. A serving of fruit consists of a medium-sized piece of whole fruit (such as an apple, pear, banana, or orange), 1/2 cup of freshly chopped, cooked, or natural juice-sweetened canned fruit (including applesauce and fruit cooked within desserts) and 3/4 cup of fruit juice (more on this later). Fruit products that don't count as a serving are jelly, fruits canned or frozen in heavy syrup, fruit drinks, fruit sodas, and the fruit juice sweetener used in some commercially made cookies and cereals.

Pesticides and Preservatives

Except for the added sugar found in several cooked fruit products, the only substances of concern you'll generally find in fruit are pesticides and post-harvest waxes that are applied to some fruits.

Because fruits are often eaten in their raw state, you should try to buy organically grown fruits as much as possible to decrease your odds of ingesting pesticide residues. Despite government claims to the contrary, not all pesticides and herbicides are checked in residue testing. Tolerance levels rarely reflect the differences in body size or the maturity or strength of immune systems. (For more information, see Pesticides in the Additives and Alternatives chapter.)

Many foreign countries do not have pesticide laws as strict as even those in the United States and may apply pesticides not allowed for use in our own country. Therefore, avoid most imported fresh fruits, limiting your fruit purchases to domestically-grown produce or from countries such as Canada and New Zealand whose pesticide policies are relatively stringent.

By law, grocery stores are supposed to label fruits and other produce that have been waxed. Vegetable wax or food-grade shellacs may be applied to fruits to seal in moisture and extend shelf life. At the same time, it seals in any agricultural chemicals which may have been used on fruits. Neither the pesticide nor the waxes can effectively be removed with washing. If you have no other choice but to buy waxed fruit, peel it before eating.

Fortunately, as of 1986, you don't have to worry about sulfites being applied to freshly cut fruit you purchase in a store or consume at a restaurant to prevent the browning of oxidized fruit. A small but significant number of people in the United States are sensitive to sulfiting agents, exhibiting symptoms ranging from shortness of breath to death. (More on sulfites in Dried Fruit.) Ascorbic acid preparations or lemon juice have been shown to be excellent alternatives to sulfites.

BUYING AND STORING

Besides buying organically grown, unwaxed fruit as much as possible, you should also make it a habit to purchase fruits in season. Not only do they taste better, they're usually much less expensive. Apples held in modified-atmosphere cold storage throughout the spring and summer months until the fall crop is harvested lack the flavor and crispness of a truly fresh apple.

Fruit at its peak of flavor and freshness has a light, sweet aroma. Unless you have the opportunity to shop for groceries on a daily basis, pick fruits that represent differ-

BAKED STUFFED FRUIT

6 pieces of your favorite fruit in season (apples, peaches, nectarines, or pears)
1/2 cup raisins
1/2 cup walnuts or pecans
1/2 tsp. vanilla
dash of cinnamon and sea salt (optional)
fruit juice (apple or whatever seems appropriate)

Preheat oven to 375° F. Prepare the fruit: If using apples, core and peel a 1" strip around the center of the apple. If using peaches or nectarines, cut in half and remove the pit. If using pears, cut in half lengthwise and remove the seeds.

Place fruit in a baking dish. Combine raisins, nuts, vanilla, and cinnamon in a blender or food processor with just enough fruit juice to facilitate blending to a coarse texture. Stuff mixture in the center of the apple or in the pit/seed area of the other fruit.

Pour apple juice into the baking dish to a depth of 1/2". Cover with foil and bake at 375° F. for 30 minutes or until just tender.

Nutrition Facts

Serving Size 1 stuffed pear (80 g)
Servings Per Container 6

Amount Per Serving	
Calories 140	Calories from Fat 60

	% Daily Value*
Total Fat 6g	10%
Saturated Fat 0.5g	3%
Sodium 50mg	2%
Total Carbohydrate 21g	7%
Dietary Fiber 2g	8%
Sugars 17g	
Protein 2g	

Vitamin C 4%	•	Calcium 2%
Iron 4%		

Not a significant source of Cholesterol and Vitamin A.
* Percent Daily Values are based on a 2,000 calorie diet.

Serve plain or with a dollop of yogurt or other favorite topping.

Serves 6.
(Pyramid Servings: 1 1/4 Fruit Group, 6 grams Fat)

---

ent stages of ripeness to avoid being stuck with an overabundance of fruit that needs to be eaten within a day or two.

You can help unripe fruit come into fullness more quickly by taking advantage of the natural ethylene gas that is released while ripening. Just place bananas, peaches, plums, nectarines, and apricots that need ripening in a loosely closed paper sack or a ripening bowl made expressly for that purpose. Within a day or two, the fruit's starch will convert to sweeter, more simple sugars. Once

refrigerated, the ripening process slows considerably.

By the way, once ripe, bananas can also be stored in the refrigerator. Their skin will turn black, but at least for a couple days, its flesh will retain the flavor and texture of a banana at its best.

Some fruits cannot be ripened at home and are sold only in their ripe state, such as apples, grapes, berries, pomegranates, and citrus fruits. While apples and citrus can be kept unrefrigerated at cool room tempera-

FROZEN BANANA CUISINE

Bananas take on a whole new persona when frozen. Besides being sweet, their texture becomes thick and creamy, making them a good, dairy-free alternative to ice cream or an exceptional thickening agent for fruit smoothies, the low-fat answer to shakes and malts.

Just peel some bananas, seal them in a plastic container or bag, and place them in the freezer until hard. Frozen banana pops can be made by first inserting an ice cream stick in the banana and, if desired, rolling it in chopped nuts. Place pops on foil and freeze until hard.

For frozen banana cream, process frozen banana chunks in a food processor or blender until smooth. Eat immediately or you'll end up with banana soup.

Use the following recipe as a basis from which to create your own fruit smoothies.

FRUIT SMOOTHIE

1 cup juice, yogurt, lowfat milk, nut milk, or yogurt
1 frozen banana
1/4 cup fresh fruit (strawberries, blueberries, peaches, etc.)

optional ingredients:
1 Tbsp. nuts or nut butter, 1/8 tsp. almond or vanilla extract, 1/2 cup yogurt (if using juice as the base)

Blend all ingredients in a blender until smooth. Serve immediately.

Serves 1.
(Pyramid serving: 3 Fruit Group, 1 gram Fat)

Nutrition Facts

Serving Size approx. 1 3/4 cup (398 g)
Servings Per Container 1

Amount Per Serving	
Calories 230	Calories from Fat 10

	% Daily Value*
Total Fat 1g	1%
Sodium 10mg	0%
Total Carbohydrate 58g	19%
Dietary Fiber 4g	15%
Sugars 51g	
Protein 2g	

Vitamin A 2%	•	Vitamin C 60%
Calcium 2%	•	Iron 8%

Not a significant source of Saturated Fat and Cholesterol.
* Percent Daily Values are based on a 2,000 calorie diet.

tures for a short period of time, they will last much longer if refrigerated after purchase. Grapes and berries should remain refrigerated at all times.

Cooking and Preparation

Raw fruits are excellent choices for snacks. If you prefer to serve them cut, process just before eating for best flavor and appearance. A sprinkling of lemon juice will help prevent the brown discoloration that accompanies oxidation of fruit.

For variety, fruits can also be simmered, steamed, baked, sautéed, or broiled. Smooth or chunky fruit sauces or stewed fruits are terrific served alone, sprinkled with a few nuts, or served over pancakes, waffles, or french toast. With the exception of very sour fruits, no additional sweetener is needed when cooking with fruits.

Fruit pies, cobblers, and crisps are familiar treats that highlight fruits, but for one of the best ways to enjoy fruit at its simple best, be sure to try apples, pears, peaches, and nectarines stuffed with nuts and dried fruits and baked in just a small amount of juice.

Exploring Your Options

In years past, it used to be that you'd be presented limited options when asking for a piece of fruit. Now, however, fruits from around the world are available in most grocery stores, joined also by new hybrids specially bred for flavor, transport, appearance, and, in some cases, lack of seeds.

Even old standbys like apples, bananas, and pears come in several varieties. Each time you shop, be sure to try a different kind. Stretch your horizons even more and experiment with the following "exotic" fruits.

ASIAN PEARS

Facts and Features

Also known as apple pears, this fruit has the juicy, sweet flavor of a pear and the crispness of an apple. Not a hybrid, this fruit was brought to the United States by Chinese prospectors during the California Gold Rush.

Eating/Cooking Guidelines

Since Asian pears are picked ripe, they are ready to eat as soon as purchased. Unlike other fruits, they store well for months when refrigerated. Their refreshing flavor and texture are best appreciated when they are eaten out of hand or added to fruit salads.

CARAMBOLA

Facts and Features

When cut horizontally, carambola slices look like a five-pointed star, accounting for its alternate name, star fruit. Yellow when ripe, its translucent flesh can be sweet, very tart, or a combination of both.

Eating/Cooking Guidelines

The texture of carambola is slightly crisp which makes it an excellent addition to add contrast to fruit salads composed of soft fruits. It is also terrific eaten out of hand.

CHERIMOYA

Facts and Features

Its rough, notched, greenish, heart-shaped exterior may not look too inviting, but cherimoya's custard-like texture and unusual, delicious flavor more than make up for first impressions. Not surprisingly, its alternate name is custard apple.

Cherimoyas are high in vitamin C. Unfortunately, cherimoyas are also one of the most expensive fruits available, due to the fact that the female cherimoya fruit must be hand-pollinated. Because they are so fragile, cherimoyas must also be hand-picked and hand-sorted. All the more reason to savor every bite.

Eating/Cooking Guidelines

When ripe, their skin turns brownish-green and yields to light pressure. Described as a combination of strawberry, banana, and pineapple, cherimoyas can be eaten right out of their own "cup" when halved or quartered or cut into chunks and added to fruit salads. Their large black seeds should be removed before eating. Don't bother cooking cherimoya; the flavor dissipates with heat.

GUAVA

Facts and Features

Guava is a small, round fruit whose outside color ranges from green to yellow. Inside its color ranges from white to deep pink. Some guavas taste like pineapple while others have a flavor reminiscent of strawberries. They are very high in vitamin C and vitamin A.

Eating/Cooking Guidelines

Guavas are ready to eat when slightly soft. Remove seeds and eat out of the "half shell" or peel and slice. Firm guavas can also be baked. They are also used in jellies and preserves.

KIWIFRUIT

Facts and Features

Kiwifruit is a prime example of how patient marketing can turn a heretofore relatively unknown, exotic fruit into one that is now widely recognized and appreciated. Originally called the Chinese gooseberry, in the 1970s it was renamed kiwifruit in honor of the native bird in New Zealand. Inside its brown suedelike skin is a bright green flesh studded with tiny black edible seeds whose flavor is often described as similar to a combination of strawberries and melon. Kiwis are very high in vitamin C.

Eating/Cooking Guidelines

When soft, it is ready to eat, a state that can be preserved for weeks when refrigerated. To prepare, cut kiwi in half and scoop it directly out of its skin or cut into slices.

Like papaya, kiwi also contains an enzyme that breaks down proteins. Accordingly, it can be used as a meat tenderizer. However, if added to gelatin, kiwi will prevent it from setting unless the enzymes are deactivated by a brief cooking. Likewise, when added to milk products in its raw state, the food or drink should be consumed immediately.

KUMQUAT

Facts and Features

Kumquats look like miniature oranges. Unlike oranges, however, both the skin and flesh are eaten since the sweet skin provides a delicious contrast to the pulp's tart flavor. Its seeds should be removed before eating.

Eating/Cooking Guidelines

Thinly slice and add to fruit salads or take advantage of its high pectin content and use to make preserves and marmalade.

Kumquats are high in vitamins A and C.

LYCHEE

Facts and Features

A fruit the size of ping-pong balls, under the bright red, rough-skinned shell of a lychee is a creamy white pulp with a jelly-like texture and flavor similar to grapes but more aromatic. In the middle is a large seed, the reason you may hear lychee sometimes referred to as a lychee nut.

Eating/Cooking Guidelines

To eat, peel off the shell, starting at the stem end and remove the seed. Eat straight from the shell or slice and add to fruit salads. Lychees are high in vitamin C.

MANGO

Facts and Features

Surprising as it may seem, mangoes are considered the most popular fruit throughout the world, widely used in areas such as India, South Africa, Brazil, Mexico, and other parts of Central America. A kidney-shaped fruit with its skin color ranging yellow to green to red, mango's flesh is golden-orange and very sweet and juicy when ripe. In the middle is a long oval-shaped inedible seed. Mangoes are very high in vitamins A and C.

Eating/Cooking Guidelines

Green, immature mangoes are used for chutneys, relishes, and pickles. Ripe mangoes can be peeled and eaten like a banana or cut into chunks for fruit salads. Some recipes include mango slices in chicken, beef, and shrimp stir-frys.

PAPAYA

Facts and Features

Originating from Central America, papaya is a large, elongated fruit with a distinctive aroma and taste. When its skin changes from green to yellow, it is ready to eat. Its flesh is golden-yellow or orange with round, black seeds in the center.

In addition to its sweet, mellow taste, papaya contains a natural enzyme, papain, which aids digestion and tenderizes meat. LIke kiwi, papaya added to gelatin will prevent it from setting. Papayas are also very high in vitamins A and C.

Eating/Cooking Guidelines

To prepare for serving, slice papaya lengthwise and scoop out the fruit, separating it from the skin. Fresh lemon or lime juice enhances its flavor. Use papaya in fruit salads, purée in smoothies, or cook it with meat or fish as is the custom in Caribbean cuisine. The seeds have a peppery taste and texture that work well as an addition to salad dressings and marinades.

PASSION FRUIT

Facts and Features

Passion fruit is egg-shaped and with a thick-skinned, purplish-red exterior. Inside, its orange-colored, juicy, seedy pulp has a sweet yet tart flavor and an alluring jasmine/honey-like aroma.

Passion fruit was named as such by early Christian missionaries stationed in South America who thought the leaves of the plant resembled the crown of thorns and nails of Jesus Christ's crucifixion. Alternative names for the fruit are granadilla or purple granadilla. It is high in vitamin A.

Eating/Cooking Guidelines

Passion Fruit is ready to eat when it becomes very wrinkled and creased. If it gets cracked or squishy, you've waited too long. Unlike many other fruits, passion fruit cannot be eaten from out of hand. Rather, the pulp is typically scooped out and used as a sauce or flavoring, either as is or lightly sweetened, over fruit salads, cakes, or frozen desserts. Passion fruit is also processed into juice. Its small black seeds are edible but, if desired, they can be strained out before using the rest of the pulp.

PERSIMMON

Facts and Features

Although there is a native American variety of persimmon, commercially two varieties originating from the Orient, Hachiya and Fuyu, are most often available.

The Hachiya persimmon has a bright orange color and is slightly pointed in shape. The Fuyu is also bright orange but flatter in shape, much like a tomato. Both have a very sweet flavor with spicy undertones. They are also very high in vitamins C and A.

Eating/Cooking Guidelines

Only eat persimmons when they are very soft, like jelly in a bag. They can be consumed raw, including the skin (use a bowl to catch the juicy pulp), or puréed for use in pies, cakes, and custards.

PLANTAINS

Facts and Features

Although longer and more pointed at its ends, there is no mistaking that plantains are a member of the banana family. However, unlike bananas, plantains are never eaten raw. Instead, they are always cooked and served as a starchy vegetable. A fair source of vitamin C, plantains are especially rich in fiber.

Eating/Cooking Guidelines

Plantains can be used at any degree of ripeness, from green and starchy through its black, sweeter, softer stage when totally ripe. Peel and slice and then bake, sauté, broil, grill, deep-fry, or simmer as you would any other vegetable. You can also bake it whole in its peel. Preheat the oven to 350° F. and bake for 45-60 minutes or until it pierces easily with a fork. Remove the skin and season, if desired, with butter or a flavorful oil.

POMEGRANATE

Facts and Features

Inside the hard, red, leathery rind of the pomegranate are many seeds surrounded by translucent sacs bursting with red, tart, juicy pulp. Larger pomegranates are best, containing the plumpest, most juicy kernels. Nutritionally, pomegranates offer small amounts of potassium and, if the seeds are consumed, some fiber.

Eating/Cooking Guidelines

While the results are worth it in the long run, a pomegranate is a fruit you probably wouldn't want to eat on a first date, due to its inevitable spurting of juice in every direction. Try cutting one about 1/4 of its length from the top and scooping out the seeds with a spoon. The seeds inside the clusters of pulp are also edible, although some people prefer to discard them. The white membrane surrounding the clusters shouldn't be eaten since it is very bitter.

The juice can also be extracted from the pomegranate by first puréeing the pulp in a food processor or blender and then straining out the seeds.

QUINCE

Facts and Features

Although quince looks similar to an apple, it's never eaten raw, due to its acidic flavor and very hard texture. Instead, it is most valued for its high pectin content, making it a perfect candidate for jams, preserves, or chutneys. Larger quince are a better buy. Perfumed quince and pineapple quince are the two varieties most commonly marketed.

Eating/Cooking Guidelines

Quince are ripe when they become pale yellow in color. Besides jams and preserves, quince are also good baked, either whole or into pies and crisps, stewed, or poached, providing they are adequately sweetened.

RHUBARB

Facts and Features

A native of Siberia, rhubarb was introduced to the rest of the world during the 18th century. In the United States, it is especially popular in the Midwest where rhubarb grown in backyards and gardens is typically used to make pies. Botanically, rhubarb is actually a vegetable, but because its extremely tart flavor needs to be balanced with plenty of sweetener, it is often characterized as a fruit.

Eating/Cooking Guidelines

Only the stalks of the rhubarb plant should be eaten. In addition to pies, rhubarb can be cooked into sauces, jams, and crisps. Most often it is combined with other fruits such as apples and strawberries.

TAMARIND

Facts and Features

Tamarinds are fuzzy, brown-colored pods, ranging in length from 2 to 8 inches, that grow on a tropical evergreen tree. Within the pods are seeds that are surrounded by a sticky pulp that has an apricot/date-like flavor. Although the pulp can be eaten raw, it is usually used in marinades or to flavor chutneys and curries. When sweetened and diluted with water, it makes a refreshing drink.

Eating/Cooking Guidelines

Tamarind can be used both when the pods are green or when brown and brittle. Crack and peel the pods to access the pulp. To make tamarind concentrate, soak the pulp from 6 tamarind pods in 1 cup hot water for 2 hours. Then strain the pulp, squeezing out the juice. Use the concentrate to flavor grains, beans, and vegetables or dilute and sweeten for a beverage.

UGLI FRUIT

Facts and Features

Originated in Jamaica as a cross between a grapefruit and a tangerine. Although its thick, bumpy, mottled greenish-yellow colored skin and odd shape are not very attractive, the fruit itself is very juicy and delicious, with a sweet, orange-like flavor.

Eating/Cooking Guidelines

Peel ugli fruit and eat out of hand or add sections to fruit salads.

WHITE SAPOTE

Facts and Features

White sapote, also known as "Mexican custard apple," is a native fruit of Central

PEAK SEASONS FOR FRUIT

JANUARY/FEBRUARY

avocado
bananas
bosc pear
comice pear
d'anjou pear
grapefruit
kumquats
kiwi

mandarins
navel oranges
papayas
persimmons
tangerines
temple oranges
valencia oranges
ugli fruit

MARCH, APRIL, MAY

avocado
bananas
berries
blood oranges
d'anjou pear
loquats

papayas
pears
pineapple
plums
strawberries
watermelon

JUNE, JULY, AUGUST

apricots
avocado
bananas
bartlett pear
blackberries
blueberries
casaba melons
cantaloupe
crenshaw melons
cherries
figs
grapes

honeydew melons
kiwis
lemons
limes
lychee
mangoes
nectarines
peaches
plums
pineapple
raspberries
watermelons

SEPTEMBER, OCTOBER, NOVEMBER, DECEMBER

apples
avocado
bananas
bartlett pear
bosc pear
casaba melons
coconuts
comice pear
cranberries
d'anjou pear
dates
figs
grapefruit
grapes

honeydew melons
kiwis
kumquats
mandarins
navel oranges
pears
persimmons
plums
pomegranate
prickly pears
quince
Santa Claus melons (Dec.)
temple oranges
ugli fruit

America that looks like a green apple without any indentation on the bottom. When ripe, it becomes soft and creamy-textured with a unique banana/papaya flavor.

Eating/Cooking Guidelines

Sapotes can be eaten out of hand as you would a peach. No peeling is necessary. They can also be eaten like a persimmon, spooning the pulp from its skin. Add to fruit salads or smoothies for a special treat.

Dried Fruits

ANOTHER WAY to enjoy fruit is in its dried, dehydrated state. Grapes become raisins or currants, some plums become prunes, and other fruits reveal sides of themselves that are merely hinted at when consumed fresh.

NUTRITION

Besides concentrating their flavors, removing the water from fresh fruit also concentrates nutrients, making dried fruits very high in potassium, iron, and, in dried apricots, peaches, prunes, and cherries, beta-carotene.

On the other hand, the dehydration process destroys any vitamin C contained in the fruit. It also concentrates the fruit's sugar content to almost 70% by weight, similar to the amount of sugar found in many candies. And, because it is so sticky, dried fruit can easily adhere to teeth, making it important to thoroughly brush your teeth as soon as possible after eating any dried fruits.

Buy organically grown dried fruit whenever possible.

Serving Sizes

Dried fruit can be considered an option to help fulfill the Food Guide Pyramid's recommendation of 2-4 servings per day. A serving size of dried fruit is 40 grams or about 1 1/2 oz. When translated to common household measures, the approximate amounts for various dried fruits are as follows:

apples: about 1/2 cup loosely packed
apricots: 10 halves
dates: 5 small whole or about 1/4 cup
    chopped
figs: 2 figs
peaches: 3 halves
pears: 2 halves
prunes: 5 small
raisins: 1/4 cup

HOW PROCESSED

Fruits are dried in the sun or mechanically dehydrated at about 125° F. for 24 hours. Even though dried fruits are very sweet, some are sprayed with a honey/water solution to soften, balance out acidity, and prevent the dried fruit from turning brown.

Sulfites

Another method to retain moisture and bright colors is to spray the fruit with sulfiting agents (sulfur dioxide, sodium sulfite, sodium and potassium bisulfite, or sodium and potassium metabisulfite. An additive used for hundreds of years to preserve all types of foods, it is also known to cause mild to serious reactions in sensitive individuals ranging from itching, gastrointestinal distress, asthma, difficulty in breathing, wheezing, hives, and possibly death.

It is estimated that 1 million Americans are sensitive to sulfiting agents, with about 100,000, primarily asthmatics, exhibiting the most severe reactions. In 1986, the FDA banned the use of sulfites on fresh fruits and vegetables but continued to allow their use in dried fruits, wines, and pickled products. Foods that contain 10 parts per million (ppm) or more of sulfites must be labeled as such. The amount set as the label declaration level was chosen not because amounts below 10 ppm won't cause harm. Rather, it's because that is the lowest amount at which sulfites can readily be measured.

Fortunately, sulfite-free dried fruits are available. Although they may have a more leathery texture and less vibrant coloring, the flavor of fruits dried without sulfites can't be beat.

COOKING AND STORING

Dried fruits are most commonly consumed in their natural state, alone or mixed with nuts in a trail mix. However, you may find you like them even better when lightly steamed for a couple minutes or soaked in a small amount of water for a few hours or overnight. Not only does it soften the fruit, plumping it up to almost its original size, the soaking water can be used as a sweet beverage or cooking liquid. Soaking the fruit also reduces the tendency to overeat the concentrated sugars in the dried fruit.

Due to the preservative action derived from their high sugar content, refrigeration of dried fruits is not necessary, but they will keep much longer if refrigerated. Store in airtight jars or plastic containers to prevent excess moisture and insect infestation. Occasionally the natural sugars in the fruit will solidify, forming harmless crystals on the surface of prunes and figs.

Exploring Your Options

The primary simple sugar found in each dried fruit is listed below. Use it as a guide to understand why some dried fruits seem to affect blood sugar levels more than others. Glucose absorbs most quickly, followed by sucrose. Fructose requires more time for your body to convert fructose to glucose, the form of sugar your cells require for energy.

Since dried fruit is so concentrated in sugars, remember to eat only moderate amounts of dried fruit at a time.

APPLES

Facts and Features

Dried apples are generally prepared from slices of cored, often peeled, Golden Delicious, Rome, or Gravenstein apples. Early Americans highly valued dried apples for their sweet flavor as well as the variety they offered their diet.

They are also very high in fiber, particularly pectin.

Fructose is the predominant natural simple sugar found in dried apples.

If the dried apples are creamy white in color and very pliable, it's a good bet they have been treated with sulfur dioxide. Untreated apples are tan to slightly brown and leathery.

Cooking Guidelines

Delicious out of hand and in trail mixes, dried apples are terrific cooked in hot cereals with a dash of cinnamon or vanilla extract. They tend to keep their shape and texture much better than fresh apples in cooked dishes. Be sure to rehydrate first before substituting them directly for fresh apples in any recipe.

APRICOTS

Facts and Features

Dried apricots are processed from pitted, halved fresh apricots. Fructose is the predominant natural simple sugar. Dried apricots are very high in beta-carotene.

If the dried apricots are bright orange in color and very moist, they're most likely treated with sulfur dioxide. Untreated apricots have a darker, rusty color and may be moist to very hard.

Cooking Guidelines

Some unsulfured dried apricots are softer than others. Eat the soft varieties out of hand or chop and use like raisins on top of cereal or in cookies.

For best results, cook or soak harder varieties. Fruit compotes based on stewed dried apricots are especially good. Raisins, coriander, nutmeg, and almonds complement the sweet, slightly tart flavor of dried apricots.

BANANAS

Facts and Features

Dried bananas can be processed into chips from sliced bananas or into sticky 6-inch strips dried from the whole.

Extremely sweet, the predominant sugar in dried banana is sucrose. Dried bananas are also very high in potassium.

Avoid banana chips that are deep fried and/or processed with added sugar. Although they may be more dry and brittle without the extra ingredients, you'll have a much more healthy snack.

Banana chips that are treated with sulfur dioxide are very light in color. Untreated chips and strips will range in color from medium to dark brown.

Cooking Guidelines

Both banana chips and dried whole bananas are usually eaten out of hand, but both can be added to hot cereals during cooking.

Another delicious variation is to "soak" a couple banana chips or pieces of chopped dried banana overnight in milk or yogurt. Process in a blender the next morning until smooth and enjoy.

CHERRIES

Facts and Features

Although not as widely known as other dried fruits, dried cherries are very sweet, maroon-colored nuggets made from either sweet or sour cherries. Unless you are endowed with a superhuman capacity for patience, look for dried cherries that are already pitted.

Dried sour cherries are often processed from Montmorency cherries that are first brined in a juice or sugar solution before drying to provide a more balanced flavor. Dried sweet cherries made from Bing or Lambert cherries need no further sweetening.

Dried cherries are also good sources of iron, fiber, and potassium.

Cooking Guidelines

Pitted dried cherries can be eaten out of hand, added to trail mixes, or soaked for a more fresh-fruit consistency. Try them also in baked goods instead of raisins.

CRANBERRIES

Facts and Features

Dried cranberries are always sold sweetened to balance the fruit's natural tartness, a flavor that is even more pronounced when dried. Typically white sugar and concentrated cranberry juice are used as sweetening agents. Accordingly, although its nutritional attributes look very similar to those of raisins, the simple sugars provided by dried cranberries are primarily from added sugars rather than naturally occurring as found in raisins.

To prevent the cranberries from sticking together, they are also often sprayed with partially hydrogenated oil.

Cooking Guidelines

Dried cranberries add color and great taste to cereals, trail mixes, sauces, and in baked goods such as muffins and quickbreads. An added bonus is that dried cranberries, unlike their fresh or frozen counterparts, do not bleed into the dough.

CURRANTS

Facts and Features

Currants are dried Zantes grapes, unrelated to the fresh berries found growing on wild or cultivated shrubs. Like raisins, currants are high in iron.

Currants are usually not treated with sulfites.

Cooking Guidelines

The tiny size of currants makes them especially good in fruit salads and in baked goods.

DATES

Facts and Features

Dates can trace their roots back to the Middle East in 2500 B.C. Grown on the date palm tree, they are sold both fresh and dried, classified according to their degree of softness and moisture contained in the fresh fruit.

Soft dates include the large and luscious Medjool date (considered by many to be the ultimate choice) and Khadrawy.

Deglet Noor, Halaway, and Zahidi are semidry. Bread dates are quite dry.

Dates are extremely sweet, with sucrose as the predominant natural simple sugar. Treat them like candy, eating them judiciously in small amounts. However, unlike candy, they also provide fiber, potassium and other nutrients.

Date pieces are made from dates whose whole appearance may not be cosmetically perfect. They are often dusted with oat flour to prevent them from forming into an unmanageable sticky clump. To prevent mold, some dates may be pasteurized. Refrigerate, tightly covered, to maintain the best flavor and to deter insects.

Cooking Guidelines

Soft dates are delicious stuffed with whole almonds or almond butter, sesame tahini, walnuts, or even peanut butter. All dates are perfect additions to fruit salads and smoothies.

Chopped dates or date pieces are excellent in cookies, muffins, and quick breads. When added to hot cereals during cooking, they impart a sweetness similar to brown sugar.

FIGS

Facts and Features

Like dates, figs have been used as a sweetener since ancient times. The drying process starts on the tree and is then followed by sun or mechanical drying. Most dried figs are further processed for use in commercially-made cookies.

There are two varieties of figs that are commonly found dried. The Black Mission fig has a purple/black skin and moist, richly flavored, golden red flesh. Grown in California, this fig was brought to the state in 1769 by Franciscan friars who planted the tree at their mission—hence, its name.

Calimyrna figs are light tan in color and very succulent. This fig variety is a descendent of the Turkish Smyrnan fig. After being introduced in California in 1880, this version was named Calimyrna to honor both its ancestry and its new roots.

Both the Black Mission and Calimyrna figs are very sweet, with glucose edging out its fructose content. They also contain a remarkable amount of fiber and calcium.

Check labels to make sure they are free of any sulfites.

Cooking Guidelines

Figs are delicious eaten plain, stuffed with nuts or nut butters, or served in fruit salads with yogurt.

The more mildly flavored Calimyrna figs are the variety most used in quick breads. Both figs make good additions to hot cereals.

MANGOES

Facts and Features

Dried mangoes are generally made by dipping the fruit in a sugar solution or its own juices. After drying, the mango strips are very sticky and have a glistening appearance. Occasionally you may find unsweetened dried mangoes that look like chopped, brittle pieces.

Look at labels carefully to avoid sulfur dioxides. Choose dried mango naturally sweetened in its own juices over added sugar varieties as they are already high in naturally-occurring sucrose. Dried mangoes also provide a good source of beta-carotene.

Cooking Guidelines

Dried mangos are usually eaten out of hand. They also make a nice addition to hot cereals.

PAPAYA

Facts and Features

Like mangoes, dried papaya may be prepared by dipping it in a sugar or honey solution. Occasionally you may find unsweetened papaya that is more brittle than the soft texture of sweetened varieties. They also provide a good source of beta-carotene.

Cooking Guidelines

Dried papaya is usually eaten out of hand or added to trail mixes. Experiment with cooking them in hot cereals.

PEACHES

Facts and Features

Dried peaches are the "sleeper" of the dried fruit industry, waiting for people to finally wake up and realize the amazing flavor it has to offer. Made from pitted halves, they are quite chewy in their dried state but come to full flavor when soaked or steamed.

The predominant natural simple sugar found in peaches is sucrose. They are also high in iron, potassium, and beta-carotene.

Avoid soft, brightly-colored dried peaches treated with sulfur dioxide.

Cooking Guidelines

Chop and add to trail mixes. Soak overnight in water or steam dried peaches for fruit salads or compotes. Almonds and walnuts are especially good accompaniments.

They are also great chopped and cooked in hot cereal.

PEARS

Facts and Features

Dried pears are very sweet and delicious. Made from cored halves or quarters of Bartlett pears, they have a soft, chewy texture when dried. They are also high in fiber and iron.

Check labels to avoid sulfur dioxide.

Cooking Guidelines

Dried pears are especially good eaten out of hand or in trail mixes. Experiment with adding chopped dried pears to baked goods and hot cereals.

PINEAPPLES

Facts and Features

Despite the fact that dried pineapple is incredibly sweet, it is usually sold presweetened since untreated pineapple tends to be sour. Available sugar-sweetened and/or dipped in honey, most preferable is the "unsweetened" version that is soaked in its own juice concentrate to increase sweetness and improve flavor.

The predominant natural sugar in dried pineapple is sucrose.

Cooking Guidelines

Dried pineapple is most often eaten like candy or added to fruit and nut trail mixes. It can, however, be soaked in water overnight to semi-reconstitute it approaching its origi-nal sweetness and texture. Some of the sweetness will transfer to the soaking water, making the pineapple more reasonably sweet.

PRUNES

Facts and Features

Prunes are the dehydrated versions of certain types of plums, a fact that is reflected in its name, the French word for plums.

California is the world's largest producer of plums since getting its start from a Frenchman who brought cuttings of the La Petite d'Agen prune plum from his native land around 1859.

Prunes are, perhaps, the most notorious of dried fruits due to their laxative effects. This effect is due to its high sorbitol content, a naturally occurring sugar that is not fully absorbed in the intestines. As the bacteria in the colon attempt to digest it, the sorbitol attracts water, stimulating elimination.

A very sweet dried fruit, prunes are also a good source of iron and potassium.

Prunes are available both with and without the pit.

Cooking Guidelines

Prunes are generally eaten out of hand or stewed for a breakfast fruit.

They are also finding new popularity as a fat substitute to replace butter, margarine, and oil in baked goods. To make 1 cup prune purée, combine 11/3 cup (or 8 oz.) of pitted prunes with 6 tablespoons of water in a food processor. Pulse on and off until prunes are finely chopped. Use the purée to replace half or more of the fat normally required in your favorite recipes. Some experiments will work very well; others may need further refinements to get the right proportion of the prune purée to fat.

CARBO COOKIES

1/2 cup raisins
3/4 cup apple juice
1/4 cup canola oil
1 1/2 cups rolled oats
1/2 cup almonds
1 cup + 2 Tbsp. whole
    wheat pastry flour
1/4 tsp. each cinnamon,
    baking soda, salt
1 1/2 tsp. vanilla extract
1/8 tsp. almond extract
1 egg, slightly beaten

Preheat oven to 350° F. Chop raisins and combine with juice in a small saucepan. Cover, bring to a boil, and simmer 5 minutes to soften raisins. Add oil and remove pan from heat to cool. In a blender or food processor, grind oatmeal and nuts to a coarse flour. Combine with remaining dry ingredients. In a separate bowl, add flavorings and egg to raisin mixture. Combine with dry mixture and form into walnut-sized balls. Flatten into 2 inch diameter cookies and place on an oiled cookie sheet. Bake for 15 minutes or until cookies are golden brown underneath.

Makes 24.

Nutrition Facts

Serving Size 1 cookie (28 g)
Servings Per Container 24

Amount Per Serving

Calories 90   Calories from Fat 40

	% Daily Value*
Total Fat 4.5g	7%
Cholesterol 10mg	3%
Sodium 40mg	2%
Total Carbohydrate 11g	4%
Dietary Fiber 2g	6%
Sugars 3g	
Protein 2g	

Calcium 2%	•	Iron 4%

Not a significant source of Saturated Fat, Vitamin A and Vitamin C.

* Percent Daily Values are based on a 2,000 calorie diet.

(Pyramid servings: 1/2 Bread/Grain Group, 1/2 Fruit Group, 4 1/2 grams Fat)

Prune purées for use as fat substitutes are also likely to be found ready-made in the sweetener or baking section of your grocery store.

RAISINS

Facts and Features

The name "raisin" is French for grape, a big clue that raisins are essentially dried grapes.

Thompson and monukka raisins are the most common varieties. Seedless Thompsons are the type most people recognize as raisins. Monukkas are a larger, more plump raisin whose slightly crunchy texture is the result of its tiny, edible seeds.

Golden raisins are not always, but most often, treated with sulfur dioxide. Check your labels.

Raisins are a good source of iron, potassium, and fiber.

Cooking Guidelines

Although raisins are most often consumed out of hand or in trail mixes, they are also delicious cooked in hot cereals, tossed in salads, and baked into cookies, cakes, muffins, and quick breads.

Fruit Juices

Fruit juices offer several of the same nutrients that are present in both whole and dried fruits.

NUTRITION

Like the other sources of fruit, juices are very high in potassium. Depending on the particular type of fruit used to make the juice, its processing method, and the length of time from its initial exposure to air, juices can be good sources of vitamins A and C as well.

However, a major nutritional drawback to juice is that it contains very little of the fruit's original fiber. As mentioned previously, the types of fiber found in fruit are especially known to help, both directly and indirectly, reduce the risk of cancer and heart disease.

Fiber also helps slow down the absorption of simple sugars in foods. Therefore, without the fiber, the sugars in fruit juice mean that the sugars will, instead, be absorbed very quickly, giving your pancreas a real workout to try to keep your blood glucose levels in balance.

So, even though fruit juice provides important nutrients, it is best consumed in moderation. The Food Guide Pyramid suggests a serving size of 3/4 cup (6 oz.). Another option is to dilute the juice with plain or sparkling water. Not only may you find it tastes almost as good, it also lessens sugar's effect on your body.

Moderate consumption of fruit juice is especially important for children. Excessive intake of fruit juice has been associated with the inability for children to grow and develop normally. Because a large quantity of juice is very filling, it dampens the appetite for higher-calorie, more nutritious foods.

Too much prune juice (and even apple) can also be the cause of chronic diarrhea in children, due to the presence of sorbitol, a natural sugar that is poorly absorbed in the digestive tract. In deference to the common practice of giving fruit juices to infants, many nutritional experts suggest that juices should not be given to children under the age of 6 months or until they are old enough to drink it from a cup. Drinking juice from a bottle is particularly bad since it bathes the mouth in sugars that can create a breeding ground for cavity-causing bacteria.

For best nutrition, always choose juice made from organically grown fruit. Because the juicing process concentrates everything in the juice, including any pesticide residues, organically produced juice prevents exposure to pesticides and toxic chemicals that may be used to grow the fruit. Buying organic is not only a vote affirming your own health, but also a vote in honor of the health of our planet.

Types of Juice and Their Effect on Nutrition

The most nutritious juices are **freshly extracted juices**, the type of juice served at juice bars or extracted from home juicers. They contain the highest amounts of water-soluble vitamins, especially vitamin C, plus minerals inherently found within the fruit.

The next most nutritious type of juice is **fresh frozen juice**. First extracted, they are then quickly frozen in bottles or cartons without prior pasteurization. Fresh frozen juice is stable until initially defrosted in the refrigerator.

Chilled juices are extracted and then packaged in cartons or plastic containers. A juice product generally sold self-service from the produce or deli departments of a store, chilled juices may or may not be pasteurized.

Pasteurized juices have a long shelf life due to the heat's destruction of microbes and bacteria that can cause juices to ferment and spoil. Water-soluble nutrients such as vitamin C decrease slightly in the process. Minerals and beta-carotene are not affected.

Frozen concentrates are the frozen solids of pasteurized juices whose water content has been evaporated. While in the freezer, the nutrients in concentrates remain stable, including vitamin C. Once mixed with water, they begin to lose nutrients with each passing day.

Reconstituted juice is made from pasteurized juice concentrates. They are sold in similar containers as chilled juices with the exception that they are labeled "from concentrates."

Canned or bottled juices are 100% juices that are pasteurized. While some juices are made from a single fruit, most are a blend of various reconstituted juices used to create flavor variety, a balance of sweetness with acidity, and to reduce production costs.

White grape juice and apple juice are most often chosen as bases due to their ability to blend unobtrusively with other juices without overwhelming the flavor.

Juices made from 100% juices may or may not have added sweetener. White grape juice is often added in lieu of white table sugar or honey.

Juices can appear cloudy or clear depending on the degree of filtering. All juices are lightly filtered to remove stems and leaves. Juices that are not further filtered are labeled as "unfiltered." These juices retain more of the pulp, pectin, and nutrients than would be present in clear, more filtered varieties.

Fruit beverages, drinks, spritzers, and cocktails contain less than 100% juice. Many are fortified with extra vitamin C and contain added sweeteners and artificial flavors. Only 100% juices should be counted as a serving of fruit.

All juices not consumed within minutes of extraction will begin to lose nutrients, particularly vitamin C, with each passing day. (Bottled pasteurized juices are stable until opened.) Because depletion of nutrients increases dramatically with exposure to air, light, and temperatures above 32° F., it is important to pour only what you need, close the container, and immediately refrigerate juices after every use.

A good gauge of the effects of time and exposure on the nutritional quality of juice can be illustrated by the levels of vitamin C that remain in orange juice following various production methods per 3/4 cup (6 oz.) serving of juice:

freshly squeezed: 93 mg. vitamin C
reconstituted frozen concentrate: 73 mg.
canned, unsweetened: 65 mg.
chilled juice: 62 mg.

COOKING WITH JUICE

Replace water or milk with juice when making hot breakfast cereals or desserts such as rice pudding, cookies, cakes, and quick breads. To take advantage of the leavening power from the combination of fruit juice with baking soda, add 1/4 teaspoon soda per 1 cup of juice used in the recipe.

Thicken juice with arrowroot or cornstarch for a sweet pancake and waffle syrup. Use juice instead of water to brew tea.

NEW JUICE LABELING LAWS

The new FDA regulations have significantly affected labeling of juices.

• Any product that purports to be a beverage containing fruit juice—either through its name, pictorial representation on the label, or its color or flavor that gives the appearance of containing fruit juice—must bear the actual percentage of juice that is contained within. This includes both carbonated and noncarbonated beverages, no matter if they are concentrated, full strength, diluted, or contain no juice whatsoever.

• The percentage of juice is calculated by the Brix levels, the minimum soluble solids content by weight for individual unsweetened juices set by the government.

For example, to be considered as 100% apple juice, the minimum soluble solids content of apple juice is 11.4% solids content and 88.6% water including trace minerals and small amounts of acid that remain after processing. If a product containing apple juice were further diluted from this minimum Brix level, it would be considered a juice beverage, cocktail, or juice drink instead of 100% juice.

• Any modified juices used in the juice cannot be calculated as part of the total percentage of juice. Also referred to as "stripped juices," a modified juice has had its color, taste, aroma, or other organoleptic proper-

BUYING A JUICER

Home juice-extraction machines remain popular even decades after they were first introduced to the American public. There are three basic types of juicers: centrifugal, centrifugal extractors, and masticating juicers.

A **centrifugal juicer** makes a clear, light, smooth juice very efficiently, creating only a small amount of pulp residue in the spinner basket. In the process, centrifugal juicers extract juice by masticating the fruit or vegetable, spinning it at high speeds in a basket, and separating the juice from the pulp.

A **centrifugal extractor** extracts juice similarly to centrifugal juicers except that the pulp is whirled over the top of the spinner basket through a pour spout into a container.

A **masticating juicer** grinds up fruits and vegetables whose juice is then extracted by being pressed through a small screen. The pulp is ejected out the front. Considering that much of the juice still remains in the pulp, masticating juicers are less efficient in extracting methods than centrifugal models. Any pulp created can be used as an addition to soups, casseroles, quick breads, cakes, and salads. If you can't use the pulp fast enough, compost it at home or collect it for a farmer.

APPLE CIDER VS. APPLE JUICE

What's the difference between apple cider and apple juice? Technically, apple cider is fermented apple juice. Any juice will begin to ferment after a couple of days with no refrigeration. In fact, until refrigeration and pasteurization became more widely spread, lightly fermented apple cider was about the only fruit beverage early settlers had available all year-round.

Now that we have access to all types of food preservation methods to prevent juices from fermenting, the only real difference is the type of apple used. Apple cider is considered tart while apple juice is sweeter.

ties processed to the extent that it no longer resembles the original juice. The term also includes juices whose nutrient profile has been diminished of any essential nutrient that is normally present in a measurable amount, to a level below the normal nutrient range for the juice. Modified juices must be listed on the ingredients panel with a short description of the exact nature of the modification.

•Multiple juices used within a product must be listed in descending order on the ingredients panel. The product's name must also indicate that more than one kind of juice has been used in the formulation. If the juice is from a concentrate, it must be labeled as such in the ingredients and, if the sole juice source, in the product's name.

•Fruit oils, essences, and pulp added in excess of the amount that would normally be present in the juice or if from a source other than the juice itself must be labeled as separate ingredients on the ingredients panel.

•A 100% juice product that contains added preservatives and sweeteners must have the fact stated on the label.

Meat, Poultry, Fish, Dry beans, eggs & Nuts Group

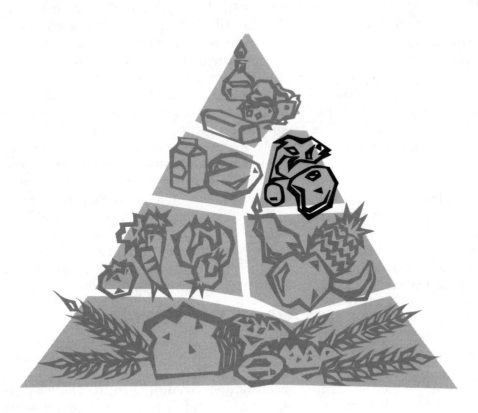

Protein

SITUATED NEAR the top of the Food Guide Pyramid on the same level as the milk group, the message is loud and clear: protein should be an adjunct to your diet, not the major component. Smaller and fewer servings are recommended with a big hint that nonanimal protein sources are just as good as meat, poultry, fish, and eggs—perhaps even better.

As illustrated by the Food Guide Pyramid, new Dietary Guidelines for Americans suggest 2-3 servings each day of foods from this group with the total amount of these servings equivalent to 5-7 ounces of cooked lean meat, poultry, or fish per day. One-half cup of cooked dried beans, 1 egg, 2 tablespoons of peanut butter, and 1/3 cup nuts each count as the equivalent of 1 ounce of meat.

This revised attitude about protein only changes the slant on its frequency and serving size, not its overall importance in our diet. Protein is made up of chains of amino acids, the building blocks of protein, made of the elements carbon, hydrogen, oxygen, nitrogen, and sometimes sulfur. It is these building blocks that the body needs from food to perform its myriad of roles in the body. Of the 22 amino acids which comprise protein, 8 must be supplied by the diet (9 for infants) while the others can be manufactured by the body. These 8 "essential amino acids" include isoleucine, leucine, lysine, methionine, phenylalanine, threonine, tryptophan, and valine.

Protein helps replace and form new tissue, transports nutrients in and out of cells, regulates the balance of water, acids, and bases, transports oxygen and nutrients in the blood, and helps form hormones and enzymes which perform the chemical reactions needed to keep your body running as it should. All in all, protein comprises about 3/4 of the weight in most human tissues.

But there's a limit; too much of a good thing can be bad for your body. Over time, a superabundance of protein can increase your odds for heart disease, osteoporosis, obesity, and cancer. Since protein is not stored in the body, excessive amounts overwork the kidneys in their attempt to excrete extra protein to maintain balance. At the same time, surplus protein increases the amount of calcium excreted, creating a potential risk for osteoporosis. And not only are many concentrated sources of protein also high in fat, but protein not utilized or excreted from the body may be converted to body fat.

PROTEIN NEEDS

We need less protein than you may imagine. In fact, the average American eats twice as much protein as is recommended in a healthy diet. According to the Daily Reference Values established by the government for adults and children aged 4 or older, average protein requirements should be calculated as 10% of total calorie intake.

For example, if based on your age, height, weight, activity level, and gender you require 2000 calories each day, 10% of 2000 calories equals 200 calories. To figure how many grams of protein you are allotted in your 200 protein calories, recall that each gram of protein equals 4 calories. Divide the 200 protein calories by 4 calories and you'll arrive at your estimated protein needs of 50 grams of protein per day.

The 10% of calories to protein guide doesn't apply to diets below 1800 calories. The minimum amount of protein recommended for all calorie levels is 46 grams.

Some nutritionists still advise modifying the Dietary Guidelines to increase protein's percentage of calories to 12-15% while at the same time decreasing the Dietary Guidelines fat allotment of 30% down to at most 20% of calories. As with any nutrient, the Dietary Guidelines are simply guidelines. Some individuals may need more, some less.

Pitches for protein periodically go in and out of vogue for athletes. It's true that maintenance of muscles, tendons, and ligaments depends on protein, but as long as athletes consume adequate calories, no additional protein is generally needed. The only exception may be some endurance athletes who may need more protein to replace what would be used under extraordinary conditions. When it comes down to it, the only way to build muscle is through training and strength-building exercise—not protein powders, protein drinks, or steaks before competition. Beyond consuming adequate amounts of protein, athletes, as with all individuals, benefit more from increased consumption of complex carbohydrates.

EATING LESS MEAT: A GROWING TREND

In 1992, 12.4 million people, 7% of the total U.S. population, were estimated to be vegetarian. This figure is double the number of people who considered themselves vegetarians in 1985 and more than 10 times the number reported in 1978.

Much of the growing trend to eat less or no animal-based proteins is linked to concerns about heart disease and cancer, the use of antibiotics and hormones in animals raised for their meat, food-borne pathogenic bacteria such as salmonella, and the overall treatment of livestock.

But considering oneself a vegetarian doesn't necessarily mean eschewing all animal proteins. **Vegans** (pronounced vee-gunz) are the only ones who actually fit the complete vegetarian model. **Lacto-vegetarians** eat plant foods plus milk products but no meats, fish, fowl, or eggs. **Ovo-vegetarians** eat plant foods plus eggs but no meats, fish, fowl, or dairy products. **Lacto-ovo-vegetarians** eat plant foods plus eggs and dairy products but no meat, fish, or fowl. **Pesco-vegetarians** eat plant foods plus dairy products, eggs, and fish but no meat or fowl.

The most recent twist on vegetarianism are **semi-vegetarians**, those who reduce but don't necessarily eliminate meat, poultry, fish, eggs, and dairy products. Eating less animal-based proteins dramatically reduces saturated fat and cholesterol. It also makes more reasonable demands on the meat industry, perhaps allowing for less efficient yet more humane methods of production. When it comes down to it, the appeal to becoming a semi-vegetarian is the freedom to make choices and experiment without making a major commitment one way or another.

It's important to remember that each person is biochemically unique. A diet that may work for one person may not work for another. While some may flourish on a vegan diet, others may find that after a time they feel better when an animal-derived protein is occasionally included. Some may need more of a certain nutrient than others, requiring vitamin or mineral supplementation. Get in tune with your own body's needs and be open to the possibilities. If you feel you need help planning your diet, consult a qualified health professional.

Nutritional Considerations

A varied vegetarian diet can supply key nutrients, such as iron, zinc, and B-12, that are abundant in meat. Iron can be found in eggs, pumpkin seeds, spinach, and all legumes. Although the type of iron found in meat is most assimilated, vitamin C from fruits or vegetables eaten at the same meal will enhance absorption of plant-based iron. Coffee and tea inhibits assimilation of iron.

Zinc can be found in eggs and whole grains. Absorption of non-meat sources of zinc is not as sensitive as occurs with iron.

Getting enough B-12 from vegetarian sources, however, is another issue. Any vegetarian who includes dairy or eggs in their diet will receive adequate amounts of B-12. However, those who avoid all animal products should take B-12 supplements, fortified nutritional yeast, or other foods fortified with the spectrum of B vitamins, including B12. Long-term deficiency can result in serious irreversible damage to the brain and central nervous system. To ensure that her infant develops properly, it is especially critical for a pregnant or lactating woman to include some source of vitamin B12 in her diet.

Kids and a Vegetarian Diet

As long as enough calories are consumed from a high quality diet including whole grains, beans, fruits, and vegetables to include all the nutrients needed for normal growth and development, a diet low in animal protein can be adequate for the average child. However, here's where the application of the complementary protein system is highly recommended.

As with any child, regardless under what type of diet they may be raised, much care should be taken to plan their meals to fulfill their special needs for optimal growth. Good sources of high quality, complemented proteins and variety are a must. Inclusion of eggs and/or dairy may make planning easier, but as long as the special nutrient considerations listed above are fulfilled, low nutrient "junk foods" are kept to a minimum, and enough calories are included in a reasonable volume of food, a vegetarian diet is possible.

COMPLEMENTARY PROTEINS

Despite the impression most of us got with the former Basic Four Food Groups that meat, fish, poultry, and eggs were the only protein foods from which to choose, eating less animal proteins or none at all can be as balanced as an animal protein-based diet. Since the beginning of time, civilizations have depended on vegetables, legumes, nuts, seeds, and grains for protein.

Much confusion rests on the fact that plant proteins, except for soybeans, quinoa, and amaranth, are considered incomplete since they may be low in one or two of the amino acids in the proportion (there is not an equal one-to-one relationship) that the human body needs. However, different plant proteins can be combined to produce a high-quality protein, as complete as that found in animal proteins. Such a relationship is the essence of the "complementary" protein system. For example, grains are low in lysine but high in methionine whereas beans are low in methionine but high in lysine. When supplied separately, the body uses the essential amino acids at the level of the poorly supplied "limiting amino acid." If the grain and the bean are consumed together, the protein quality is increased dramatically and is biologically the same as eating a complete protein.

The book that made "complementary protein" a household phrase for vegetarians, Frances Moore Lappe's *Diet for a Small Planet* (Ballentine Books) published in 1971, gave the impression that to get enough protein on a meatless diet, considerable attention was needed in choosing foods in the right combinations. In her completely revised and updated version, she has since claimed that studies have shown that it is much easier than previously thought. **As long as adequate calories are consumed from a wide variety of nutritious foods**, you can get more than enough of all the essential amino acids from plant foods that are necessary to keep the body in top condition.

Curiously, whether consciously or unconsciously, different cultures have used the protein complementary system for centuries. Caribbean black beans and rice, Middle Eastern garbanzo bean hummus and bulgur wheat tabouli, East Indian rice and wheat chapatis with lentil bean dahl, Japanese tofu stir-fry over rice, Mexican anasazi beans and corn tortillas, and even the American peanut butter sandwich illustrate the basic principles of complementary proteins. In fact, when most people create menus, they automatically combine their proteins because the combination simply tastes good.

The complementary protein system does not preclude the use of animal products, nor is it only for vegetarians. Small amounts of protein can supplement a plant protein to make it more complete—the way most traditional cultures throughout the world cook with animal proteins.

Even though there is no need to be overly preoccupied with complementary

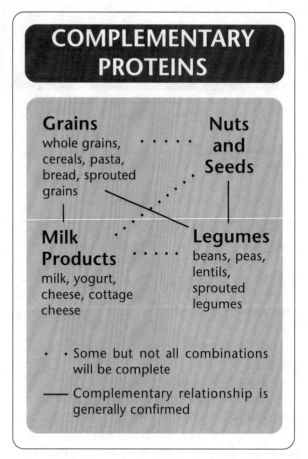

COMPLEMENTARY PROTEINS

Grains
whole grains, cereals, pasta, bread, sprouted grains

Nuts and Seeds

Milk Products
milk, yogurt, cheese, cottage cheese

Legumes
beans, peas, lentils, sprouted legumes

· · Some but not all combinations will be complete

—— Complementary relationship is generally confirmed

proteins if you are getting enough calories, the system still has value. Knowledge of the general principles provides a comforting buffer for those who would like to experiment with meatless meals but are concerned about getting enough protein. It also illustrates the concept of variety. Eating the same few foods day after day may create imbalances in your diet. Awareness of complementary proteins can make planning for a varied diet much easier, reminding you of the several possible menus that can be devised through its mix and match format.

Meat

GRILLED HAMBURGERS on the Fourth of July, hot dogs with the works at the baseball game, parsleyed leg of lamb at Passover, and brown-sugar-glazed ham at Easter...no matter what the holiday or event, a meal featuring red meat is often at center stage. Even with everyday meals, it's the most commonly consumed protein food in the United States.

However, concerns with the amount of fat and cholesterol found in meat, the use of synthetic growth hormones and other drugs, food safety, the effect of meat production on the environment, and animal welfare have placed its dominance on shaky ground since the mid-1970s. As a result, the meat industry has been scrambling to change meat's eroding health image through low-fat breeding and production techniques as well as through advertising campaigns expounding the virtues of meat as a convenient, easy-to-prepare, nutritious food.

NUTRITION

Besides being very high in protein, beef, pork, and lamb are also good sources of B vitamins and highly assimilable forms of zinc and iron. Although iron can be obtained from green leafy vegetables and dried beans and peas, the type of iron found in meat, called "heme" iron, is more easily absorbed by the body.

While its cholesterol matches that of roasted, skinned chicken, the bad news is that meat is the largest source of saturated fat in the American diet. Research has found a strong correlation between diets high in saturated fats and increased risk for heart attacks as well as colon, breast, and prostate cancers.

The most incriminating evidence against meat was the result of a Harvard University study tracking about 89,000 registered nurses ages 30-59 from 1980-1986. Researchers found that women who ate beef, pork, or lamb as a main dish every day had 21/2 times the risk to develop colon cancer as women who ate meat sparingly or not at all. In January 1992, colon cancer in men was also attributed to a diet which included red meat.

In the fall of 1993, scientists from Harvard University and the Mayo Clinic announced the results of studies which tracked the eating habits of 47,000 men, linking the consumption of red meat with increased risk of prostate cancer. Those who ate high amounts of red meat were twice as likely to be diagnosed with advanced cases of prostate cancer.

Cardiologist Dr. Dean Ornish has made waves by proving that a meat-free, high-fiber, low-fat diet combined with stress reduction and exercise can halt and even reverse heart disease.

In response to rising fears about the fat

in meat, many producers are now using genetics to breed their animals to be leaner and slaughtering them at an earlier age when their muscle-to-fat ratio is at its peak. As a result, today's beef is generally about 25% leaner and pork about 50% less fat than in the past. While it's a good start, meat still needs to be consumed in moderation.

What's a serving?

Taking into account all the positive and negative nutritional aspects of meat, the Food Guide Pyramid suggests we eat smaller and fewer portions of meat than typically served in the United States. Serving size should be limited to 2-3 ounces of lean cooked meat. In practical terms, four ounces of raw meat will yield a 3- ounce cooked portion, about the size of a deck of playing cards.

Total amount of protein per day should be the equivalent of 5-7 oz. of cooked lean meat, poultry, or fish per day. However, this is not to say that the use of meat or even poultry or fish is mandatory. Rather, much of the protein allotment should frequently be provided with cooked dry beans and peas, small amounts of nuts and seeds, and even the occasional egg.

It's best to follow the advice of our country's third president, Thomas Jefferson: "I have lived temperately, eating little animal food and that...as a condiment for the vegetables which constitute my principal diet."

Change your perspective on meat by considering it an adjunct to the meal rather than the main focus. Minimize your intake by adding small amounts in stir-fries, pasta dishes, and casseroles and keep the frequency to once per week or a couple times per month.

BUYING MEATS

Ironically, meat is graded by the U.S. Department of Agriculture not by nutritional value but by appearance, texture, and the amount of marbling—the white flecks of fat within the muscle. The more fat, the more tender and flavorful the meat, the higher the grade. However, designating the most fatty meat as top grade, or *Prime*, seems a bit contrary to current nutritional research that preaches the value of a low-fat diet.

At the other end of the spectrum, *Select*, the least fatty and flavorful of the three grades, has about 1/2 the fat of Prime. Right in the middle in terms of fat, flavor, and tenderness is *Choice*. All things considered, Choice is the most preferable of the three and, luckily, the most readily available grade of meat found in supermarkets.

Higher fat content is not the only way meat can be tender and flavorful. Some beef and lamb are specially aged to improve their characteristics. While stored for several weeks at temperatures between 34°-38° F., the meat shrinks, thereby intensifying the flavor, and natural enzymes break down the connective fibers within the meat. Some meat is aged within cryovac bags, a special type of polyethylene bag that is often used to hold meat in a hermetically sealed environment for 3-4 weeks. While traditional methods of aging will produce optimum results, some enzymatic changes still occur in the cryovac bags.

No matter the grade, all contain about the same amount of cholesterol since cholesterol is found primarily in the muscle tissues of an animal rather than the fat.

Preservatives on Fresh Meat

As of April 18, 1994, five natural preservatives—ascorbic acid, erythorbic acid, citric acid, sodium ascorbate, and sodium citrate—

TOP LEAN CUTS

BEEF

Choice or Select Grade:
top round
eye of round
round tip
sirloin
top loin
tenderloin
bottom round
chuck arm
pot roast

Prime Grade:
top round
eye of round
round tip

Select Grade:
ribs: small end

PORK
tenderloin
center loin
whole ham
boneless ham (regular or extra lean)
Canadian bacon

LAMB

Choice Grade:
leg shank
leg sirloin
whole leg
loin
foreshank

can be applied to the surface of fresh beef, lamb, and pork cuts to delay discoloration. To retain their "natural" status, no other preservatives such as BHT or nitrites are allowed.

Buy it Lean

Even within the same grade, different parts of the cow, hog, or lamb naturally contain different amounts of fat. Meat from the areas most exercised, such as the shoulder, leg, and rump, are most lean.

You can also choose lower-fat cuts by noting the nutrient claim listed on some meats. Each claim has specific guidelines for maximum amounts of total fat, saturated fat, and cholesterol that must be met considering a 3 oz. cooked serving of meat or, if referring to lunch meat or canned meat, by a 2 oz. serving.

Ground beef

Ground beef has special labeling rules. It is labeled as a percentage of lean to fat **by weight** (i.e., 85% lean, 15% fat), not by the percentage of calories from fat. By law, ground beef has a maximum fat by weight content of 30%.

Whereas previously there were no standard definitions to designate ground beef as lean or extra lean, new labeling laws now require that it comply with the same fat claim guidelines as other meats. Therefore, only ground beef that is no more than 90% lean/10% fat by weight may be called lean. Extra lean ground beef must be less than 95% lean/5% fat by weight.

A more realistic picture of fat content is to translate the percentages of lean to fat by weight into the grams of fat and percentage of total calories from fat you'll actually get from various selections **based on a 3 oz. medium broiled portion**. Comparable percentage of fat levels in ground pork and lamb will yield similar results.

NUTRIENT CLAIMS ON MEAT

Term	Total Fat	Saturated Fat	Cholesterol
"Lean"	< 10 grams	< 4 grams	< 95 mg.
"Extra Lean"	< 5 grams	< 2 grams	< 95 mg.
"Fat-Free"	< 0.5 grams		
"Low Fat"	< 3 grams and	< 30% calories from fat	
	(If the product meets the requirements for "low fat",		
	__% of lean may also be listed on the label)		

"Reduced Fat"	at least 25% less fat compared to typical product
"Light or Lite"	at least 1/3 fewer calories or 50% less fat than typical product

FAT CONTENT OF GROUND BEEF

Sold As	% Calories from Fat	Grams Total Fat
73% lean/27%fat	79%	18 grams
80% lean/20% fat	71%	15 grams
85% lean/15% fat	64%	12 grams
90% lean/10% fat	53%	9 grams
95% lean/5% fat	34%	5 grams

You may also find ground beef designated by its source. Ground beef is generally ground from the trimmings of various cuts of meat to yield. Ground chuck is from the shoulder area, yielding ground beef that can usually be sold as extra lean. Ground round, from the hip area, is leaner than ground chuck. Ground sirloin, from the back area, is even leaner but also the most expensive. Some of the extra lean ground beef is made with hydrolyzed oat flour or carrageenan to compensate for the reduced fat which otherwise would not permit it to hold together well when making burgers or meatballs.

CURED MEATS

Cured meats include bacon, ham, sausages, and luncheon meats. Instead of curing for preservation as was done out of necessity in the distant past, meats are now cured for flavor. Although tasty, cured meats are also high in fat and sodium. Foods high in saturated fat stack the odds for heart disease and cancer. Excessive consumption of salt-preserved food has been linked to stomach cancer. Therefore, cured meats are best eaten infrequently and in moderation.

The meat industry has been trying to win back a few deserters by introducing lower-fat alternatives. Read labels carefully, noting the grams of fat per serving size to make sure you're really getting something lower in fat. To decipher the percentage fat-free claims, keep the previous ground beef fat conversion chart in mind. If the label doesn't claim at least 95% lean, you're not getting that great a deal. The closer to the top water or broth is on the list of ingredients, the less fat (and meat) it will contain.

Bacon is cured in salt brine and may or may not be smoked. Canadian bacon, cured, smoked pork from the loin area of the hog instead of the belly, has about 40% less fat. Make sure you buy only nitrite-free brands.

Ham may be cured by one of two methods. With the traditional "dry-cure," the hind leg portion of a hog is coated with salt, sodium nitrite, sugar, and spices. For at least 2 months, it is allowed to cure during which the meat dehydrates to the point where no bacteria can grow. It is then smoked and aged but requires cooking before consumption.

"Wet-cured" ham is soaked in brine or injected with a solution of water, salt, sodium nitrite, and sugar. It is then smoked until partially or fully cooked.

Ham is labeled according to its protein content, an indirect way of indicating how much added water and additives it contains. "Ham" contains at least 20.5% protein after the fat has been removed. "Ham with natural juices" contains at least 18.5% protein. "Ham—water added" is at least 17% protein. Hams labeled as "Ham and water product" must list the percentage of weight that constitutes added ingredients.

Sausages can be divided into four categories:

1. Fresh, uncured, uncooked sausage in casings or in bulk, i.e., bratwurst, pork sausage

2. Uncooked smoked sausages that must be cooked before eating, ie. country-style pork sausage, kielbasa

3. Cooked sausages that are ready to serve or merely need reheating, i.e., hot dogs, bologna, braunschweiger

4. Dry and semidry sausages that may be smoked or air-dried but require cooking before eating, i.e., salami, summer sausage, pepperoni.

Sausages and hot dogs labeled as "all meat" may contain only skeletal meats such as pork shoulder, beef chuck, brisket, flank, and loin. No organ meats are allowed to be used under this designation.

Casings for sausages may be naturally derived or artificial. Depending on the diameter needed, natural casings are derived from beef, hog, or sheep intestines.

Most commonly used collagen-type casings are made from sinews or the flesh side of split cowhides heat-processed into long tubes.

Cellulosic-type casings are made from cotton linters or wood pulp that is chemically dissolved and extruded into its shape. Often used on large salamis, this reddish-brown casing is inedible. Another variety of inedible casings are the red plastic casings used for bologna and the white for liverwurst.

Luncheon Meats are cooked meats that are prepared for slicing, including fully-cooked, ready-to-serve sausages and variations on ham. Fat and sodium content varies considerably, so read labels carefully. Avoid brands with more than 500 mg. sodium per 2-ounce serving.

Common Ingredients

Basic ingredients for cured meats are salt and sodium or potassium nitrite with smoking optional, depending on the desired finished product. Additional ingredients may include sugar, spices, binders and fillers, and phosphates.

Salt acts as a preservative, inhibits bacterial growth, and adds flavor.

Sodium nitrite is primarily used to maintain the pink or red colors in meats and to enhance flavor by inhibiting rancidity. Additionally, sodium nitrite helps protect against bacterial growth, specifically clostridium botulinum, the bacterium that produces botulism.

Also known as saltpeter, sodium nitrite has been used for curing since Roman times, but now its use is very controversial. When meat containing nitrite, especially bacon, is heated at high temperatures, nitrites can combine with protein substances called amines to form nitrosamine, a very potent carcinogenic compound.

More than 1/3 of the nitrite found in the typical American diet comes from cured meat. Nitrites are produced naturally in our own saliva and occur naturally in baked goods, cereals, and vegetables. Since studies have shown that your odds of getting stomach cancer triple with each extra milligram of nitrite in your diet, it makes sense to eliminate any nitrite source that is deliberately added and could be eliminated.

U.S.D.A. regulations now mandate a reduction in the amount of nitrite used to cure meats plus the addition of some form of vitamin C such as sodium ascorbate or sodium erythorbate. As an antioxidant, the vitamin C not only helps preserve the color of the product but also scavenges nitrite so less, if any, is available to convert to nitrosamine.

Several varieties of cured meats including bacon, sausage, ham, and lunch meats are available processed without nitrites. They may not have as rich a color, but they are very safe to eat and free of any probability for nitrosamine formation. You'll usually find them in the frozen meat section of your supermarket. Make sure to thaw them in your refrigerator, not on the kitchen counter, and use within 4-7 days.

Sugar, whether in the form of white sugar, honey, or maple syrup, is used to improve texture and flavor. It balances the flavor of the salt found in the cured product and counteracts the salt's tendency to dehydrate meat fibers, making them more tough.

Spices used to make sausage may include black pepper, cloves, ginger, rosemary, or sage. Besides the good flavor they impart, these particular spices also contain natural antioxidants.

Binders and fillers make the sausage more moist, easier to slice, and less prone to shrinkage during cooking. Binders such as isolated soy protein, dry whey, or sodium caseinate help keep the sausage from falling apart by binding both fat and water in the sausage.

Fillers work similarly but hold only water. Common fillers include cereals and corn syrup solids. Lower-fat versions of sausage, hot dogs, and lunch meat often contain vegetable and food starches to replace some of the fat.

Government regulations stipulate a maximum of 2% corn syrup solids for hot dogs, bologna, and similar types of cooked sausage and a maximum of 30% fat by weight. To allow for production of lower-fat hot dogs, new rules stipulate that combined total fat and added water must be less than 40% by weight.

Phosphates help retain moisture during processing and home preparation to make the cured meat more juicy and flavorful. While a small amount may be acceptable, some of the weight you may be paying for could just be water.

Some dry and semidry sausages also contain **BHA & BHT** as antioxidants to inhibit off-flavor development. Studies linking them as possible carcinogens have been inconclusive. As doubt remains, take the safe route and avoid products with BHA & BHT.

GAME MEATS

Venison, water buffalo, and buffalo, game meats occasionally available in meat markets, are all lower in calories, fat, and cholesterol than beef. The added advantage is that they generally are free of antibiotics and synthetic hormones. Marinating, removing excess fat, and cooking at moderate, not high, temperatures will help reduce overly strong flavors.

FOOD SAFETY CONCERNS

According to the Centers for Disease Control, meat and poultry products are the primary cause for the huge number of foodborne illnesses reported each year. Beef, pork, and lamb can carry harmful bacteria such as salmonella and other microbiological pathogens that can cause illness if consumed in raw, contaminated, or undercooked food.

The source of the problem is multifaceted. Poor conditions and procedures in some slaughterhouses and processing plants are partly to blame. Because thorough cooking will destroy these bacteria on raw products, improper food handling is also an issue.

Processing Problems

Since meat inspection was first instituted in 1906, procedures have changed little, relying primarily on an inspector's sight, smell, and touch to identify contamination. However, microbial pathogens cannot be seen, smelled, or felt. Therefore, under our current inspection system, there's always a chance contaminated meat can enter the food supply.

In May 1993, stories reminiscent of the unsanitary conditions found in meatpacking plants at the turn of the century as revealed in Upton Sinclair's book, *The Jungle*, hit the newspapers and broadcast news. More than half of the 90 beef slaughterhouses that underwent surprise inspections had major violations of code that could be the source for bacterially contaminated meat.

Since 1985, several reports by the National Academy of Science and the U.S. General Accounting Office to Congress have concluded that only a scientific, risk-based inspection system using routine microbiological testing of equipment surfaces and raw meat would determine whether sanitation and processing controls were working properly and whether the meat was free of contamination.

Fortunately, many slaughterhouses and processing plants have taken their own initiative to establish the Hazard Analysis Critical Control Point system (HACCP) within their operations. The HACCP system identifies the points in processing where problems could occur. These points are then systematically monitored to prevent hazards being created or allowed to persist.

A good example is Coleman Natural Meats, Inc. of Denver, Colorado. Twenty-seven separate control points include feed, water, and urine analysis at the ranch or feedlot and pre-evisceration testing at the slaughter plant in addition to sight, smell, and touch inspections. Records on each animal are maintained through a bar-code identification number ear-tagged to each calf or lamb shortly after birth. The tags can be electronically scanned with hand-held scanners and the I.D. numbers are stored in a computer database, allowing for a permanent record all the way from where the animal was born and raised, to the feedlot, and through slaughter, packing, and marketing. After slaughter, each quarter of meat from the animal is tagged with its identification number and sent to a retail store with additional tags to place in packages, providing an easy tracking system should any problem occur.

Tight monitoring and detailed record-keeping should be prerequisite to be licensed as a meat producer and processor. In fact, a good HACCP program in place at the processing plant coupled with proper cooking techniques could likely have prevented the food poisoning tragedy that occurred in January 1993 when 475 people became seriously ill and 3 children died as a result of eating fast-food hamburgers tainted with Escherichia coli 0157:H7.

A rare and very dangerous form of E. coli, Escherichia coli 0157:H7 can be transmitted through contact with fecal matter during the processing of animal foods or because of improper food handling.

Since it doesn't cause illness in animals, current inspection procedures can't detect contaminated carcasses. However, microbial testing at the plant would likely have discovered it before it was too late.

While E. coli 0157:H7 can survive refrigeration and freezer storage, like other bacteria, it is easily killed by pasteurization or when cooked to medium doneness with an internal temperature at least 155° F., preferably 160° F. Unfortunately, the contaminated hamburger meat at the fast food restaurants was cooked only rare, to an internal temperature of 140°F. While steaks and roasts can safely be cooked rare, in the process of grinding meat into ground beef, the surface bacteria are distributed throughout the product, thus requiring higher cooking temperatures to ensure that all the bacteria are destroyed.

DRUGS IN MEAT PRODUCTION

Some drugs are inevitable. Federal law requires all heifers sold in interstate commerce must be immunized by six months of age for brucellosis, a highly contagious disease which can lead to an epidemic of spontaneous abortions or delivery of dead or weak offspring.

Depending on problems associated with their specific region, ranchers, even those who market naturally raised beef, also innoculate for various other contagious diseases such as blackleg (fatal toxemia), a respiratory infection called IBR (infectious bovine rhino-trichinosis), and for the prevention of "shipping fever" complications which may arise after calves are weaned and shipped to their next destination. Internal and external parasites are controlled with a broad spectrum parasiticide injected subcutaneously.

Drug-resistant Bacteria

The use of the same antibiotics as used by human beings in animal feed and to treat sick animals has created a unique potential human health hazard.

In 1949 scientists discovered that small doses of an antibiotic fed to chickens and piglets caused them to gain 10-20% more weight than normal. This led to years of routine use of antibiotics in animal feed to not only control diseases common in crowded livestock conditions but to fatten cattle, sheep, and hogs more quickly through improved feed efficiency.

While it may have helped cut overall costs, the high use of subtherapeutic doses of antibiotics has resulted in the emergence of antibiotic-resistant bacteria. When meat containing these drug-resistant pathogenic bacteria, particularly resistant strains of salmonella, is consumed, severe gastrointestinal infections may develop which are untreatable by commonly used antibiotics.

Several studies linked the surge of antibiotic-resistant bacteria and outbreaks of illnesses with cattle fed antibiotics in their feed.

The FDA proposed the restriction of antibiotics in animal feeds in 1977. While Congress called for more research, widespread use continued. High material costs, the need to respond to rising consumer concern, and irritation over FDA inactivity on the matter led the National Cattlemen's Association, representing the largest producers of beef, to urge members in 1986 to discontinue the use of antibiotics in feed for growth promotion and inject them solely on a per animal basis to treat disease.

According to the National Cattlemen's Association, now less than 10% of cattle are likely treated with antibiotics. As the beef industry runs on a slim profit margin, practical business sense dictates that it is more advantageous for the beef industry to maintain good preventative health practices rather than rely on expensive medical treatment.

Even so, the National Academy of Science reports in their comprehensive study, *Alternative Agriculture* (National Academy Press), published in 1989 that about 9.9 million pounds of antibiotics are fed to all types of livestock each year, not only as a way to improve feed efficiency but to control many of the disease problems that come with strict confinement and intensive management of animals.

Synthetic Hormone Use

Injection of growth promotants is widespread, encompassing about 60-65% of the cattle slaughtered in the United States.

Beef producers inject hormones to save money and resources and to get leaner meat. The average cow is said to consume 4 fewer bushels of corn and gets to market weight 18 days sooner with 50 lbs. more lean muscle tissue than an untreated animal. Industry-wide, hormone implants save producers about $650 million per year. The added bonus is that a hormone implant makes for more docile animals that are easier to confine.

But how safe is it? Five hormones are allowed to be used to make cattle grow faster, larger, and leaner. Testosterone, estradiol, and progesterone are found naturally in animals and humans. Zeronal and trenbonone acetate are synthetically produced. Regulations require that the hormone pellet be implanted behind the animal's ear in muscle tissue that won't be eaten. Small amounts of these drugs are released into the animal's bloodstream on a continuous basis.

Most apprehension about injected growth hormones seems related to concerns about estrogen as high levels have been associated with endometrial and breast cancers and increased cardiovascular risk. A synthetic hormone called diethylstilbestrol (DES) was used in livestock for over 20 years before it was banned by the FDA. Unfortunately, the ban occurred only after several women were diagnosed with uterine cancer and other reproductive disorders. Despite the fact that the hormones used today are chemically different than DES, it's a story that's hard to forget.

The European Economic Community ban on hormone-treated beef in 1989 brought the safety issue of hormones into the limelight. Critics of the ban claimed that in 35 years of use, no risk has been demonstrated to either cattle or individuals consuming the beef from cattle treated with these products. They also cite the minute difference between the amount of estrogen found in 3 oz. of meat from a hormone-treated animal—1.85 nanograms (1 billionth of a gram) in contrast to a untreated animal—1.01 nanograms.

Nonetheless, concerns haven't been entirely abated. The FDA claims that doses are so small that, even if used improperly, a health hazard wouldn't be too likely. And yet a 1986 study by the USDA found evidence that several feedlots in the Southwest were illegally implanting hormones in the neck or breast of the animal. High residues were found that even the FDA admitted could result in "adverse effects." While abuse may be rare, even the possibility raises some concern.

Recent reports on the dangerous side effects experienced by athletes also raises the question why growth hormones are tolerated in cattle. While the amount in beef is very minute compared to those used in sports, in essence, its purpose is the same: to accelerate growth much quicker than would occur naturally.

When it gets right down to it, meat from hormone-treated beef may not even be as tasty. Whether growth hormones present potential risks or not, some producers don't like to use hormone implants simply because they believe the meat is often consistently tougher and less flavorful than beef truly matured according to natural life cycles.

Illegal Drugs

Growth hormones aren't the only way producers can increase muscle tissue in their cattle. A memo from the USDA's Food Safety and Inspection Service (FSIS) and the FDA in April 1991 warned producers of the initiation of residue testing for clenbuterol in an attempt to stop illegal application of the drug.

Clenbuterol is used to increase muscle mass in meat-producing show animals such as cattle, pigs, and sheep. Individuals in Spain who consumed beef liver containing clenbuterol residues were hospitalized with symptoms of increased heart rate, muscular tremors, headache, nausea, fever, and chills. Similar incidents have occurred in France

and illegal use of the drug has been revealed in Ireland.

It doesn't stop with Clenbuterol. Several types of animal drugs are available without needing a veterinarian's prescription. Many have not been approved by the FDA for the particular application for which they are actually used.

HUMANE TREATMENT OF FARM ANIMALS

While many people are eating less meat for health considerations, concern over the disrespectful treatment of farm animals, including the extensive switch to controlled confinement systems and the subsequent increased administration of drugs, has convinced many people to stop eating meat entirely.

Until the end of World War II, most farms were diversified crop-livestock operations in which farmers produced forage and feed grains for their animals that, in turn, provided manure for fertilization of the land. Today, however, to maximize efficiency and provide a more tender product, much beef, lamb, and pork are raised in a different manner. Steers and heifers are range-fed during calfhood and then transferred to a feedlot where they eat high-energy rations until fat enough for slaughter, between 15-24 months of age. Lambs are also sent to a feedlot for final fattening while pigs are raised in ultra-confinement units for intensive management.

Unlike pasture or low-confinement systems where animals have plenty of room to move and express their normal patterns of behavior, high-density confinement systems, in effect, treat animals merely as agricultural commodities with no other purpose for being except to put on weight and be slaughtered.

Many people are either oblivious to what is going on (out of sight, out of mind) or fail to see the need for concern, arguing that whether humanely raised or not, the animals will be eventually slaughtered anyway. However, even if one could see no further than one's plate, the fact of the matter is that various stressors, including close confinement or isolation and reprehensible conditions while being transported to market can not only lower the animal's immune system, thus requiring more drugs, but also adversely affect the quality of the meat.

To be fair, many producers probably consider their methods very humane, providing ample food and shelter to their animals. And, since many humans don't think twice about popping a drug for one reason or another, for some consumers the issue of drugs and livestock may appear insignificant. However, the denial of social interaction, normal behaviors, and untethered movement is painful and cruel, leading to depression (yes!) and increased susceptiblity to disease.

Veal

Veal calves are a classic example. While the consumption of veal is hardly a new idea, the current practice of raising surplus dairy calves in confinement solely on a liquid diet began in 1962 when the Provimi Corporation introduced a unique formula feed which revolutionized the industry. Not only did this new method solve the problem of what to do with the unwanted male calves born into dairy herds, it was a way to utilize the ongoing surplus of skim milk and whey from butter and cheese production.

Calves are separated from their mothers as early as one or two days after birth, often before having the opportunity to nurse and receive colostrum, the antibody-rich milk that helps protect them from disease. The calves are trucked to auction barns where they are sold and delivered to veal barns. For the next 4 months, they are con-

fined to tiny, unbedded, slat-floored, wooden stalls only slightly larger than their bodies. Normal behaviors such as turning around, lying down in a natural position, stretching their limbs, and grooming themselves are severely restricted—all for the purpose of developing super-tender meat.

To maintain the white flesh and mild flavor synonymous with "prime" veal in the eyes of consumers, the calves' diet consists solely of a liquid milk replacer purposely deficient in iron, which would otherwise give the muscle its normal reddish hue. To encourage maximum consumption of the formula, the calves have no access to water.

The denial of solid food leads to abnormal development of the calf's digestive system and thwarts their natural urge to ruminate (chew their cud). As calves normally suckle from their mother an average of 16 times per day and begin eating solid food at 2 weeks of age, confined veal calves display neurotic behaviors such as sucking and eating the boards of their stalls and rolling their tongues.

Anemia and the stress of confinement make the animals more prone to disease. Accordingly, they are routinely fed antibiotics, administered up to 5 times the amount over their short life span as comparably aged calves allowed to pasture.

It's hard to imagine that the fleeting enjoyment of eating bland, white-fleshed tender meat is truly worth putting a young animal through 4 months of sheer torture. This total disregard for the physical and behavioral needs of milk-fed veal is bizarre, barbaric, and appalling.

The Use of Confinement Systems

Veal calves aren't the only ones raised in an unnatural environment. Pigs are increasingly taken away from their mothers shortly after birth to live in crowded confinement systems. Stress and respiratory problems are rampant with veterinary and medical costs twice those in comparably productive "pasture and hutch" systems. Breeder sows are individually tethered in narrow "gestation crates," allowing virtually no movement, visual contact, or any other sort of stimulation or normal behavior.

Like cattle, sheep are fattened and finished off at feedlots. Some operations provide plenty of room to move; others tend toward crowded conditions and are anything but picturesque.

Does efficiency mean higher profits for the producer? Ironically, in the long run, considering aging of facilities and equipment, labor costs for repair and maintenance, and increased medical expenses, producers who use controlled environment confinement facilities are rarely any better off financially on their investment than those who use pasture or low-confinement systems.

Lack of Substantive Anti-Cruelty Laws

Farm animal protection laws in the United States are minimal. In 1906, the Twenty-Eight Hour Law required railroad companies to provide facilities on their lines where animals could obtain feed, water, and rest every 28 hours of transportation time. Since most animals are shipped by truck, currently the law does little good. Some states have extended the law to protect animals transported by truck; however, overcrowding and exposure to varying weather conditions aren't covered.

The Humane Slaughter Act was passed in 1979, requiring that livestock (except for chickens and ritually slaughtered animals) be handled humanely in the livestock pens and while being driven to and from the pens.

Metal pipes and sharp, pointed objects are forbidden to prod the animals. If livestock are to be held more than 24 hours before slaughter, they are to be given food, water, and enough room to lie down. Animals are supposed to be stunned into unconsciousness (usually done with a shot from a penetrating bolt or concussion stunner) before slaughter.

Hopefully, these regulations are being observed more than the one which states that disabled, weak, or sick sheep, pigs, calves, and cows (called "downers") are supposed to be humanely treated and are not to be dragged from the truck or left to die from lack of water or exposure. In the fall and winter of 1991/92, investigators from the Humane Society of the United States visited 31 livestock markets in 7 states. They found that "downer" animals were abused and neglected in 73% of the markets where they were present. Actions observed included a cow being dragged out of a truck by a chain wrapped around one leg, resulting in ligaments and joints tearing from the stress of the weight of its 1,100 pound body. A paralyzed sheep was dragged onto an aisleway and allowed to be trampled by other animals. A half-dead calf was dragged by its ear and left by a dumpster without food, water, or veterinary care. Investigators were told that if it were alive the next day, it would be slaughtered.

Hope on the Horizon

Fortunately, humane solutions are being created and implemented worldwide that not only consider farm animals' basic physical and behavioral requirements but also consumer health.

Typically referred to as "humane sustainable agriculture," the intent is to produce adequate amounts of safe, wholesome food in a manner that is ecologically sound, economically viable, equitable, and humane.

Europe has taken the lead in developing humane husbandry practices that incorporate natural animal behavior. Several countries have also adopted animal welfare legislation.

Swiss law forbids permanent tethering and battery cages for laying hens, and requires government approval of all animal housing systems. Sweden passed legislation in 1988 that requires adequate space for each animal, proper bedding material, reasonable air quality, limitations on total animals per unit, access to pasture for cows in the summer, and a ban on battery cages for poultry. Restrictions are also placed on castration, dehorning, and tail-docking while breeding, slaughtering, and transportation methods are closely regulated.

In the United States, anti-animal cruelty legislation is often dismissed. However, isolated segments of the meat industry are trying to make some headway. For example, some stockyards have stopped accepting "downer" animals. Some state cattlemen's associations, as well as The National Pork Producers' Council, are also working to resolve the downed animal problem. Many other ranchers have made the commitment to humane treatment for animals in every aspect of the animal's life, from birth through slaughter.

Naturally Raised Meat

To further develop and promote humane rearing of all livestock (including poultry), the Humane Society of the United States and the International Alliance for Sustainable Agriculture collaborated in 1990 to form The Humane Sustainable Agriculture Project. In 1993 they published *The Humane Consumer and Producer Guide*, a comprehensive national listing of 437 farmers and ranchers representing 44 states who market products based on humaneness and sustainability as well as names of restaurants and stores that use and sell products from these producers.

Naturally raised meat is readily available wherever you live. Many small local farmers and ranchers offer naturally raised alternatives and larger operations, such as Coleman Natural Beef, Inc., provide natural beef and pork nationwide.

Several ranchers are raising natural, humanely raised veal in which calves are untethered and fed a nutritious, balanced diet free of added hormones or antibiotics. Because grass and other foods high in iron are not restricted, naturally raised veal meat is pink in color and more flavorful. For many chefs who feature veal dishes in their restaurants, it's become the preferred type of veal, both for ethical and gastronomical reasons.

But don't depend on beef simply labeled "natural." According to the USDA, "natural" merely describes meat that is minimally processed and free of artificial additives such as preservatives, artificial flavors, or colors. Since most meat already meets this criterion, look instead for labels with the phrase "raised without antibiotics or growth hormones."

Individual companies can file a "Memorandum of Understanding" with the USDA establishing an audit trail to verify that no antibiotics, growth hormones, or any other drugs except vaccinations have been used on individual animals through time of slaughter. The USDA is also given the right to make unannounced checks and inspections at any phase of production.

While beef, lamb, and pork naturally raised without antibiotics or growth hormones is an excellent choice, meat from animals fed organically grown feed is even better. Nearly half the total pounds of pesticides applied in the nation are used in corn production, the primary grain fed to livestock. Soybeans, another common constitu-

HOW MUCH MEAT TO BUY PER PERSON

Boneless cuts ——————————————————— 1/4 lb.
(ground meat, boned roasts and steaks, stew meat)

Meat with some bone ——————————— 1/3 lb.
(rib roasts, unboned steaks, chops)

Bony cuts ——————————————— 3/4 -1 lb.
(ribs, shanks)

RECOMMENDED INTERNAL TEMPERATURES FOR MEAT

medium rare	145-150° F.	beef, lamb
medium	160° F.	beef, pork, lamb, ground meats
well-done	170° F.	beef, pork, lamb

ent of animal feed, receives about 25% of all herbicides. To be certified as organically fed, not only must the grain be certified organic, but the water must also be free of any pesticide, fertilizer, and herbicide runoff.

If you enjoy eating meat, it is your responsibility to respect and honor the lives of those who serve your own needs. Insist on buying only naturally raised meat, even when ordering at restaurants. Your demand will encourage others to make the extra effort, expanding the awareness of humane sustainable agriculture, thus creating more demand for more ethically treated animals.

HOW TO PREPARE AND COOK MEAT

Meat is easy to prepare. Choosing what cooking method to use depends on the tender-ness of the particular piece of meat. Tender steaks, chops, roasts, and burgers can be roasted, broiled, panbroiled, panfried, or stir-fried. Less tender pot roasts, stew meat, and some steaks can be braised or cooked in liquid as a stew.

To keep fat to a minimum, trim visible outside fat before cooking and inside fat before eating. When roasting, broiling, or grilling, place meat on a rack to allow the fat to drain. To easily remove fat from cooked soups and stews, chill them in the refrigerator before serving and skim off the fat that rises to the top.

To marinate meat for flavor, marinate 15 minutes to 2 hours. If using a marinade for tenderizing lower-fat cuts, marinate 6-8 hours or overnight.

Preparation Methods

Roast: Preheat oven to 325° F. (Tenderloin and bottom sirloin should be roasted at 425° F.) Place roast straight from the refrigerator, fat side up, on a rack in a shallow roasting pan. Season and insert a meat thermometer into the thickest part of the roast without touching bone or fat. Do not add water and keep pan uncovered. Roast 5-10° below desired doneness. Allow roast to stand 15-20 minutes before serving.

Broil: Set oven to broil. Place meat on the broiler pan. Cuts 3/4-1 inch thick should be placed 2-3 inches from the heat source. Thicker cuts should be placed 3-6 inches from the heat. Broil for half the recommended time for the desired doneness, keeping the broiler or oven door open slightly. Season, turn the meat over, and finish cooking.

Panbroil: Place thin steaks or patties in a preheated skillet. Do not add oil or water and do not cover. Use medium to medium-low heat for cuts thicker than 1/2 inch and turn occasionally. Use medium-high heat for thinner cuts and turn only once. Season and serve.

Panfry: Brown tender meat cuts on both sides in a small amount of oil. Season and continue to cook over medium heat until done, turning occasionally. Do not cover.

Stir-fry: Slice meat into thin, uniform slices, strips, or pieces. Marinate if desired while preparing vegetables. Stir-fry beef first in a small amount of oil. (You may need to stir-fry half of it at a time.) Cook over medium-high to high temperature, stirring meat continuously until done. Set aside and stir-fry vegetables. Return beef to the wok to mix with vegetables and briefly reheat. Serve over cooked whole grains or pasta.

Grill: Place cuts of meat that cook quickly (steaks, burgers, kabobs) directly on the grill grid above medium coals. The grill can remain open or covered. Roasts and larger steaks should be placed on a grid over a dip pan with coals on each side of the pan. Cover the grill and cook with the vents open.

Braise: Brown meat on all sides in a small amount of oil. Pour off drippings and season meat. Add a small amount of liquid. Cover pan tightly. Simmer over low heat or bake in a 300-325° F. oven. Add vegetables towards the end of cooking.

Cook in liquid: Coat meat with flour and brown all sides in a small amount of oil in a pan. Pour off drippings. Cover meat with liquid, season, and cover tightly. Simmer on top of stove until done. Vegetables, if desired, should be added towards the end of cooking.

FOOD SAFETY TIPS

Proper handling of meat at home, as well as thorough cooking, can eliminate illness from food-borne pathogens.

Cleanliness

• Always wash hands thoroughly in hot soapy water before preparing foods and after handling raw meat.

• Don't let raw meat juices touch ready-to-eat foods either in the refrigerator or during preparation

• Don't put cooked foods on the same plate that held raw meat.

• Wash utensils that have touched raw meat in hot, soapy water before using them to serve cooked foods.

•Be sure to wash counter tops, cutting boards, or any other surfaces raw meats have touched. Wood cutting boards have been shown to be better at preventing bacterial growth than plastic surfaces. You can sanitize them with a solution of 2-3 Tbsp. of household bleach in 1 quart of water.

Defrosting frozen meat

• Defrost meat only in the refrigator, not at room temperature or in warm water. Most food-borne pathogens thrive at room temperature.

• You can also thaw meat in a microwave; however, the meat must then be cooked immediately after thawing.

Cooking

• Never eat raw beef.

• Always marinate meat in the refrigerator. Do not reuse the marinade as a sauce unless it is first brought to a rolling boil. You can also reserve some of the marinade before adding it to the meat.

• Since surface bacteria are transferred to the interior meat during grinding, ground beef should always be cooked medium or well-done, at a temperature of at least 160° F.

• Steaks, roasts, and other cuts of beef have lower risk of carrying food-borne pathogens when cooked rare since the bacteria, which exists only on the outside surfaces, are destroyed in the cooking process.

• To prevent the possibility of trichinosis, be sure to cook pork to an internal temperature of at least 160° F.

• When baking, set the oven no lower than 325° F.

Leftovers

• Refrigerate leftovers quickly. Don't wait until the foods have cooled down. Refrigerators are designed to accommodate changes in temperatures.

• Pack in shallow containers to ensure that the food will cool quickly, preventing hot spots that can breed bacteria.

• Meat gravy and broth are very perishable. Store in the refrigerator no longer than 1-2 days. Before using, boil them for a few minutes to kill any bacteria.

• Use or freeze cooked meat within 3-4 days.

• Store frozen ground meat no longer than 3-4 months; cooked meats no longer than 2-3 months.

Brown bag lunches and picnics

• Leaving food unrefrigerated for more than 2 hours is risky. To keep foods cold, freeze a small ice pack, a carton of juice, or a plastic container of water and add to the lunchbox.

continued

FOOD SAFETY TIPS CONTINUED

•Get in the habit of using mustard in your sandwiches instead of mayonnaise or other egg-based spreads which present a higher risk of going bad when unrefrigerated.

•Pack a cooler with ice or ice packs for picnic foods.

•Only pack foods that are already thoroughly chilled.

•Wash hands with soap and water after handling uncooked meat.

Parties

•Keep hot foods hot and cold foods cold.

•Use chafing dishes or other heated servers that keep the foods at a temperature of at least 140° F.

•Set cold foods on top of ice.

•Never mix fresh foods with foods that have already been out and served.

TEXAS FAJITAS

1 1/2 lbs. skirt steak
2 fresh lemons
unseasoned meat tenderizer
lemon pepper
2 onions, sliced into rings
2 green peppers, cut in
    1/2" strips
1/2 lb. mushrooms, sliced
1 Tbsp. butter or canola oil
1/4 cup white wine
12 whole wheat flour
    tortillas
Optional condiments: salsa,
    pico di gallo, guacamole,
    sour cream, grated
    cheese, black olives

Trim excess fat and place meat in a large baking dish. Squeeze one lemon over meat and sprinkle lightly with meat tenderizer and lemon pepper. Turn meat over and repeat process with other lemon. Cover and marinate in the refrigerator 8-12 hours.

Preheat the oven to 350° F. Just before the grill is ready to use, sauté onion, green pepper, and mushrooms in butter. Splash on white wine and cook a minute or so until the liquid has been absorbed. Warm tortillas in a tortilla warmer or in a covered baking dish in the oven for 10 minutes.

Meanwhile, place meat on the grill close to the coals and cook quickly, 3 minutes per side. Cut meat across the grain into 1/4" strips. Place on a large platter with sautéed vegetables. Serve with tortillas and condiments.

12 fajitas.

(Pyramid servings: 1 Bread/Grain Group, 1/4 Veg. Group, 1 Meat/Protein Group, 7 grams Fat)

Nutrition Facts

Serving Size 1 fajita (157 g)
Servings Per Container 12

Amount Per Serving	
Calories 220	Calories from Fat 70

	% Daily Value*
Total Fat 7g	11%
Saturated Fat 3g	16%
Cholesterol 40mg	14%
Sodium 230mg	10%
Total Carbohydrate 24g	8%
Dietary Fiber 3g	12%
Sugars 2g	
Protein 19g	

Vitamin A 2%	•	Vitamin C	30%
Calcium 2%	•	Iron	15%

* Percent Daily Values are based on a 2,000 calorie diet.

Poultry

FROM 1955-1987, the amount of poultry the average American ate tripled while red meat consumption declined. With 1/3 the saturated fat content of beef, poultry's popularity is little surprise. However, its claim to being low-fat depends on the type of poultry, the particular part being consumed, the cooking method, and whether the skin is consumed along with the meat.

NUTRITION

Just because it's poultry doesn't mean that it's necessarily low-fat. In general, however, you can count on game birds (especially from the wild) and white breast meat to be most lean. Because their unencumbered movement can work off extra fat, free-range poultry allowed to roam freely in both an outdoor pen and poultry house are lower in fat than poultry raised in confinement.

Duck, goose, dark meat from stewing hens, the back meat and thigh from chicken, and any bird or its individual parts that are consumed with its skin will be highest in fat. Everything else is in-between.

Even when you're in the mood for higher fat selections, simply removing the skin can cut fat content almost in half. For example, 3 1/2 oz. of roasted duck eaten with the skin provides 28 grams of fat, with 76 % of its calories from fat. Without the skin, the numbers plummet to 11 grams of fat and 50% fat. Since the skin is mostly fat and satu-rated at that, discarding also lessens the odds for fat-related heart disease and cancer .

Studies show that fat content remains the same regardless whether the poultry skin is removed before or after cooking. Retaining the skin also helps keep the poultry juicy. But if cooking poultry with its skin remains too tempting when it comes to eating, it makes sense to discard the skin before you proceed with cooking.

Pan-juices from chicken cooked in its skin will contain a great deal of fat so, before using them to make gravies and sauces, be sure to skim off the fat with a fat separator cup, baster, or refrigerate ahead of time to congeal the fat.

Roasting, grilling, braising, broiling, steaming, and stir-frying are all low-fat ways to cook poultry. Deep-frying or pan-frying should be used rarely, if at all.

Ground Poultry

Ground chicken and turkey are both good substitutes for ground beef. They can be ground exclusively from dark meat or from a blend of both dark and white meat. Typically, ground poultry is 85% lean/15% fat by weight (64% calories from fat).

Obviously, poultry ground without the skin is your best bet for lean meals. Ground skinless chicken contains approximately 6% fat by weight while ground skinless turkey is about 5% fat by weight, putting it on a par with extra lean ground beef.

For the freshest-tasting ground poultry, grind your own in a food processor just before preparation time. Remove the skin and bone from a chicken or turkey breast. Freeze it for 20 minutes to get it firm. Slice the meat into cubes and process it until you create a fine, but not mushy, texture.

Cured and Processed Poultry

Turkey and chicken luncheon meats and sausages are now just as common as beef- and pork-based versions. But don't assume they are more nutritious. Chicken or turkey bologna, hot dogs, and salami are often quite high in fat and sodium. Limit your purchases to varieties with less than 2 grams of fat and 500 mg. sodium per 2 oz. serving. Roasted chicken or turkey breast, pastrami, and turkey ham (from thigh meat processed and flavored to simulate ham) are generally good choices.

Ingredients used to process cured poultry are little different than those used in beef- and pork-based cured meats: salt, sodium nitrite to preserve color and enhance flavor, sugar for flavor and texture, spices, and binders and fillers to form the final product. Sodium nitrite is most controversial since the nitrites added to the meats can react during the cooking process and be converted into nitrosamine, a potent carcinogenic compound. (For more details, see page 171.)

Several varieties of sausage, hot dogs, and lunch meats are available processed without nitrites. They may not have as rich a color, but they are very safe to eat and free of any probability for nitrosamine formation. You'll usually find them in the frozen meat section of your supermarket. Make sure to thaw them in your refrigerator, not on the kitchen counter, and use within 4-7 days.

What's a Serving?

The Food Guide Pyramid suggests we get 2-3 servings of protein foods per day. A cooked serving of poultry is considered 2-3 ounces (4 ounces in its raw state), the amount of meat on half a medium-sized chicken breast or one chicken leg and thigh. A standard serving size of luncheon meat or sausage is 2 ounces.

Be sure to also include other sources of protein in your diet besides poultry. While it generally is lower in saturated fat than red meats if consumed without the skin, cooked dried beans and peas are much lower in all types of fat.

FOWL FOOD SAFETY

As much as poultry has been praised for its relatively low saturated fat content, concern about its food safety has kept it humble. Much of poultry's problems originate with new processing and slaughter methods, developed primarily as a way to keep up with rising consumer demand.

Most changed is the method in which poultry are raised on the typical large poultry farm. Instead of having the option to peck around outside of their fairly spacious coop for grubs and worms to supplement their feed, most chickens are confined in crowded houses that allow only 0.7-0.8 square feet per bird when grown to market weight, making fresh clean air the exception. Despite their large size, turkeys only get an average of 2 square feet per bird.

All poultry, including naturally raised poultry, receive various drugs and vaccinations to prevent the occurrence of specific poultry-prone diseases. A coccidiostat prevents the proliferation of a parasite that can scar a bird's stomach wall so nutrients cannot be absorbed. At the hatchery chicks are vaccinated when one day old against bronchitis, leucosis—a serious disease of the nervous system, and a common virus called Marek's disease. Since vaccinations are administered to produce natural antibodies to the diseases, they go through the poultry's system quickly without leaving a trace in the meat.

Antibiotics are an entirely different matter. Feeding low levels of antibiotics on a routine basis not only helps prevent diseases from running rampant throughout the crowded flocks, it also promotes growth and improves the efficiency of feed conversion. While naturally raised birds receive on the average 2.3-2.5 lbs. of feed to produce each pound of chicken, antibiotics enable birds to reach the same weight with only 1.95 lbs. of feed. Even though the difference in feed requirements may seem minimal, when multiplied by the number of birds found in many typical large commerical operations, the savings can be astronomical.

Larger doses of antibiotics may be administered when a disease becomes evident within the flock. Seven-day withdrawal periods are mandatory, and yet transmission of the antibiotics themselves is not so much the problem as the drug-resistant, antibiotic-altered bacteria which can breed in meat and possibly make people ill. The constant exposure to the same antibiotics also administered to humans can also cause a person to become immune to their effects when antibiotics may be a necessity. Most heavily abused during the 1960s and 70s, antibiotics are still in full force today.

Due to selective breeding and feed revisions, hormones haven't been used in the poultry industry since the mid-1960s. Originally used to help in developing larger breasts in birds and for calming their temperment, hormones have been replaced by genetics. Today's poultry can get to market faster, heavier, and better-looking than it could over 30 years ago without any increase in feed.

But genetics haven't always considered the comfort of the bird. For example, the Beltsville white turkey was developed to be a heavy-breasted, compact bird to satisfy the increased desire of the American public to eat more breast meat. Unfortunately, they didn't figure in adequately sized legs to carry the heavy burden of its body. The Beltsville turkey has difficulty walking and, in some cases, can't walk at all.

Flavor isn't all it could be either. Poultry forced to market faster lacks some of the good taste that comes with normal maturity. As a result, many turkeys are pumped with artificial basting solutions to add flavor and moistness that, given the way they are raised, isn't there naturally.

The best commercial feed for poultry is all-vegetarian, consisting of a mix such as soybeans, corn, milo, oil, and supplements. More often than not, however, it contains not only antibiotics but animal by-products or animal fat derived from a rendering process of cooking and grinding chicken meat, offal, heads, feet, blood, and feathers. There has been some concern that feed with animal by-products may help increase the likelihood of salmonella in poultry.

Salmonella

The U.S. Department of Agriculture (USDA) estimates that about 40% of raw poultry is contaminated wtih salmonella. Used to describe a group of related bacteria that cause symptoms similar to the intestinal flu, salmonella is a major source of food poisoning in the United States. In addition to the direct transmission of the bacteria from a hen to its eggs, fecal contamination arising from crowded housing conditions, as well as from procedures used in the processing plant to process poultry as quickly as possible, are primarily responsible for the rising spread of salmonella.

Processing procedures at the various slaughterhouses are fairly universal. Chickens are first removed from the truck and hung upside down by their feet on hooks to decrease their activity. A conveyer belt carries them to an area where they are electrically stunned before their jugular veins are slit by an automated knife. After being bled, they are then conveyed to a scalding tank to loosen feathers. Since the tank can get contaminated with mud and feces, bird after bird can be exposed to bacteria. The hot water also opens pores on the skins, allowing the bacteria to enter the skin. Defeathering machines with rubber finger-like projections beat the carcasses to remove feathers, a procedure that can pound feces out of the bird and into its skin.

Many large processing plants use automatic eviscerating machines to remove internal organs, including the chicken's intestines. While hand-eviscerating has the potential to be more exacting, machine-eviscerating has a higher likelihood to puncture the bird's intestines, further spreading contamination.

Federal inspectors then check each eviscerated bird before further processing, but in some plants, up to 91 chickens may pass through each minute, making it difficult, to say the least, to see much of anything. According to the National Academy of Science's 1987 report on the reliability of inspection systems used by the poultry industry, current procedures are old-fashioned and unscientific. Microorganisms such as salmonella cannot be seen by the naked eye; they must be evaluated by microbiological testing.

After the minimal inspection, birds are dropped into chill tanks to reduce their temperature to 40°F., thus introducing another opportunity for bacteria from one chicken to be transferred to others.

Stricter inspection rules were set for the poultry industry in 1994 to reduce the proliferation of salmonella. A "zero tolerance" standard was set for raw birds, allowing no visible feces to remain on poultry carcasses. Inspectors will have to reinspect every contaminated bird to make sure the feces have been removed. Processors will also be required to use a bacteria-reducing rinse before the bird is placed in the cold water bath that is used to quickly chill the birds after slaughter.

Food irradiation was approved by the FDA to kill bacteria on poultry. However, concerns of the general public over the potential formation of unknown radiolytic products has made the poultry industry shy away from irradiating their poultry.

In 1993, it was reported that scientists at the U.S. Department of Agriculture found that spraying trisodium phosphate on raw chicken and turkey before they leave the processing plant dramatically reduces the poultry's salmonella count. An additive used for years as an emulsifier in processed cheese, trisodium phosphate affects neither texture, taste, nor color of the poultry. Because it leaves little or no residue, it isn't required to be listed as an additive on the label.

HUMANE TREATMENT OF FARM ANIMALS

Despite the fact they may use hand-evisceration rather than by machine, there are no guarantees that naturally raised poultry is necessarily less likely to harbor salmonella. But there are several other aspects that make it a worthwhile option.

Except for the standard coccidiostat and initial vaccinations, natural poultry is never administered antibiotics. (Check your sources carefully. Some brands that advertise themselves as natural still use low levels of antibiotics to prevent intestinal infections in very young chicks.) If a flock does get sick and requires antibiotics to keep them alive, the entire flock is then sold on the commercial market.

Considering the optimum growing conditions producers of naturally raised poultry allow their flocks, antibiotics would rarely be needed in the first place.

Free-range poultry have access to both an enclosed poultry house that allows over twice the square footage per bird as provided in typical poultry production and an outdoor pen in which to freely roam and forage. Not only does the opportunity to engage in their natural behaviors result in less stress, the exercise makes for a leaner bird. A noticeable flavor difference can be attributed to longer maturation time and their ability to eat, in addition to their normal feed, tasty morsels they may find in the yard.

Housed but uncaged poultry are given similar amount of room within the poultry house, including roosts and the opportunity to scratch in rice hulls or shavings on the floors of the house. However, they do not have access to the outside, presumably to protect them from extreme variations in weather.

The success of naturally raised poultry demonstrates that poultry can and should be raised according to methods that allow for expression of their natural behaviors. Granted, while production for naturally raised poultry may not be as efficient in time and costs, it ultimately provides a better product for the consumer. Since we have access to several low-cost protein alternatives besides poultry, it wouldn't hurt us to pay a bit more for humanely raised poultry.

Retired caged laying hens that are used for stewing meat or for processed foods don't even get the privilege to be stunned before slaughter. Because their confinement to small cages usually makes the bones of laying hens too brittle from lack of exercise, retired laying hens are often not stunned

DON'T EAT PÂTÉ

In 1992, the United States imported 23 of the 10,000 tons of duck and goose liver pâté produced each year. Consumption of this very fatty "delicacy" might not be so high if consumers realized what it took to get the pâté on their plate.

About 25% of the geese raised for their down are also used for pâté production. In order to make sure the geese expend as few calories as possible, they are crowded 12 to a pen smaller than 2 square yards or 1 to a 10 x 15-inch cage to prevent movement, including stretching their wings or preening. Four times per day over a 3-week period, each goose is restrained between a worker's legs to shove a 12-16 inch tube down its throat. Huge amounts of salted fatty maize are then crammed down the tube via a pressurized pump. Some producers put an elastic band around the bird's neck to prevent regurgitation.

Ducks are similarly treated including the possibility of having their bills cauterized to minimize fighting injuries caused by the stress of overcrowding.

Eliminate the demand for liver-based pâté by refusing to buy it at your meat market, gourmet shop, or favorite restaurant. Instead, reach for the vegetable pâté or those made from chicken livers. It's hard to believe anything could taste so good that it was worth torturing a goose or duck in the process.

before slaughter for fear that the stunning will cause their bones to shatter, thus decreasing the economic value of their meat. Since the bones of retired free-range layers remain dense due to their ability to exercise, uncaged layers can be stunned before slaughter like other poultry raised for its meat—yet another reason to insist on eggs from uncaged hens.

HOW TO PREPARE AND COOK POULTRY

A general rule of thumb is to cook young birds with dry heat: roasted, broiled, grilled, or stir-fried. Older, less tender birds should be cooked with moist heat: braised or stewed. Be sure to cook raw poultry within 2-3 days.

Unlike beef, poultry is always cooked well-done to an internal temperature of 180 to 185° F. to ensure that all harmful bacteria are destroyed. A meat thermometer inserted into the bird's thigh or breast is the most accurate way of testing for doneness. Otherwise, cook until the juices run clear and the texture appears tender when the flesh is pierced with a fork. Cooked poultry can be stored in the refrigerator up to 4 days.

Preparation Methods

Roast: Place whole poultry breast side up or halves or parts skinside up in a shallow pan or roasting pan. Prick the skin of duck or goose with a fork to let fatty juices run out. On other poultry, brush skin with a light coating of oil. Rub the cavity with salt and dried herbs such as sage, thyme, or basil. Stuff or place quartered onion and celery in cavity. Cover loosely with foil, removing it 20 minutes before poultry is done in order to brown the meat. Roast at 325-350° F. for approximately 40 minutes per pound for poultry less than 8 lbs. and 20 minutes per pound for larger poultry.

Broil: Cut poultry into halves, quarters, or pieces, leaving the skin on to prevent excessive drying. Prick the skin on ducklings and parboil to allow fatty juices to escape and reduce the chance of flaring while broiling. Brush other poultry with oil or butter. Place them skinside down on a lightly oiled broiler rack several inches from the heat to permit slow cooking. During broiling, turn the pieces 2 or 3 times, brushing them with fat or barbeque sauce. Allow 20-30 minutes to broil chicken and 60-75 minutes for turkey and duckling.

Grill: For best results, use a covered grill. Remove part or all of the skin to reduce the chance of flare-ups due to fat dripping onto the coals. Marinades and frequent basting enhance flavor and tenderness.

White meat cooks quicker than dark, so put the dark meat on the grill about 15 minutes before adding wings or breasts. Count on 12-15 minutes per side for both leg/thigh pieces as well as bone-in breasts. Chicken wings and boneless breasts take the least amount of time to cook, only about 5 minutes per side. Cook chicken or turkey burgers 4-6 minutes per side, until no pink is visible in the interior.

Stir-fry: Slice meat into thin, uniform slices, strips, or pieces. Chicken tenders are perfect. Marinate, if desired, while preparing vegetables. Stir-fry poultry first in a small amount of oil. (You may need to stir-fry half of it at a time.) Cook over medium-high to high temperature, stirring meat continuously until no pink is visible in the interior. Set aside and stir-fry vegetables. Return cooked poultry to the wok to mix with vegetables and briefly reheat.

Steam: Place young, tender poultry on a rack or steaming basket above 1 inch of steaming water. Cover the pot and steam parts for 45 minutes and whole birds for 11/2 hours. Add extra boiling water, if necessary.

Braise: Braise whole or cut-up poultry, onions, carrots, and desired seasonings in a heavy pan placed in a 325° F. oven or over medium heat on the stove. Cover with a tight-fitting lid to allow it to steam in the juices that will be released during cooking. To brown: sauté pieces in a small amount of oil before cooking on top of the stove. If braising in the oven, you can also remove the lid during the last 30 minutes of cooking.

Stewing: Place poultry in enough water to cover and season with onions, celery, and herbs. Cover, bring to a boil, and then reduce heat, simmering approximately 2 hours until tender.

Cooking With Ground Poultry:

Recipes such as lasagna, spaghetti, chili, and casseroles that traditionally use ground beef can easily be substituted with ground poultry with little difference in flavor, appearance, or preparation. Although ground turkey can be used with no modifications necessary, recipes using the milder-flavored ground chicken may benefit from more seasoning and perhaps a sauce or seasoning mix to mask its light color.

Both ground turkey and chicken can also be used made into patties or meat loaves. However, since they are so low in fat, pans and skillets need to be greased with extra oil or butter to prevent sticking.

Exploring Your Options

The term poultry includes not only chicken and turkey, but also Rock Cornish hen, duck, goose, and various game birds. Types within each classification are categorized according to their sex, age at slaughter, and size.

Grading is optional, rating only cosmetic features of the poultry such as conformation, lack of pinfeathers, cuts, tears, blemishes, as well as disjointed or broken bones. Grade A poultry is meaty with unbroken skin. Grade B poultry is more bony with slightly flawed skin.

CHICKEN

Facts and Features

There's no doubt that chicken is the most popular of all poultry. The younger the chicken, the more tender the results. Look for naturally raised, free-range chickens in your grocery store or buy them dressed, directly from farms that raise their chickens in a humane manner.

Varieties and Cooking Guidelines

A **broiler/fryer** chicken is about 7-9 weeks old of either sex, weighing between 3 and 41/2 lbs. As its name implies, it is best broiled or fried but can also be roasted, steamed, or poached.

A **capon** is a castrated male chicken about 4-5 months old, weighing 5-9 lbs. Due to its higher fat content, it is delicate and tender. Roast for best results.

A **roaster** chicken is about 3-5 months old of either sex, weighing between 41/2 and 8 lbs. With more meat per pound and more fat under the skin to make it juicy, roasting is the best cooking method.

HOW MUCH POULTRY TO BUY PER PERSON

Chicken
broiler/fryer, bone-in	3/4-1 lb.
bone-less	1/3-1/2 lb.
capon	1/2 lb.
roaster	1/2 lb.
Rock Cornish hen	1 bird

Turkey
fryer/roaster	3/4-1 lb.
hen/tom	1/2-3/4 lb.

Ground Poultry
	1/4 lb.

Duck/Goose
	1 lb.

A **Rock Cornish hen** is 5-6 weeks old of either sex, weighing 1-2 lbs. It is a cross between the Plymouth Rock chicken and Cornish gamecock, developed to be small but extra meaty. Roast, split and grill, or broil.

A **stewing hen** is a retired laying hen (female, of course) 10 months of age or older, weighing 3-7 lbs. Although it is the most flavorful of the bunch, the meat is tough, requiring long, slow, moist cooking or stewing to tenderize.

TURKEY

Facts and Features

Turkey is no longer just for the holidays; you'll find it in good supply throughout the year, particularly frozen. Look for naturally raised turkeys that have never been administered antibiotics. Pay special attention to labels to avoid turkey that is injected with basting solutions.

Varieties and Cooking Guidelines

A **fryer/roaster** turkey is about 10-16 weeks old of either sex, weighing 5-8 lbs. The most tender of turkeys, fryer/roasters are also the most expensive per pound.

A **young hen** (female) or **young tom** (male) are 4-7 months old, weighing between 8-20 lbs. Both are tender and well suited to roasting.

A **yearling tom** is a 6-12 month old male turkey, weighing more than 20 lbs. Due to its age, its meat is more tough. Roast or simmer.

Rolled turkey roast is boned and tied white or combination dark/white turkey meat.

GOOSE

Facts and Features

Although goose is most plentiful around the holidays, you'll likely find it frozen throughout the year. The younger the goose, the more tender the results.

Varieties and Cooking Guidelines

A **mature goose** is more than 6 months old of either sex, weighing more than 14 lbs. Less tender than a gosling, it is best braised.

A **young goose (gosling)** is less than 6 months old of either sex, weighing between 5-12 lbs. Best roasted.

DUCK

Facts and Features

Like goose, duck is most plentiful around the holidays but usually available frozen throughout the year.

FOOD SAFETY TIPS

The use of proper cooking, cleanliness, and storage methods at home can control the spread of salmonella and other harmful pathogens. Just follow these simple rules:

•Keep foods refrigerated. Be sure the interim time from purchase to home refrigeration is minimal and consider transporting them in an ice chest during the hot weather.

•Thaw frozen poultry only in the refrigerator, never at room temperature. Use the chart below to plan how much time you'll need before your actual preparation can begin.

•Be sure to thoroughly wash your hands, kitchen counter tops, utensils, dishes, and cutting boards with soap and hot water after contact with raw proteins.

•Do not allow foods to stand at room temperature for more than two hours after cooking. Bacteria thrive at temperatures between 45-115° so keep foods either below 40° or above 140°.

Stuff poultry immediately before roasting, not ahead of time. Otherwise, bacteria from the raw poultry juices inside the cavity can cause bacteria to begin to grow within the stuffing. After cooking, remove the stuffing and serve or refrigerate separately.

TYPE OF POULTRY	REFRIGERATOR THAWING TIME
Chicken:	
less than 4 lbs.	12-24 hours
more than 4 lbs.	1-1 1/2 days
Rock Cornish hen	12 hours
Turkey:	
4-12 lb.	1-2 days
12-20 lb.	2-3 days
20-24 lb.	3-3 1/2 days
halves, quarters, breasts	1-2 days
cut up pieces	3-9 hours
Duck, Goose:	1-1 1/2 days

Varieties and Cooking Guidelines

A **broiler/fryer Pekin or Long Island duck** is 7-8 weeks old of either sex, weighing less than 3 lbs. Very tender, it is best broiled or fried.

A **roaster duck** is 8-16 weeks old of either sex, weighing 3-6 lbs. Roast or braise.

GAME BIRDS

Facts and Features

Game birds are imported wild or domestically raised. By law, wild birds caught in the United States cannot be sold directly to consumers or restaurants.

Varieties and Cooking Guidelines

Guinea hen (female) are sold when 2-3 lbs. Tender, delicate, and very lean, they are good roasted, braised, or poached.

Partridge are smaller than pheasant, about 1-3 lbs. and more strongly flavored. Young partridge, weighing 1-1 1/2 lbs., can be roasted or sauteed. Older partridge are best braised or stewed.

Pheasant, usually farm-raised and sold

CHICKEN TERIYAKI

2½-3 lb. chicken thigh/
leg quarters (remove
skin to reduce fat)
1/4 cup tamari shoyu
1 inch ginger root, grated
1 Tbsp. honey or rice
syrup
2 Tbsp vinegar or lemon
juice
1/3 cup water
2 cloves garlic, minced
2 tsp. arrowroot
2 Tbsp. cold water

Wash chicken and cut into serving pieces. Combine shoyu, ginger, rice syrup, vinegar, water, and garlic. Place chicken in a mixing bowl and mix in marinade. Cover bowl and refrigerate overnight or at least 6 hours. Just before cooking, preheat oven to 325°. Remove chicken from bowl and place in a baking dish, skin side up, reserving marinade. Bake uncovered for 1½ hours, basting with 1/4 of the marinade every 20 minutes until marinade is used.

To thicken marinade for a gravy, dissolve arrowroot in cold water. Pour hot marinade into saucepan and add diluted arrowroot. Bring to a boil, reduce heat, and stir constantly until thickened.

Nutrition Facts

Serving Size 1/4 recipe (346 g)
Servings Per Container 4

Amount Per Serving

Calories 380   Calories from Fat 100

	% Daily Value*
Total Fat 11g	17%
Saturated Fat 3g	14%
Cholesterol 235mg	78%
Sodium 1190mg	49%
Total Carbohydrate 8g	3%
Sugars 5g	
Protein 58g	

Vitamin A 4%	•	Vitamin C 8%
Calcium 4%	•	Iron 15%

Not a significant source of Dietary Fiber
* Percent Daily Values are based on a 2,000 calorie diet.

Pour marinade over chicken or transfer to a gravy boat and allow guests to serve themselves.

Serves 4
(Pyramid servings: 3 Meat/Protein Group, 11 grams Fat, 3 grams)

when 2-4 lbs., are very lean, flavorful birds best roasted or braised.

Quail of either sex are very small, about 6-8 oz. Roast, grill, braise, or saute, being careful not to overcook.

Squab are 4-week-old pigeons of either sex, weighing less than 1 lb. Not even old enough to fly, squab is very tender. Roast or braise.

BASIC TURKEY BURGERS/SAUSAGE

1 lb. ground turkey
1/2 tsp. pepper
1 tsp. sage
Optional condiments:
    sautéed onions, pesto,
    salsa, grilled peppers,
    mustard, grilled
    mushrooms, etc.

Combine all ingredients and mix well. Refrigerate for a few hours or overnight to let the flavors mingle and develop. Shape into 4 patties. Lightly oil a skillet and cook over medium heat until done.

Variations: Replace sage with Italian seasoning or any other favorite combination. Zip it up with 1/4 tsp. cayenne pepper. Add garlic for depth.

    Patties may be formed, wrapped individually without precooking, and frozen until needed.

Nutrition Facts

Serving Size 1/4 recipe (114 g)
Servings Per Container 4

Amount Per Serving

Calories 170   Calories from Fat 80

	% Daily Value*
Total Fat 9g	14%
Saturated Fat 2.5g	13%
Cholesterol 90mg	30%
Sodium 390mg	16%
Total Carbohydrate 0g	0%
Protein 20g	

Calcium 2%	•	Iron 8%

Not a significant source of Dietary Fiber, Sugars, Vitamin A and Vitamin C.

* Percent Daily Values are based on a 2,000 calorie diet.

Serves 4.
(Pyramid servings: 11/2 Meat/Protein Group, 9 grams Fat)

Fish and Seafood

Seafood consumption has soared within the last several years. While its ease of preparation and versatility no doubt have played a large part in its widespread acceptance, its nutritional attributes are equally responsible for much of seafood's acclaim.

NUTRITION

Tops on the list is its high protein, low saturated fat content. Seafood is also a good source of vitamins B_6, B_{12}, and niacin, selenium, zinc, and (in saltwater types) iodine.

As a general rule, seafood contains moderate amounts of cholesterol, slightly lower than meat and poultry. Some shellfish, however, such as shrimp, crab, oysters, may contain up to twice as much cholesterol. Fortunately, they are also extremely low in saturated fat, creating a balance to negate what could have made them sure fuel for heart disease. The presence of a unique kind of fat in seafood, omega-3 fatty acids, reduces the odds even more.

Omega-3 Fatty Acids

As one of two essential fatty acids we must obtain from food, the omega-3 variety or alpha-linolenic acid serves as building blocks for hormone-like compounds (prostaglandins) that influence several important functions within the body. Of particular interest is the ability of one of the omega-3 fatty acids, eicosapentenoic acid (EPA), to cancel out a prostaglandin called thromboxane that promotes clotting of blood.

While the blood's ability to clot is important to stop the flow of blood when we are injured, a blood clot can also attach to a damaged artery wall and combine with white blood cells and cholesterol to form plaque, gradually growing until it cuts off the flow of blood. When it lodges in an artery of the heart, the result is a heart attack. When it affects an artery in the brain, it is known as a stroke.

EPA interferes with thromboxane by making the blood platelets less sticky so that it takes longer for blood to clot. Therefore, it's likely that a diet that includes foods high in omega-3 fatty acids, such as seafood, could help decrease the incidence of heart attacks and strokes.

And there's more benefit to omega-3 fatty acids. EPA also appears to boost the immune system. Another one of the omega-3 fatty acids, docosahexaenoic acid (DHA), is found in high amounts in the brain and retina, further emphasizing how essential it is for us to eat foods that are good sources of omega-3 fatty acids for proper development.

Cold deep-water fish, including sardines, salmon, mackerel, tuna, and herring contain the most omega-3 fatty acids. In cold fresh water fish, look to rainbow trout. Leaner fish like cod, flounder, and haddock contain small amounts.

What's a Serving?

According to the Food Guide Pyramid, 2-3 ounces of fish constitutes a serving. Four ounces of raw boned fish will yield approximately 3 ounces cooked.

Technically, your protein requirements could easily be met if you consumed 2 to 3 servings of fish per day for a total equivalent amount of protein as found in 5-7 ounces of cooked lean meat, poultry, or fish. However, for best overall nutrition, vary your protein sources, including cooked dried beans, peas, and even some nuts and seeds within your menus.

CANNED FISH

Canning is an effective way to preserve and store fish, a system typically used for processing tuna, salmon, anchovies, sardines, clams, and crab meat. Optimum shelf life is one year. Stored any longer, the fish may take on a strong flavor and odor. Once opened, canned fish should be stored in a tightly covered container and used within 3-5 days.

Canned **tuna** is most apt to be in the pantry of anyone who includes fish in his/her diet. Most desirable is tuna packed in water, with or without salt. While water-packed tuna has only 1 gram of fat per 3 oz. serving, tuna packed in oil and drained contains 7 grams of fat for the same amount.

Tuna can also be processed in vegetable broth and hydrolyzed vegetable protein to enhance flavor. Except for adding a great deal of sodium to the tuna, neither are necessarily bad additives, but neither are they necessary if the tuna is of good quality in the first place. Individuals allergic to soybeans may have difficulty with hydrolyzed vegetable protein as it is a highly refined additive generally made from soy.

It takes 20 lbs. of fresh tuna to make about 24 cans. Light chunk tuna can include two or more species of tuna. More expensive albacore, sold as "solid white or chunk white tuna, is suitable for substituting in dishes that call for cooked chicken breast.

Although over 90% of tuna is caught where dolphins are not threatened by the commercial tuna industry, fishermen in the Eastern Tropical Pacific who took advantage of the companionship that exists between dolphins and yellowfin tuna nearly made, for many individuals, the purchase of tuna a thing of the past.

For reasons still unknown, schools of spotted dolphins, spinner dolphins, and common dolphins travel in company with yellowfin tuna in a six million square mile area that includes the warm waters west of Mexico, Central America, Columbia, Ecuador, Peru, and northern Chile. When a school of dolphin was sighted, speedboats were lowered from the side of the large tuna vessels. Aided by noisy underwater explosives to frighten and disorient the dolphins, the speedboats corraled the dolphins into a circle. The ship then surrounded the exhausted and confused dolphins with a huge purse seine net. Four hundred fifty feet deep and up to a mile long, the net is equipped with floats on the top and weights and rings along the bottom edge. A cable called a purse line runs through the rings. With the cables drawing the bottom closed, similar to pulling the drawstrings of a purse, the dolphins were trapped along with the tuna. Helplessly entangled in the nets underwater and deprived of the fresh air they require to breathe, the dolphins would drown, be badly mutilated, or crushed.

Since 1959, 6.5 million dolphins have been ensnared and needlessly killed in nets intended to catch yellowfin tuna. Attempts to legally protect dolphins met with limited success. In response to public outrage, the Marine Mammal Protection Act was passed by Congress, placing a moratorium on the deliberate killing of dolphin and other marine mammals. Yearly quotas were introduced with the intent to reach zero mortality.

Unfortunately, many of the tuna boats formerly under the flag of the United States re-flagged under another country to avoid restricting regulations and high operating and labor costs. Recognizing the trend, Congress reauthorized the Marine Mammal Protection Act in 1988, stipulating that by 1991, any company who exports tuna to the U.S. must have dolphin mortality less than 1.25 times the U.S. rate.

In 1989, consumer and environmental groups waged a nation-wide moratorium on the purchase of all brands of canned chunk light tuna and a massive letter-writing campaign denouncing the practice of major tuna companies buying tuna caught by the purse-seining method.

In the spring of 1990, Starkist Tuna succumbed to public pressure and announced that they would stop buying any tuna caught in association with dolphins in the Eastern Tropical Pacific. In addition, they would not buy any tuna caught by gill or drift nets, fishing methods that are known to be dangerous to dolphins and many types of marine life. The other tuna companies followed suit soon after.

Thanks to the power of consumer demand, any canned tuna you buy from any major tuna company is now dolphin-friendly. For extra assurance, look for the telltale dolphin-friendly insignia on the can. You'll probably also notice the "solid light" or "chunk light" tuna you buy is darker in color. That's because tuna fishermen will likely avoid the lighter-colored yellowfin tuna in favor of the darker varieties that don't swim with the dolphins.

Sardines are usually packed in salted or unsalted brine, oil (olive, cottonseed, non-descript vegetable oil, or soybean oil), or in sauces (tomato, mustard, garlic, curry, and chili). To avoid extra fat as well as solvent-extracted oils, go for the brine or sauce-packed varieties.

It's a little-known fact, but there is no such fish specifically named sardine. Derived from the name of a Mediterranean island, Sardinia, it is a term used to refer to various kinds of small fish once they are processed and canned.

Sardines from Denmark and Norway generally use brislings and silds. Those from France, Portugal, and Spain use pilchards, a smaller and fatter relative of herrings. Maine and Eastern Canadian sardines are derived from small herrings. All are an excellent source of omega-3 fatty acids.

SMOKED FISH

Curing fish with smoke and salt has been used for centuries as a way to preserve fish for months. Now, with refrigeration readily available, most smoked fish is cured with a different process that concentrates on flavor rather than preservation.

The fish is first salted down or placed in brine to bring out flavor as well as help preserve the fish. Sodium nitrites may also be used by some producers to give their fish a desired color and moistness. The flip side of its use, however, is that under certain cooking conditions, nitrites are converted to nitrosamines, introducing a potentially carcinogenic situation. Your best bet is to look for smoked fish free of nitrites.

After brining, the fish is hung in breezy, cool air to allow excess brine to drip from the flesh and to make the surface look glossy. Then it is ready for either cold or hot smoking.

Cold smoked fish is processed at temperatures between 70° and 90° F. for 6-16 hours, yielding a moist, flavorful result.

Hot smoked fish is processed at temperatures between 120° to 200° F. for up to 12 hours. As this essentially cooks the fish, the moisture content is reduced, yielding a more firm, dry texture with a slightly less rich flavor.

Since they are not processed enough to allow them to be fully preserved, fish smoked either way must be refrigerated like other fresh seafoods. Because they are soaked in a salt brine before smoking, they will last for as long as 2-3 weeks in the refrigerator.

Smoked fish sent through mail-order specialty houses need no refrigeration until their special packaging is opened. Although it may be hard to imagine how the fish inside could be safe to eat, they are processed similar to canned fish except the "can" is a thin metallic pouch.

SURIMI

Somewhat new on the market is surimi, imitation crabmeat, scallops, and lobster made from lean white fish, sugar, sorbitol, salt, water, egg whites, starch, natural and artificial colors, and natural and artificial flavors. Once made into a paste, it is then molded, cooked, and cut into the desired shapes.

Since they are precooked they are ready to eat, hot or cold. Open packages should be used within 3-5 days.

However, given the presence of sugars, artificial colors, and artificial flavors, it's hard to understand why anyone would even bother buying such a fabricated food. If its convenience is the reason you may choose to buy surimi, do yourself a big favor and stick to canned, smoked fish, or any of the many good-quality frozen fish sticks or medallions that are based on fish, grains, and natural seasonings.

FOOD SAFETY CONCERNS

Unfortunately, the positive nutritional aspects of seafood are often overshadowed by media reports concerning the polluted waters from which seafood is fished, microbiological hazards, the natural toxins associated with some species, and parasites.

Polluted Waters

Runoff from industry and agriculture as well as accidental and illegal dumping of the more than 65,000 chemical compounds used worldwide has contaminated and, in many cases, annihilated several species of seafood. Fish from lakes and rivers have a higher probability of chemical contaminants than ocean fish since the ocean's great expanse helps dilute the effects of pollution. However, the "cleaner" attributes of ocean fish correspond only to seafood from areas hundreds of miles from shore. Ocean species caught near shore in industrial areas are best avoided.

Toxic substances from industrial pollution have persisted within our environment, entering the food chain at its most basic level, photosynthetic producer organisms. At each successive stage of the food chain, from small plant-eating fish to larger fish who eat them, to humans who consume the various types of seafood, the toxins progressively accumulate in fatty tissues. Sometimes the effects are so toxic that symptoms manifest upon ingestion. Most of the time, it goes unnoticed until one's immune system reaches the saturation point.

A prime example is **polychlorinated biphenyls (PCBs)**, synthetic fluids once used in electrical equipment such as transformers and condensers. Although banned in 1977 as a toxic substance, their legacy continues in waters polluted by the many industries that used them. Accidental leaks of PCBs into the food supply in the past left those contaminated with fatigue, headache, nausea, skin eruptions, and liver disorders. Chronic exposure to PCBs has been linked with cancer and fetal abnormalities. Because PCBs tend to concentrate in the fatty tissues, species of fish relatively higher in fat such as salmon, swordfish, bluefish, and lake whitefish fished near industrial areas are most suspect.

Another product of industrial pollution is the discharge of **mercury** into some waterways. Initially released as inorganic mercury, bacteria in the water convert it into its more readily absorbed and toxic form, methylmercury. High exposure can adversely affect the maturation and maintenance of the nervous system, impairing vision, coordination, and intellectual development. Longer-lived fish, such as swordfish and tuna that tend to accumulate a higher concentration of mercury from their consumption of organisms lower in the food chain, are most often implicated.

Contamination from **agricultural chemicals** has also wreaked havoc in our lakes, rivers, and streams. Insecticides, herbicides, fungicides, and rodenticides were initially developed for maximum persistence to be able to withstand rain, sunlight, and time. Unfortunately, what may have seemed to be a good idea has left present and future generations with lifetime exposure to the biological effects of pesticides: nerve damage, liver toxicity, and cancer.

Despite being banned for use in 1972, DDT continues to show up not only in farmland and waterways but also in the fatty tissues of birds and fish and even human breast milk. But DDT is only one example. More and more commonly used pesticides are undergoing toxicity testing that should have been done long ago. Unfortunately, the results aren't too comforting. What's been used on the land often ends up in the water and, ultimately, in fish.

Microbiological Hazards

Also linked to polluted waters are the bacteria and viruses found in molluscan shellfish that are harvested from coastal waters contaminated by untreated sewage. Consumption of raw or undercooked clams, mussels, and oysters harvested from these waters can result in hepatitis, cholera, typhoid, and general gastroenteritis.

Oysters, mussels, clams, and scallops are also susceptible to microorganisms originating from the dramatic increase of certain types of phytoplankton during late summer and early autumn. Known as "red tide," it produces toxins in the shellfish that eat them. Individuals who then consume the affected shellfish set themselves up for paralytic shellfish poisoning (PSP) which attacks the nervous system, particularly breathing and muscle control.

Listeria monocytogenes is a common bacterium found in soil, water, and raw molluscan shellfish. Infections rarely occur except in pregnant women (causing spontaneous abortions, miscarriages, and stillbirths) and in individuals with weakened immune systems. Since thorough cooking destroys the bacterium, shellfish should never be consumed raw by these groups, or, to be very safe, by anyone.

Vibrio vulnificus is another bacterium that appears in some waters during April through October. The immune systems of most healthy individuals can destroy these infections; however, those with weakened immune systems suffering from cancer, AIDS, alcohol abuse, liver disease, chronic kidney disease, or inflammatory bowel disease are at high risk for a serious infection which can be fatal. Like Listeria monocytogenes, thorough cooking kills the Vibrio bacteria, another reason why eating raw shellfish may not be the best idea.

While the microbiological hazards listed above are linked only with molluscan shellfish, finfish can also be carriers of harmful bacteria. Cinguatera is an illness associated with the consumption of coral reef fish such as barracuda, amberjack, and some grouper and snapper species. Occurring only sporadically in these fish, it is caused by the accumulation of toxins originating from the fish's consumption of dinoflagellate algae as well as smaller fish that may have consumed the same. Symptoms can last for weeks, including nausea, vomiting, and numbness around the mouth and lips. Cooking does not destroy the toxin.

Scombroid fish poisoning is caused by a bacteria found in fish that naturally contain high levels of the amino acid histidine in their flesh, including mackerel, bonito, skipjack, tuna and swordfish. Unlike other types of natural fish toxins, scombroid poisoning only appears when these fish are held at warm temperatures for several hours after capture. Therefore, occurrences are indicative of poor handling practices. Symptoms such as nausea, headache, dizziness, diarrhea, and flushing usually last no more than 24 hours. Cooking does not destroy the toxin.

Parasites

Roundworms, tapeworms, and flatworms can be found in many species of fish, particularly in swordfish, cod, black sea bass, and calico scallops.

Before you completely write these and other seafood off your list in fear of parasites, it is important to note that all parasites can be destroyed either with thorough cooking or thorough freezing at 0° F. for a week.

Good seafood packing houses also routinely "candle" fillets by holding fillets in front of a light. Parasites that are sighted can easily be removed.

Most problems people have had with infections or illness from seafood parasites have been from eating raw seafood, including sushi, sashimi, gravalax, and seviche. If you want to continue eating these entrees made from raw fish, make sure whoever has prepared them has used fish that has previously been thoroughly frozen.

How to Choose Safe Seafood

As pervasive and frightening as environmental and microbiological contamination may seem, high-quality, safe seafood is readily available. But you need to know what questions you should ask before buying a particular type of seafood and what to expect in regard to cleanliness and food safety standards.

Because the effects of pollution linger in our waterways, it's critical that you inquire about the source of the fish you choose to eat. This is especially true when buying molluscan shellfish: oysters, clams, and mussels. As filter feeders, they sit in one place and eat whatever they can filter from the water in which they live each day, including toxins, sewage, and residual pollutants. No matter whether you're buying finfish or shellfish, your best bet is to buy seafood that is harvested as far away as possible from industrial or agricultural areas.

Eat a variety of fish rather than concentrating on one type. The smaller and younger the fish, the less toxins they likely will have accumulated. Consumption of species that may be candidates for PCB or mercury contamination should be limited to once per week. Pregnant and lactating women should avoid them entirely to protect developing nervous systems in fetuses and infants which are most sensitive to the effects of PCB or mercury accumulation.

Buy shellfish only from reputable dealers who buy from harvesters licensed with the National Shellfish Sanitation Program (NSSP). This certification program is a cooperative venture between the FDA, the shellfish industry, and the states in which shellfish is harvested. Each state is responsible for adopting laws and regulations that ensure sanitary control over the growing, harvesting, shucking, packing, and interstate transportation of shellfish. Likewise, waters must meet certain purity standards before certified shellfish can be harvested. The FDA then sends out a monthly list of all shellfish shippers certified by states that comply with the standards. The program also includes a tagging system to provide an audit trail that makes it easy to track back to the source any problems, should they occur in distribution and handling.

In an attempt to improve the food safety record of seafood, the FDA now requires all seafood processors, packers, and warehouses, both domestic and foreign, to implement a written quality-assurance plan. Called the Hazard Analysis Critical Control Point program, or HACCP (pronounced **ha**-sup), it includes an analysis of potential hazards, identification of the critical control points that must be controlled to minimize the risk, itemization of the procedures to monitor each of the critical control points, and a record-keeping system to document the monitoring of the critical control points. At least one staff person must have completed a course in the application of HACCP principles to seafood processing.

A good fish market will also have adopted a thorough HACCP plan for good sanitation and handling procedures. While few of us have the opportunity to inspect the boats and processing plants that produce the fish we buy, the conditions at your local fish market can give a good clue as to the quality they demand from their suppliers. Odor within the department should be mildly seaweedy, not a strong, fishy smell. The display case should look spotlessly clean with no signs of old, encrusted pieces of seafood in the corners. Whole fish should be mixed with ice that has been changed and replenished every day. Rather than placed directly on ice, fillets should be in clean metal or plastic containers to protect their texture and appearance. Cooked fish products should be separated from raw fish.

Clerks should wear clean aprons, gloves, and hats. Utensils used to serve the fish should be immaculate and used only for one particular type, unless washed after each use. Knives should be washed immediately after each use to prevent cross-contamination.

Each of these criteria can and should be fulfilled by any size of seafood retailing operation. Don't settle for less.

HOW FRESH IS FRESH?

Technically, "fresh" fish has never been frozen or subjected to any heat treatment. Using that criterion, fresh fish is very abundant. However, when most people ask for fresh fish, they are expecting to get fish freshly caught and marketed in its optimum, unspoiled condition. On this basis, "fresh" fish is often the exception.

Under proper temperature control, between 30-32° F., lean fish have a maximum refrigerated life of 10-12 days. Oily fish have an even shorter span: 6-8 days. When you consider that most fish are caught by crews who spend several days at a time out at sea, along with another 2-3 days in the distribution network, not to mention time spent on display in the retail store, that "fresh" fish can be over a week old before you buy it and very close to being over the hill in terms of taste and appearance.

Errors or fluctuations in temperature control at any step in the process will reduce "freshness" even more. Each 4° F. increase in temperature beyond the ideal 32° F. ages the fish an equivalent of another 1/2 day. Considering that the average temperature in a home refrigerator is between 35-40° F., it's extremely important to buy very fresh fish and use it within a day.

In addition to knowing how many days it has been since the fish has been caught, another guide to freshness is the appearance of the fish. Whole fish should have eyes that are convex, not sunken, and the skin should be shiny. Fillets should be translucent and light in color, not yellowed or dark. The flesh should be firm and springy when pressed. Clams, mussels, and oysters should be alive with shells that are tightly closed or close upon handling.

Unfortunately, fish are often dipped in chemical solutions to enhance the appearance of freshness. Some scallops and fillets are soaked in sodium tripolyphosphate to reduce moisture loss that occurs as the fish begins to age. While relatively harmless to one's health, the sodium tripolyphosphate soak can cause a gain in water weight to the point that you may be paying more for water than fish. It also tends to whiten surface color, making some fish appear fresher than they may be. Too much sodium tripolyphosphate can make the fish tough in texture and even cover up the odor of a too-old fish.

Chlorine and water dips may also be used to brighten the color and hide the odor of old fish. Although its appearance may look renewed, once cooked, one taste will reveal its true age. Obviously, fish markets that engage in this practice should be avoided. Since no vendor would proudly advertise the use of chlorine dips, it's important to ask before buying.

Sulfites (sulfur dioxide, potassium or sodium bisulphite, potassium or sodium metabisulfite) are often used to help prevent or bleach out a black pigment on shrimp shells called melanosis or "black spot." This discoloration is the result of a natural chemical reaction that occurs in warm water shrimp if not properly rinsed and iced once their heads are removed. Melanosis is harmless, similar to the blackening of a banana peel as it ripens; however, its presence could indicate poor handling from the shrimp being left out too long in warm temperatures after being caught.

The legal limit of sulfites on shrimp is 100 parts per million, high enough to cause allergic reactions in sensitive individuals.

HOW MUCH FISH TO BUY PER PERSON

whole fish (unprepared, as taken from water)	3/4-1 lb.
dressed fish (gutted & scaled w/ head, fins, and gills removed)	1/2-3/4 lb.
steaks (sliced crosswise w/ a section of back-bone and skin)	1/3-1/2 lb.
fillets (boneless sides of fish)	1/4-1/3 lb.

Asthmatics are particularly at risk. Symptoms may include hives, shortness of breath, cramps, abdominal pain, diarrhea, anaphylactic shock, and, in those most sensitive, possibly death.

Frozen shrimp are more likely to be sulfited than fresh or farm-raised shrimp that are processed quickly after harvest, so look closely at the package label before buying. If thawed previously-frozen fish is displayed for sale in your fish market's cooler case, ask to see its original packaging before purchasing. Clams, scallops, lobsters, and dried cod may also be sulfited.

A NEW LOOK AT FROZEN FISH

Although in years past frozen fish was considered low-quality and second-rate, the realities that "fresh" seafood may be several days old and, in some cases, treated with preservatives to extend "cooler life," has led to a newfound respect for properly frozen fish.

Many modern fishing boats are equipped with state-of-the-art freezing equipment to enable crews to freeze fish on board within minutes of being caught. New technologies have greatly enhanced the quality of frozen fish, such as the IQF (individually quick frozen) method which freezes each fillet as individual units rather than freezing several into a block.

Freshly frozen fish retains most of its fresh flavor. Fish that has been frozen several days after capture has already deteriorated in flavor and often has a tough and rubbery texture.

When purchasing frozen fish, look for solidly frozen, tightly wrapped packages free of discoloration and excessive ice buildup.

If freezing fish at home, freeze only fish you are absolutely sure is very fresh. If your fish market uses specially coated paper designed to retain moisture, keep it in its original wrapper.

Raw lean fish such as catfish, cod, flounder, haddock, halibut, monkfish, ocean perch, pike, orange roughie, shark, and snapper can be frozen up to 6 months.

Since their fat can turn rancid if stored too long, raw fish with moderate or high fat content such as barracuda, bluefish, bonito, mackerel, mahi-mahi, salmon, striped bass, sturgeon, swordfish, lake trout, rainbow trout, tuna, and whitefish should be frozen no longer than 3 months.

Previously cooked fish, whether from lean or fatty fish, should be used within 3 months.

Raw shrimp can be frozen for up to 6 months while previously cooked shrimp (as well as lobster and crayfish) should be used within 2 months after freezing. Other types of shellfish, squid, and frogs' legs, can be stored in the freezer for up to 3 months.

Thaw frozen fish only in the refrigera-tor, NOT AT ROOM TEMPERATURE. Allow about 24 hours for a 1 lb. package. To retain more juices and moisture, do not thaw frozen fish completely. If a quick thaw is needed, place the fish in a "zipper-lock" type plastic bag and place in a pan of cold water in the refrigerator. Use thawed frozen fish within 24 hours.

Fish under 2" thick doesn't even need to be thawed before preparation. Just allow twice the cooking time.

AQUACULTURE

Aquaculture is the cultivation of seafood in ponds, cages, or pens anchored in natural bodies of water or in man-made tanks supplied with filtered and oxygenated water. Although aquafarming has been practiced for centuries in other cultures around the world, its use is just beginning to catch on in the United States as a viable way to deal with polluted waters and the diminishing natural supply of seafood due to overfishing.

There are several benefits to aquaculture. Most aquaculture seafood is delivered to the processing plant alive, thus eliminating the timing and freshness problem prevalent in harvesting and processing "fresh," wild-caught fish.

Areas unsuitable for other types of food production can be used for aquaculture. Many farmers are switching to raising fish since they convert feed to body tissue more efficiently than cows, sheep, and pigs.

They can also be selectively bred for flavor, texture, and nutrition, including omega-3 fatty acid content. When compared nutritionally to wild fish, the farm-raised varieties are normally somewhat higher in both saturated and unsaturated fat due to the feed they are deliberately fed.

Seafood commonly "farmed" in the United States includes catfish, tilapia, rainbow trout, crawfish, shrimp, mussels, clams, oysters, striped bass, and salmon.

However, there are some drawbacks to the aquaculture process. Since the fish are confined to a small area, they produce a greater density of wastes than do their counterparts in the wild, creating a special challenge to deal with it effectively and environmentally. Related is the excessive use of precious area water supplies by some operations.

The confinement of fish in a small, unnatural environment as found in some operations may also present a form of cruelty and lead unnecessarily to the use of chemicals, similar to intensive livestock agriculture. In fact, over thirty chemicals are allowed in production, including antibiotics, disinfectants, fungicides, parasiticides, chemicals to control algae blooms, and, sadly enough, anesthetics to reduce stress on fish resulting from crowded conditions.

Dyes to improve the flesh color in fish are also used. Salmon naturally obtain their deep pink flesh color from eating microcrustaceans. In contrast, farmed salmon is commonly fed a synthetically derived source to emulate the desired color.

Several unique aquaculture operations have addressed most of the negative aspects that plague many other aquafarms. AquaFutre in Montague, Massachusetts, grows salad greens and herbs hydroponically above their fish tanks, using a special medium that uses 1/3 of the fish waste for fertilizer. The water in which fish are grown is recycled 30 times per day through physiological and biological means. Bacteria similar to those found in compost piles that break down plant material into humus are used at AquaFutre to decompose the fish waste. The water is also oxgenated and ozonated to provide not only a better environment for the fish, but to purify the water as well. No antibiotics, hormones, pesticides, or other chemicals are needed.

Nor are they used at Sea Run Steelhead Salmon in Kennebunkport, Maine. Their

HOW TO DECIPHER SHRIMP SIZING

Shrimp is sized by the number per pound. Larger sizes are more expensive, worth the price depending on how you plan to serve the fish and on how patient you are with shelling. Nevertheless, after they are cooked and peeled, you'll get the same amount of edible shrimp once they are cooked and peeled, no matter what size you buy. In general, gauge on buying 1/4 lb. per person.

Size	Number of shrimp per pound
extra colossal	under 10
colossal	under 15
extra jumbo	16-20
jumbo	21-25
extra large	26-30
large	31-35
medium large	36-40
medium	41-50
small	51-60
extra small	61-70
tiny	over 70

hatchery relies on three natural water sources that constantly recirculate. At any early age, the salmon are exposed to natural diseases common to fish to build up their immune systems. Maturation takes place in special net cages that are moored in waters offshore at Eastport, Maine, where they are fed a blend that matches their natural diet to supplement what they get naturally from the ocean.

With consumer demand, hopefully more aquaculture operations may follow suit.

WHAT COOKING METHOD TO USE

whole fish:	bake, poach, steam, grill
steaks & fillets more than 1" thick	bake, poach, steam, grill, stir-fry strips or cubes
steaks & fillets 1/2" -1" thick	broil, poach, steam, grill stir-fry strips or cubes
fillets ess than 1/2" thick	broil, pan-poach (for delicate fish), steam, sauté, stir-fry strips
shrimp	broil, poach, steam, sauté, boil, stir-fry, grill

HOW TO PREPARE AND COOK SEAFOOD

Fish is one of the easiest and quickest protein foods to cook. Since fish has little connective tissue, it is cooked not to tenderize but to develop its flavor. Cook briefly at moderate temperatures to retain moistness. Overcooked fish falls apart into pieces and develops a tough texture, tasteless flavor, and fishy odor.

As a general guide, use the "10 minute per inch of thickness" cooking time guide developed by the Department of Fisheries in Canada. Measuring the fish at its thickest point, add or subtract 2 minutes for each 1/4 inch above or below the standard 1 inch. The fish is done when it turns opaque and **just begins** to flake when pierced with a fork in its thickest part.

Depending on its size, shrimp cooks in 3-5 minutes. It is done as soon as it becomes pinkish/white in color, whether cooked in or out of its shell. For best flavor and richer color, cook shrimp in its shell.

Subtle seasonings can make a remarkable difference when preparing seafood. Use 1/2 teaspoon dry herbs or 1 teaspoon fresh per 1 pound of seafood. Marinades can enhance mildly flavored fish and mellow strong varieties. Experiment with mayonnaise, wine, mirin (rice wine), tomato sauce, vinegar, tamari shoyu soy sauce, or prepared salad dressings. Keep marinating time from 10 minutes for thin, delicate fillets to 30 minutes for thick steaks.

After seasoning or marinating, the particular cooking method you use should be appropriate for the form and size of the fish you are serving. The following directions illustrate how easy any method of cooking fish can be.

Bake: Preheat oven to 400° F. Rub oil on 1 side of steaks or on the skin side of fillets. Place oil or skin side down in a baking dish. Brush with oil, extra marinade, or lemon juice, if desired. Gauge the baking time according to the thickness of the fish.

Poach: In a pan large enough to hold the fish in a single layer, pour in enough vegetable or chicken stock, water, or dry white wine/water combination to cover the fish by 1". Bring the liquid to a boil, add fish, reduce the heat, cover, and cook according to the thickness of the fish.

Pan-poaching: The method is similar to regular poaching except the liquid is usually a sauce that will be served with the fish. It

OVEN "FRIED" FISH

3/4 lb. firm fish fillet
pinch of sea salt
1/2 tsp. dried garlic
1/2 cup corn meal, fine
    bread crumbs, or even
    mashed potato flakes
1 egg, beaten (optional)
2 Tbsp. canola oil

Preheat oven to 500°F. Rinse fish under cold water. Mix together sea salt, garlic powder, and flakes or crumbs. Dip fish into beaten egg, if desired, and then into the breading mixture, coating well. Place fish in 8" X 8" baking dish. Drizzle oil over fish. Put in preheated oven on middle rack for 10-12 minutes. Serve with pasta, cooked whole grains, or grilled potatoes.

Serves 2.
(Pyramid servings: 1 Bread/Grain Group, 3 Meat/Protein Group, 18 grams Fat)

Nutrition Facts

Serving Size 1/2 recipe (237 g)
Servings Per Container 2

Amount Per Serving	
Calories 380	Calories from Fat 160

	% Daily Value*
Total Fat 18g	28%
Saturated Fat 2g	9%
Cholesterol 130mg	43%
Sodium 290mg	12%
Total Carbohydrate 24g	8%
Dietary Fiber 2g	9%
Protein 30g	

Vitamin A 8%	•	Calcium 6%
Iron 10%		

Not a significant source of Sugars and Vitamin C.

* Percent Daily Values are based on a 2,000 calorie diet.

---

also doesn't need to cover the fish. In a covered frying pan, bring the sauce to a boil, add the fish, spoon sauce over fish, cover, and cook 3-5 minutes.

Steaming: Add about an inch of plain or seasoned water to the bottom of a pan in which a bamboo steamer, expandable metal steamer, or steamer insert can be placed. Bring liquid to a boil, add fish, cover, and steam 6-8 minutes per inch thickness.

Broil: Preheat broiler. Adjust oven rack so the fish will be 3-4" from the heat. Brush both sides of fish and lay on broiling pan. Broil according to the thickness of the fish.

Grilling: Steaks grill best. When using fish that is not big or firm enough to be made into steaks, fillets can be used; however, they must have the skin attached to prevent falling apart while grilling. Make 1/4" deep diagonal slashes in fillets to keep the fish from curling and shrinking.

Small, whole, thick-skinned, scaled and gutted fish can also be used. If weighing between 2-3 lbs, they should be scored diagonally across the thickest portion to permit uniform heat penetration. Whole, scaled and gutted fish over 3 lbs. require a grill cover and slow cooking over a low fire. To avoid losing natural juices over the long duration of cooking, large whole fish should not be scored.

Preheat the grill for a fire that is moderately hot, enough to sear the surface of the flesh but not too hot that the outside is charred before the fish is cooked all the way through. Place fish on grill perpendicular to the grill bars to minimize contact of the fish with the grill. Brush fish with melted but-

LEMON CURRY MAHI-MAHI

2 Tbsp. toasted sesame
    seeds
1 1/2 lbs. mahi-mahi
4 cloves garlic
juice of 1 large lemon
2 Tbsp. sesame oil
1 tsp. curry powder
1 Tbsp. tamari shoyu
    (natural soy sauce)
fresh parsley

Heat a skillet and toast sesame seeds over moderate heat for about 5 minutes, stirring constantly to prevent burning. Cut mahi-mahi into 4 serving pieces and place in a baking dish. Cut each clove of garlic lengthwise in quarters. Make four 1/4" slits in each piece of fish and insert garlic slivers. Combine lemon juice, sesame oil, sesame seeds, curry powder and soy sauce and pour over the fish. Cover and marinate fish in the refrigerator 2-8 hours, turning the fish occasionally. Remove fish from marinade. Grill on one side for about 4-5 minutes. Turn over, baste with the reserved marinade, and grill an additional 4-5 minutes or until fish begins to flake when tested with a fork.

Nutrition Facts

Serving Size 1/6 recipe (136 g)
Servings Per Container 6

Amount Per Serving

Calories 160   Calories from Fat 60

                                          % Daily Value*

Total Fat 7g	11%
Saturated Fat 1g	5%
Cholesterol 85mg	28%
Sodium 260mg	11%
Total Carbohydrate 3g	1%
Dietary Fiber 1g	2%
Sugars 1g	
Protein 22g	

Vitamin A 4%	•		Vitamin C 8%
Calcium 6%	•		Iron 10%

* Percent Daily Values are based on a 2,000 calorie diet.

Transfer the fish to plates and garnish with parsley before serving.

Serves 4.
(Pyramid servings: 2 Meat/Protein Group, 7 grams Fat)

---

ter, oil, or oily sauce to prevent fish from sticking to the grill. Baste frequently with a pastry brush while cooking to seal in the natural juices. Test with a small bamboo or metal skewer in the thickest part of the fish and feel the resistance of the flesh. Since fish continues to cook after it leaves the heat, remove from the grill as soon as it just begins to flake.

Stir-fry: Cut steaks or fillets into thin strips or 1/2" cubes. Shrimp and scallops can stay whole. Preheat wok to medium-high heat. Add 1-2 Tbsp. oil for each 1 lb. of seafood. Add a small amount of fish, stir-fry until cooked, remove from wok, and adding and stir-frying more fish until done.

Sauté: Preheat frying pan over medium-high heat. Cook 2-3 minutes per 1/2" thickness on one side until lightly brown. Then turn fish over and cook the second side for another 2-3 minutes until done.

EASY FISH CHOWDER

1 Tbsp. safflower or
   canola oil
1 large onion, chopped
5 medium-sized potatoes,
   large cubes
4 cups water
1/2 tsp. salt
1 bay leaf
3 stalks celery
1/2 pkg. frozen peas or 1
   cup fresh peas
1/2-3/4 lb. firm fish (cod,
   snapper, orange
   roughy), cut in bite-
   sized chunks
black pepper to taste

Heat oil in soup pot. Add onion and sauté until translucent. Add potatoes, water, salt, bay leaf, and celery and bring to a boil. Reduce heat to medium-low and simmer 15 minutes. For a creamy texture, blend some of the cooked potatoes and soup liquid in a blender and return to soup pot. Add peas and fish and continue to simmer 10 more minutes.

Season with black pepper and serve.

Serves 3-4.
(Pyramid servings: 2 Veg. Group, 1 Meat/Protein Group, 6 grams Fat)

Nutrition Facts

Serving Size 1/3 recipe (782 g)
Servings Per Container 3

Amount Per Serving

Calories 370	Calories from Fat 50

	% Daily Value*
Total Fat 6g	9%
Saturated Fat 0.5g	3%
Cholesterol 20mg	6%
Sodium 540mg	23%
Total Carbohydrate 59g	20%
Dietary Fiber 9g	35%
Sugars 9g	
Protein 21g	

Vitamin A 10%	•	Vitamin C 70%
Calcium 8%	•	Iron 10%

* Percent Daily Values are based on a 2,000 calorie diet.

Dry Beans

ONCE CONSIDERED plain, humble peasant food, beans have finally won our long-overdue admiration. Not only are we eating more of them in our daily meals, beans are also appearing on the menus of the country's hottest restaurants.

Interest in ethnic and regional cooking account for much of beans, new found respectability. Red beans and rice, Middle Eastern garbanzo bean hummus, New England baked beans, Indonesian tempeh, Japanese tofu, Southwestern enchiladas and tacos...virtually every cuisine features beans in one way or another.

Beans also are the logical choice for cholesterol-free, low-fat, high-fiber meals. Like whole grains, beans are seeds—storehouses of nutrition to fuel the needs of upstarting plants. Accordingly, they have a lot to offer when cooked.

NUTRITION

Beans are the best plant source of protein. In the Food Guide Pyramid, 1/2 cup of cooked dry beans equals the amount of protein found in 1 oz. of lean meat.

Unlike meats, poultry, seafood, and dairy, the protein in beans is incomplete, with lower levels of the amino acid methionine than found in an ideal pattern of protein. However, when grains, seeds, dairy, or small amounts of meat are eaten either in combination with the beans at the same meal or at some other time during the day, the lacking amino acid is supplied, transforming beans into a high-quality protein.

Beans are one of the best sources of soluble fiber, the kind that has been shown to lower serum cholesterol and stabilize blood sugar levels. They also contain some insoluble fiber, which helps maintain regularity and prevent certain types of cancer. Another benefit of its high fiber content is that it helps reduce the tendency to overeat, by making you feel full faster and satiated for longer periods of time.

Good sources of B vitamins, beans likewise are rich in many essential minerals, including calcium, iron, potassium, and zinc. For the best absorption of iron, beans should be consumed with foods high in Vitamin C, such as bell peppers and broccoli. Along with the fact that beans contain no cholesterol and, except for soybeans, little fat, it's no wonder that traditional diets throughout the centuries have included beans as the major source of protein.

DIGESTION

While beans are both delicious and nutritious, they also maintain a reputation as being difficult to digest. This is due to the complex sugars collectively referred to as oligosaccharides found in beans. We humans don't possess the digestive enzymes to deal with them as we would most complex carbohydrates. Therefore, they pass intact through the digestive tract until they reach the large intestine. Bacterial enzymes then go to work to break down these sugars. While their intent is noble, in the process methane, hydrogen, and carbon dioxide are produced as waste products, leaving us with you know what—intestinal gas.

Fortunately, there are several ways to alleviate any potential problems.

1. Soak the beans and discard the soaking water prior to cooking.

Soaking serves to rehydrate the beans, making them easier and quicker to cook. It's also the sure-fire way to get rid of a significant portion of their hard-to-digest sugars. But merely soaking them for a matter of hours isn't enough. The trick is to first bring them to a boil for 3 minutes. This softens the plant cell walls to allow for the complex sugars to leach into the soaking water.

After the initial boiling, the beans should be removed from the heat, covered, and allowed to soak for a few hours. Four hours is plenty. Beyond this, beans don't absorb much more water. After soaking, discard the water which now contains up to 80% of the complex sugars. Rinse the beans, add fresh water, and proceed with cooking.

2. Cook beans with a bay leaf, cumin, or epazote.

Various cultures have found that certain herbs have carminative (gas-reducing) properties. Epazote is one of the most effective. This strongly scented plant, native to the tropics of Mexico and South America, can now be found growing in the Southern United States. Add 2 teaspoons dry or 6 fresh leaves of epazote per pot of beans just before you start them cooking.

3. Cook the beans thoroughly.

Well-cooked beans can be easily mashed with a fork. Thorough cooking softens the starch and fibers, requiring less work throughout the digestive process.

By virtue of its naturally occurring monosodium glutamate, kombu, a sea vegetable, helps tenderize the beans while enhancing their flavor. It also helps replace minerals that are lost down the drain when the bean's soaking water is discarded. Use about a 2-inch strip per pot of beans.

4. Avoid beans that are cooked with sweeteners.

Some people who have little difficulty digesting most beans have trouble with sweetened beans, presumably because it adds more carbohydrate fuel for the large intestine bacteria to digest in addition to the oligosaccharides. Experiment. If the after-effects of baked beans sweetened with brown sugar, honey, maple syrup, molasses, or apple butter make life a bit uncomfortable, opt for plain beans. Or cook them with naturally sweet, but gentle, root vegetables such as carrots.

5. Eat smaller quantities of beans until your body adjusts to digesting them.

People who eat beans regularly often find their digestive system gradually adapts, making for easier eating. Start off by limiting yourself to about 1/2 cup at a time a couple times per week, gradually increasing the amount and frequency.

6. Focus on legumes that are easier to digest.

Navy beans, limas, and whole cooked soybeans are the most difficult to digest. Anasazi beans, azuki beans, black-eyed peas, lentils, and mung beans have the least amount of the problematic complex carbohydrates and therefore are the least gas-forming. Tofu and tempeh are also easy to digest since the individual processes of making them eliminate or break down most of the oligosaccharides.

Sprouted beans may be your best bet. Since oligosaccharides in beans act as stored fuel to provide energy when or if the seed (bean) is germinated, the process of sprouting beans uses up virtually all the oligosaccharides. While some people serve sprouted beans raw in salads or sandwiches, light steaming, stir-frying, or sautéing is preferred for ultimate digestibility.

7. Sprinkle a few drops of BEANO™ on your beans.

Beano™ is a liquid additive that supplies a natural digestive enzyme to break down the oligosaccharides before they get down to the bacteria in the large intestine, thus eliminating or greatly reducing the probability of intestinal gas. All it takes is 3 to 8 drops sprinkled on the first bite of a 3/4 cup serving. While cooking beans with Beano™ may sound like a good idea, don't. High heat makes it ineffective.

Note: Since Beano™ is made from a safe food-grade mold, individuals allergic to mold or penicillin may want to avoid it. Diabetics may need to account in their diets for the fact that Beano™ makes vegetable sugars more available.

HOW TO BUY AND STORE

Not only are beans nutritious, they are inexpensive and readily available. Virtually every grocery store will sell dry beans packaged; several sell them in bulk. You'll likely find packages of mixed beans specially formulated for soups and stews, too.

Select beans with smooth surfaces and bright colors. Beans that are too old or too dry will have cracked seams or dull, wrinkled surfaces.

Canned precooked beans are lifesavers when you want a meal in no time. While it's hard to beat the flavor of freshly cooked beans, a bit of seasoning can perk up canned varieties. Look at the Nutrition Facts information panel on the can to compare sodium levels between brands. The beans can also be drained into a colander and quickly rinsed to reduce the sodium before proceeding with your recipe.

Instant beans are equally convenient. Precooked, dried, ground and mixed with seasonings and vegetable oil, most require boiling water and 5 minutes to rehydrate. You may find they digest better if allowed to simmer over low heat or at least sit for 10-15 minutes to allow for more rehydration.

Dried beans will last up to a year when stored in airtight glass or plastic containers away from heat. The older the bean, the longer the cooking time, so try to use beans within 2-3 months of purchase.

Cooked beans will keep 5 days in the refrigerator and up to 6 months in the freezer. Planning ahead, cooking a quantity of beans at a time, and freezing extras is a very worthwhile investment.

HOW TO PREPARE BEANS

Prepare beans by sorting through them for small pebbles that could linger from harvest. Wash them several times under cold water, discarding any that float to the surface.

Except for lentils, split peas, and split baby garbanzos, all beans should be soaked before cooking. Add fresh, cool water to sorted beans, covering them with about 3 inches to spare or in 3-4 times their volume in water. Bring beans to a boil for 3 minutes and set them aside for 2-4 hours off the heat. In hot weather, refrigerate beans when using the long-soak method to prevent fermentation.

When ready to cook, discard the soaking liquid to remove most of the hard-to-digest complex starches that are responsible for bloating and intestinal gas in some individuals. (As the soaking water contains some vitamins and minerals, you may prefer to cook the beans in their soaking water if you

COOKING TIMES FOR COMMON BEANS

Cooking time is determined by several factors: simmering temperature, soaking time, the size and age of beans, the variety of bean, and the altitude at which you live. Beans destined to be whole in salads are usually cooked less than beans cooked into soups. Whatever the case, well-cooked beans should be easily mashed with a fork.

BEANS (1 cup dry)	TIMING Simmering	Pressure Cooking
aduki beans	1 1/2 hours	25 minutes
anasazi beans	1 1/2 hours	25 minutes
baby limas	1 hour	not recommended
black beans	1 1/2 hours	25 minutes
black-eyed peas	1 1/4 hours	25 minutes
garbanzos	2 1/2 hours	30 minutes
great northern	2 hours	25 minutes
kidney beans	1 1/2 hours	25 minutes
lentils, green	45 minutes	20 minutes
lentils, red	25 minutes	not recommended
lima beans	1 1/2 hours	not recommended
mung beans	1 1/4 hours	25 minutes
navy beans	2 hours	25 minutes
pinto beans	2 hours	25 minutes
split peas	1 1/4 hours	25 minutes

have little difficulty digesting beans.)

Add fresh water to the beans and prepare according to any of the following methods. For best flavor and nutrition, cook the beans in enough, but not too much, water. About an inch of water above the beans is usually plenty once they have been pre-soaked.

Chopped onion, garlic, herbs, or spices may be cooked with the beans for added flavor. But lay off the salt, fats, sugars, tomatoes, wine and other acidic ingredients until the end of cooking. Otherwise, your beans will take forever to cook.

Some cooks and books have suggested that baking soda should be added to beans while cooking. Unless your water is exceedingly hard and would benefit from baking soda's alkalinity to cook beans faster, it's best to forego it. Excess alkalinity can break down the cell walls. Not only will you be left with a mushy texture, valuable protein and vitamins will leach into the cooking water as well. Baking soda can also deplete thiamin (vitamin B_1). If you still decide you need/want baking soda in your beans, keep it to 1/8 teaspoon per cup of dry beans.

Boil/simmer: In a large covered pot, combine beans and water, using 4 cups water for each cup of beans. Bring the beans to a boil, then reduce to a simmer until the beans are tender and most of the liquid is absorbed. Simmer gently to prevent the skins of the beans from bursting. Check them frequently to prevent overcooking and to ensure an adequate amount of water while cooking.

Pressure-cooking: A pressure cooker can help prepare beans in almost half the time. Because less water escapes as steam, you'll only need to add water to a depth of about one inch from the surface of the beans. Since some beans tend to foam and clog pressure release vents, keep the amount of beans and water to no more than 2/3 of the pressure cooker's capacity. Another trick to prevent this problem is to add a tablespoon of oil before bringing the beans to pressure.

Baking: For each cup of beans, boil for 15-20 minutes in 41/2 cups water. Then transfer beans and water to a covered baking dish. Bake beans at 350° for about 31/2 hours.

Slow-cooking: An electric crock pot enables you to cook beans while you're away from home. Use the same ratio of water to beans as for baking. Cook at the high setting for 1 hour, then on low for up to 8 hours. Perfect cooked texture may require some experimenting with timing.

Exploring Your Options

Within the vast family of beans emerge eight major categories (genus and species) classified according to like flavors and features. One of the categories, Arachis hypogaea, commonly known as the peanut, will be dealt with in the "Nuts & Seeds" chapter. The remaining seven will be individually subdivided into several sections.

In addition to commonly consumed beans, both heirloom beans and hybrid beans are included. Heirloom beans are beans popular in times past that are now experiencing a resurgence. Some lost favor due to low yields; others simply fell victim to newly developed varieties. Now these heirloom beans are being reintroduced for their remarkable flavors and nutritional contributions.

Hybrid beans are developed for several reasons: resistance to fungi and insect infestations, reduced amount of oligosaccharides for easier digestion, as well as for their beauty, texture, and flavor.

While many of our commonly consumed beans are hybrids in one way or an-

other, only the most recently developed will be indicated as hybrids.

CHICKPEAS
(Cicer arietinum)

Facts and Features

Chickpeas, also known as garbanzos or Italian cece beans, resemble, upon close scrutiny and with a good imagination, the head and beak of a chicken. If you think that's stretching it, consider that ancient Romans thought it looked like a ram's head with its curling horns. In fact, its species name (the second word in Cicer arietinum) means "ramlike."

Whatever you think this roundish, cream-colored bean looks or doesn't look like, you'll appreciate its hearty, yet mild, flavor and the fact that chickpeas keep their unique shape when cooked.

In addition to being a good source of protein, and calcium, chickpeas are particularly high in iron. Even though chickpeas are somewhat higher in fat than other beans except for soybeans, they contain only about 12% calories from fat, primarily unsaturated.

Varieties and Cooking Guidelines

Whole chickpeas are featured in traditional Middle Eastern, Mediterranean, and East Indian cuisines served in several ways: marinated and served alone or in a salad, mashed and combined with sesame tahini and garlic into a dip called hummus, cooked with vegetables and pasta into minestrone, and mixed with spices and formed into patties or meatball shapes for falafel.

Boil/simmer: 21/2 hours. Pressure cook: 25-30 minutes.

Chana dal are split and polished baby chickpeas that look and taste like small kernels of sweet corn. They are at their best in soups, salads, and rice dishes.

No pre-soaking is necessary. Boil/simmer: about 30 minutes. Pressure-cook: not recommended.

Flavor Enhancers: Curry powder, basil, oregano, onion, garlic, cumin, cayenne pepper.

LENTILS
(Lens esculenta)

Facts and Features

Lentils are the world's oldest cultivated legume, domesticated around 7000 B.C. Its name is derived from its small, round, flat shape, looking much like a lens. Colors range to greenish-brown, brown, reddish orange, and coral.

Beyond their delicious flavor, lentils' popularity can be attributed to their short preparation time and versatility. Because they hold their shape after cooking, lentils make an excellent soup. They are also a favorite bean to mash and mold into loaves and patties.

A good source of protein and fiber, lentils are also high in iron.

Varieties and Cooking Guidelines

Domestic green lentils are grown in the northwestern United States. A very flavorful variety, they look like flat, greenish-brown disks.

Boil/simmer: 45-60 minutes. Pressure-cook: 20 minutes.

Petite French green lentils are about 1/3 the size of domestic green lentils, darker in color, and slightly peppery in flavor. Since they hold their shape very well when cooked, they are often used as a side dish or as a base for meats, fish, or game.

Boil/simmer: 45-60 minutes. Pressure-cook: 20 minutes.

Brown lentils are smaller, more plump, and more brown in color than green lentils. Cook similarly to green lentils.

Spanish pardina lentils are also known as Spanish brown lentils or continental lentils. About 1/3 the size of regular lentils, Spanish pardina lentils also have a delicious nutty flavor. Like other brown and green lentils, they hold their shape when cooked. Cook similarly to green lentils.

Whole red lentils have a beautiful coral color that turns golden when cooked. When rinsing red lentils prior to cooking, they will tend to clump together and appear soapy when moistened- a result of the release of starch. Since red lentils also like to foam during cooking, it may be advisable to cook them with the lid slightly ajar.

Unlike their green and brown cousins, red lentils tend to lose their shape during cooking. Soups made with red lentils are,

ITALIAN RED LENTIL SOUP

1 Tbsp. olive oil
1 onion, diced
1 cup red lentils, quickly rinsed
5 cups water
3 medium carrots, cut in 1" chunks
3 stalks celery, cut in 1" chunks
1 tsp. Italian seasoning herbs or 1/2 tsp. oregano and 1/4 tsp. each basil and thyme
1/2 tsp. salt
parsley for garnish

Heat oil in a soup pot and sauté onion for 5 minutes, stirring frequently. Add lentils, water, vegetables, and Italian seasoning. Bring slowly to a boil, reduce heat, and simmer 45 minutes or until lentils are very soft. Add salt and continue cooking for 5 minutes. Serve garnished with chopped parsley.

Serves 4.
(Pyramid servings: 1 Veg. Group, 2 Meat/Protein Group, 31/2 grams Fat)

Nutrition Facts

Serving Size 1/4 recipe (453 g)
Servings Per Container 4

Amount Per Serving

Calories 220   Calories from Fat 30

	% Daily Value*
Total Fat 3.5g	6%
Sodium 360mg	15%
Total Carbohydrate 36g	12%
Dietary Fiber 10g	38%
Sugars 7g	
Protein 12g	

Vitamin A 300% • Vitamin C 15%
Calcium 8% • Iron 8%

Not a significant source of Saturated Fat and Cholesterol.
* Percent Daily Values are based on a 2,000 calorie diet.

---

therefore, creamy. They also make terrific vegetarian pâtés when allowed to bake and cool in a baking dish or loaf pan.

To help them keep their shape for salads and side dishes, add salt or acidic ingredients such as tomatoes, citrus, or vinegar immediately after they become tender.

Boil/simmer: 20-25 minutes. Pressure-cook: not recommended.

Petite crimson lentils are about 1/3 the size of regular lentils and reddish-orange in color that turns golden once cooked. Since they have their outer seed coat removed, they cook even quicker than whole red lentils, but disintegrating just as readily.

Boil/simmer: 15-20 minutes. Pressure-cook: not recommended.

Flavor Enhancers: Curry powder, sage, basil, oregano, garlic, onion, chives, and dill.

ASIAN-BASED BEANS
(Vigna radiata, unguiculata, and sinensis)

Facts and Features

Originating in India and finding its way to China and Africa, the Vigna family of beans includes mung beans, black-eyed peas, cowpeas, and pigeon peas. Ranging from small to medium in size, all have a flavor often described as "vegetable-like."

Like all beans, they provide a good source of protein, iron, and fiber that is very low in fat.

Varieties and Cooking Guidelines

Mung beans are small, round, olive-green beans commonly sprouted for use in Chi-

LENTIL ALMOND SOUP

1 tsp. canola oil
2/3 cup green lentils
1 small onion, diced
2 cloves garlic, minced
1 large or 2 medium
    rutabagas, cut into 1"
    cubes
2 bay leaves
1/4 tsp. whole peppercorns
4 cups water
1/4 tsp. almond extract
1 tsp. umeboshi vinegar
roasted chopped almonds
    for garnish

Heat oil over medium heat in a soup pot. Add lentils, onion, and garlic and sauté for 5 minutes, stirring constantly. Add cubed rutabagas, bay leaves, peppercorns, and water. Bring to a boil, cover, reduce heat, and cook for 40-45 minutes until lentils are soft. Turn off heat and add almond extract and umeboshi vinegar. Allow flavors to mingle for 5 minutes before serving. Garnish bowls of soup with roasted chopped almonds.

Serves 4.
(Pyramid servings: 1 Veg. Group, 1 Meat/Protein Group, 1 1/2 grams Fat)

Nutrition Facts

Serving Size 1/4 recipe (325 g)
Servings Per Container 4

Amount Per Serving

Calories 140   Calories from Fat 15

	% Daily Value*
Total Fat 1.5g	2%
Sodium 90mg	4%
Total Carbohydrate 23g	8%
Dietary Fiber 11g	44%
Sugars 5g	
Protein 10g	

Vitamin A 4%	•	Vitamin C	20%
Calcium 4%	•	Iron	20%

Not a significant source of Saturated Fat and Cholesterol.
* Percent Daily Values are based on a 2,000 calorie diet.

---

nese stir-fries and egg rolls. When cooked they play an important part in Indian curries and dahls.

Very easily digested, they cook quickly without the need to presoak. Boil/simmer: 1-1 1/4 hours. Pressure-cook: 20 minutes.

Black-eyed peas are a familiar bean to southern regions in the United States and Latin America, traditionally cooked with rice and greens. This bean can be identified by its creamy-white oval shape and black "eye." A must for southern New Year's celebrations, they are often marinated and transformed into "Texas Caviar."

Boil/simmer: 1-1 1/4 hours. Pressure-cook: 25 minutes.

Cowpeas are similar to black-eyed peas yet smaller in size and somewhat darker in color. Despite the difference between them, cowpeas and black-eyed peas are often considered as one and the same.

Since cowpeas are smaller than black-eyed peas, they will cook even quicker. Boil/simmer: 45 minutes. Pressure-cook: 30 minutes.

Pigeon peas are most commonly used in Caribbean-style cooking. They are small and grayish brown with an elongated eye on its flat side. Pigeon peas have tougher skins than black-eyed peas. Boil/simmer: 1 1/2 hours. Pressure-cook: 30 minutes.

Flavor Enhancers: Assertive seasonings: curry powder, ginger, garlic, chilis, tomatoes, and plenty of sauteed onions.

FAVA BEANS
(Vicia faba)

Facts and Features

Fava beans, also known as broad beans and Windsor beans, have a history reaching far back to antiquity, about 3000 B.C. Particularly popular in Europe, fava beans are beginning to find their way into American cuisine.

Oval-shaped and light brown in color, fava beans are also quite large, about 11/2" long. When cooked they have a creamy texture and nutty, earthy flavor.

Varieties and Cooking Guidelines

Whole fava beans must have their tough skins removed before cooking. Fortunately, they can be peeled off fairly easily after soaking. Use in soups, salads, and puree into pates.

Boil/simmer: 40 minutes. Pressure-cook: not recommended.

Peeled and split fava beans save you time, both in peeling and cooking—they're ready in about 20 minutes. Since they don't hold their shape very well, for best results purée or use in soup.

Flavor Enhancers: Fresh herbs, tomatoes, garlic, and black pepper.

DRIED PEAS
(Pisum sativum)

Facts and Features

Dried peas have been cooked since 6000 B.C., no doubt for soup. They are not just a dried version of the peas we generally consume as a vegetable. Instead, they are known as field peas, higher in starch content.

Varieties and Cooking Guidelines

Whole green peas can be used in casseroles, as a side dish, or puréed and made into spreads, dips, croquettes.

Soak before cooking. Boil/simmer: 1-11/2 hours. Pressure-cook: not recommended.

Split green peas have their skins removed by a machine before another one splits the pea in half. No presoaking is necessary, although if you soak them for at least 30 minutes, they'll keep their shape after cooking. Generally, however, it's their creamy texture that is most appealing.
Boil/simmer: 1-11/2 hours. Pressure-cook: 25 minutes.

Split yellow peas are milder in flavor than split green peas. Boil/simmer: 11/2 hours. Pressure-cook: 25 minutes.

Flavor Enhancers: Garlic, onion, dill, curry, ginger, bay leaf, thyme, and basil.

COMMON BEANS
(Phaseolus angularis, coccinus, limensis, lunatus, vulgaris)

Facts and Features

Originating in Central America, the Phaseolus family of beans is the most extensive. Included are the seemingly very diverse varieties such as Asian azuki beans, lima beans, pinto beans, black beans, and even navy beans.

As a group, the Phaseolus beans are very low in fat and high in fiber, protein, and iron.

Varieties and Cooking Guidelines

Anasazi beans are an heirloom variety cultivated in the American Southwest since about 130 A.D. Production lagged considerably around 1200 A.D., leaving most of its survival to the wild and a few gardens of Native Americans in the Four Corners region of Colorado, Utah, Arizona, and New Mexico. Commercial production was rekindled by agronomist Bruce Riddell and Ernie Waller, an entrepreneur, both sharing a common interest in this native bean. In 1987 they named it "anasazi" from the Navajo Indian language meaning "the ancient ones." From their work collecting the beans from local sources, anasazi beans have been reestablished botanically and confirmed as an heirloom variety.

Anasazi beans are as striking as they are delicious. Similar in size and shape to pinto beans, they are mottled burgundy and white, markings that, unfortunately, fade with cooking. Both sweeter and more flavorful than pinto beans, they also hold their shape better once cooked.

Much of the anasazi bean's popularity can be attributed to its ease of digestion. Many people report less problems with intestinal gas, a belief that is well grounded in reality. The levels of hard-to-digest complex carbohydrates are 25% less than found in other beans.

Use in recipes where pinto beans are often used.

Boil/simmer: 1 1/2 hours. Pressure-cook: 25 minutes.

Appaloosa beans are a new hybrid bean, two-toned black and white on the diagonal with a long, thin shape. Not surprisingly, the beans are named after the Appaloosa pony whose coloring is quite similar. During cooking their markings fade somewhat.

The flavor of appaloosa beans is remarkable, like an incredible black bean. Accordingly, you can substitute appaloosa beans for any recipe containing black beans.

Boil/simmer: 1 1/2 hours. Pressure-cook: 25 minutes.

Azuki beans (aduki, adzuki beans) are small, burgundy-colored round beans traditionally used in Japanese cuisine. Their low fat content makes them more easily digested than other beans.

Slightly sweet in flavor, azuki beans are often used in Japanese desserts. However, they are equally delicious when served with rice or barley. Add cubes of winter squash the last half-hour of cooking and season with tamari soy sauce for an exceptional dish. Stretch tradition and try azuki beans in Southwest cuisine, too. They make a beautiful contrast with corn tortillas.

Boil/simmer: 1 1/2 hours. Pressure-cook: 25 minutes.

Black beans (black turtle beans) are small, oval-shaped, and, of course, black in color. Particularly high in magnesium, black beans are also low in fat and high in fiber.

Their rich, earthy flavor is a perfect foil to the spicy seasonings used in Mexican and South American dishes. Black beans are often accompanied by rice and tomatoes, cooked into a delicious soup, or served in or with enchiladas, burritos, and chapatis.

Boil/simmer: 1 1/2 hours. Pressure-cook: 25 minutes.

Calypso beans are hybrid beans bred for their beauty. Amazingly, they look like the Chinese yin/yang symbols in black and white, complete with a black polka dot.

Considered similar to black beans, they are more bland in flavor and cook much faster. If cooked too long, they lose their shape and considerable coloring.

Boil/simmer: 45 minutes-1 hour. Pressure-cook: 15 minutes.

Cannellini beans (white kidney beans) are heirloom beans best known as an essential ingredient in Italian minestrones. Considering their smooth texture and nutty flavor, cannellini beans are delicious in any soup, especially tomato-based varieties, or served simply with a dash of olive oil and freshly ground black pepper.

Boil/simmer: 1-11/2 hours. Pressure-cook: 25 minutes.

Christmas lima beans are an heirloom variety of lima beans that are as beautiful as they are delicious. Similar in shape to regular lima beans, Christmas limas are larger and more colorful, mottled maroon and creamy white. Once cooked, their markings become even darker and richer-looking. Most exciting of all, they taste remarkably like roasted chestnuts, making this one of the top "must-try" beans.

Use Christmas limas as a main dish entrée, in casseroles, and in salads. They are particularly wonderful combined with onions, portabello mushrooms, and kale sautéed in sesame oil and tamari soy sauce. For the crowning touch, serve with baked kobocha winter squash and millet or rice.

Boil/simmer: 11/4- 11/2 hours. Pressure-cook: 20 minutes

Cranberry beans are heirloom beans traditionally used in New England for succotash as well as in Italian and Portuguese dishes. While they very closely resemble the pinto bean in size and shape, cranberry beans are more pink in color streaked with cranberry-red markings that fade when cooked.

Cranberry beans have a more delicate flavor than pintos. Use in soups, casseroles, or pasta dishes seasoned with moderate amounts of aromatic fresh or dried herbs.

Boil/simmer: 1-11/4 hours. Pressure-cook: 20 minutes.

Flageolets are heirloom beans popular in French country cuisine, often served as a side dish for meats, especially lamb, and poultry.

Looking like very pale green, miniature kidney beans, flageolets are actually immature kidney beans removed from their pods. Their delicate flavor is enhanced with aromatic vegetables and herbs such as onion, celery, carrots, garlic, bay leaf and thyme. For an Italian variation, try mixing pesto into flageolets as soon as they become tender.

Boil/cook: 1 hour. Pressure-cook: 15 minutes.

French navy beans are small heirloom navy beans that appear white with just a hint of green. Like regular navy beans, they are perfect for soups and salads, slightly bacon-like in flavor.

Boil/simmer: 1 hour. Pressure-cook: 15 minutes.

Great northern beans are white, medium-sized beans that look and taste much like navy beans, generally cooked in soups or baked bean casseroles. Their delicate flavor gives you the option to go assertive or mild when seasoning. When substituted for chickpeas, great northern beans also make a delicious twist with a traditional hummus recipe.

Boil/simmer: 11/2-2 hours. Pressure-cook: 25 minutes.

Jacob's cattle beans, also known as trout beans, are heirloom beans popular in New England and Germany. Speckled maroon and white, these beans are long, slim, and kidney-shaped.

Their robust flavor makes for a terrific soup.

Boil/simmer: 45 minutes-1 hour. Pressure-cook: 15 minutes.

Kidney beans are deep reddish-brown beans shaped like you-know-what. They are often used in chili, soups, and salads due to the fact they keep their shape so well.

Subtly sweet in flavor, kidney beans can be cooked with spicy Southwestern spices or with mild, aromatic seasonings. For a salty/sweet, creamy base, mix in a tablespoon of diluted white miso per 2 cups cooked kidneys instead of salt.

Boil/simmer: 11/2 hours. Pressure-cook: 25 minutes.

Lima beans (butter beans or fordhooks) are large, creamy white, disk-shaped beans. Their neutral yet buttery flavor and starchy texture make them particularly good for soups and stews. Baby lima beans are another variety of lima beans, more buttery in flavor. Since they are smaller, flatter, and thinner than regular lima beans, they cook more quickly.

Soaking the limas helps loosen some of their skins before cooking. More skins will loosen during cooking, illustrating why pressure-cooking limas is not a very good idea since they are the perfect fuel to clog the pressure-vent.

Boil/simmer: 11/2 hours—large limas, 1 hour—baby limas.

Marrow beans are heirloom navy-type beans that were popular during the 1850s for baked bean casseroles. They are more round and plump in shape than navy beans and much more flavorful.

Use marrow beans in soups or baked bean casseroles.

Boil/simmer: 11/2-2 hours. Pressure-cook: 25 minutes.

Navy beans are small, white oval-shaped beans considered a staple for soups, stews, and baked bean dishes. As their name implies, sailors aboard ships and submarines were more than familiar with the many ways navy beans could be served.

Boil/simmer: 2 hours. Pressure-cook: 30 minutes.

Pea beans are an even smaller version of navy beans. Use and cook similarly as above.

Pink beans are small, salmon-colored beans that are used extensively in Caribbean cooking. Their flavor is mild, similar to pinto beans, and they can be used interchangeably with pintos in Southwestern-style recipes.

Boil/simmer: 2 hours. Pressure-cook: 25 minutes.

Pinto beans are salmon-pink and brown speckled oblong- shaped beans that are typically the bean of choice in Southwestern cuisine. Its mealy texture makes particularly good refried beans.

For pintos at their best, cook with seasonings such as garlic, bell peppers, green chilis, cilantro, cumin, and oregano.

Boil/simmer: 2 hours. Pressure-cook: 25 minutes.

Prince beans (Spanish tolosanda beans) are heirloom beans introduced in the late 1920s. Although smaller in size, they are shaped like kidney beans and have a mottled cinnamon and brown color that lightens slightly when cooked.

Take advantage of their creamy texture in soups or add to salads. Prince beans are also used in Mexican and Spanish cuisine.

Boil/simmer: 45 minutes-1 hour. Pressure-cook: 15 minutes.

Rattlesnake beans are a hybrid variety much like pintos in shape and flavor but darker in color. Its name is derived from the fact that their growing pods twist like snakes.

Cook in recipes that usually depend on pintos, especially chili.

Boil/simmer: 2 hours. Pressure-cook: 25 minutes.

Red beans are small, pea-shaped, dark red beans used extensively in Southern cooking. Many New Orleans restaurants feature red beans and rice for Monday lunches, a tradition that supposedly helps rebalance those who enjoyed the weekend a bit too much.

Their delicious, rich, full flavor makes red beans with anything any day of the week a welcome dish.

Boil/simmer: 2 hours. Pressure-cook: 25 minutes.

Rice beans are heirloom beans hailing back to the 1860s in Germany. As their name implies, they look like a plump version of cooked rice. Imagine…a way to possibly fool those who won't eat beans.

Delicate and slightly sweet in flavor, rice beans are delicious additions to soup, casseroles, or vegetable dishes. Quick-cooking, too.

Boil/simmer: 30 minutes, uncovered. Pressure-cook: not recommended.

Scarlet runner beans are an heirloom variety that can be traced back to the 1750s. Fairly large in size and sweet in flavor, they have a deep magenta and black color and are shaped similarly to kidney beans.

Mix with new potatoes or use in salads and side dishes.

Boil/simmer: 2 hours. Pressure-cook: 30 minutes.

Soldier beans are an heirloom bean originally used in early New England for baked beans. They are long and white with red markings that look curiously like the outline of a toy soldier.

Experiment with soldier beans in your favorite soup recipe.

Boil/simmer: 1 hour. Pressure-cook: 15 minutes.

Swedish brown beans are heirloom beans that were introduced about 100 years ago by Scandinavian immigrants. These small, tan-colored beans are the beans of choice for old-fashioned baked beans.

Boil/simmer: 11/2 hours. Pressure-cook: 25 minutes.

Tongues of Fire (Borlotto Lingua di Fuoco) is an heirloom Italian version of the cranberry bean distinguished by its mottled beige and brown markings. Its delicious, full-bodied flavor is good in Italian pasta dishes and soups. They bake well, too.

Boil/simmer: 11/2 hours. Pressure-cook: 25 minutes.

White emergo beans (sweet white runner beans) are hybrid beans that are white, slightly larger than lima beans and irregular in shape. Their sweet, creamy flavor is good in soups and salads.

Boil/simmer: 2 hours. Pressure-cook: 30 minutes.

Yellow-eye beans ("Molasses Face") are heirloom beans dating from the 1860s in Maine and Vermont. These beans are white with a large yellow "eye."

In the Northeast, yellow-eye beans were used for baked beans. In some parts of the South they were used as a substitute for black-eyed peas in "hoppin' john", a traditional beans and rice dish. Both dishes remain the best way to take advantage of yellow-eye beans' flavor.

Boil/simmer: 11/4 hour. Pressure-cook: 25 minutes.

WHITE BEAN CELERY SOUP WITH FRESH SAGE

1¼ cups French navy, Great Northern, navy, or marrow beans
6 cups water
4" piece of kombu (sea vegetable)
1 tsp. sesame oil
1 medium onion, diced
6 stalks celery, chopped
3 Tbsp. chopped fresh sage (not packed) or 1/2 tsp. dried rubbed sage
1 Tbsp. tamari or tamari shoyu soy sauce
2 tsp. grated lemon peel
1/2 tsp. salt

Soak beans in water 6-8 hours. Discard soaking water and replace with 4 cups fresh water or enough to cover the beans plus an additional 1" depth above the surface. Add kombu and pressure-cook beans for 25 minutes (or cook on the stovetop for 2 hours). Meanwhile, heat oil in a skillet and sauté onion, celery, and sage, seasoned with tamari, for 20 minutes. Add vegetables and any accumulated cooking liquid to the cooked beans. Stir in grated lemon peel and salt and allow flavors to mingle for 10 minutes before serving.

Nutrition Facts

Serving Size 1/4 recipe (514 g)
Servings Per Container 4

Amount Per Serving

Calories 250   Calories from Fat 20

	% Daily Value*
Total Fat 2g	3%
Sodium 600mg	25%
Total Carbohydrate 44g	15%
Dietary Fiber 17g	69%
Sugars 6g	
Protein 16g	

Vitamin A 2%	•	Vitamin C 15%
Calcium 15%	•	Iron 25%

Not a significant source of Saturated Fat and Cholesterol.
* Percent Daily Values are based on a 2,000 calorie diet.

Serves 4.
(Pyramid servings: 1 Veg. Group, 2 Meat/Protein Group, 2 grams Fat)

SOYBEANS (GLYSINE MAX)

Facts and Features

Soybeans are the only beans containing the proper proportion of all 8 essential amino acids to be recognized as a complete protein.

Besides being high in protein, they have the distinction of containing significantly more fat than any other bean. Most, however, is unsaturated, causing less of a potential problem with blood cholesterol buildup than the saturated fat content found in many other high-protein foods. Soybeans are also a good source of Omega-3 fatty acids, the type of essential fatty acid found to reduce production of thromboxane, the prostaglandin that promotes blood clotting, leading to decreased risks for strokes and heart attacks.

Research has linked the lower incidence of breast cancer in Japan with increased consumption of soybean products, due to the presence of antiestrogenic compounds.

And, to top it off, soybeans are inexpensive. With all these good things going for it, it's too bad they're so hard to digest. But that's only in its cooked whole form. Traditional methods of preparing soybeans into tofu, miso, tempeh, soy milk, and soy sauce either break down or remove components that inhibit digestion and assimilation.

Varieties and Cooking Guidelines

Black soybeans, characterized by their round, shiny black appearance, are much more tasty in their whole form than the yellow variety. When fermented, they are the basis of Chinese black bean sauce, a strong, salty condiment used in many Chinese dishes.

Boil/simmer: 3-4 hours. Pressure-cook: 1 1/2 hours.

Yellow soybeans are the basic variety of soybean used for cooking and processing. When cooked in its whole bean form, they must be cooked very thoroughly.

Boil/simmer: 3-4 hours. Pressure-cook: 1 1/2 hours.

Soy grits are coarsely ground soybeans, occasionally used in recipes as a protein booster. Like whole soybeans, any product or recipe containing soy grits should be thoroughly cooked to facilitate digestion. Since many recipes using soy grits only suggest minimal cooking times, you're probably better off adding the more digestible tofu or tempeh to casseroles or "burgers". Otherwise, cook with twice the amount of water as to grits and cook a minimum of 30 minutes alone or with a stew.

Miso

Miso is a fermented soybean paste made by mixing cooked soybeans with koji (grain inoculated with aspergillus mold), salt, and water. Depending on the type of miso, the mixture is then fermented from 2 months to 3 years, It can be used in soups or sauces instead of bouillon or as a base for stews, gravies, salad dressings, dips or spreads. For a change in pace from salt or tamari shoyu, season beans or grains with miso.

Miso is a good source of protein and digestive enzymes. It has also been reported to alkalize the blood and to neutralize the effects of smoking and environmental pollution.

Flavors vary according to the type of miso. Basically, misos can be divided into 2 types, short-term misos and long-term misos. Each miso has its own unique ratio of ingredients and proper fermentation time.

A **short-term miso**, aged for about 2 months, is fermented with more koji and less salt than longer-term misos. Because its color can be white, yellow, or beige, short-term miso is sold by names such as mellow miso, sweet miso, or sweet white miso. All are appropriate for summer cooking, dips, sauces, and salad dressings. The high carbohydrate content in the short-term miso yields a sweet flavor. It also contains twice the niacin (B_3) and 10 times the beneficial lactic acid bacteria of dark salty miso.

Long-term miso is aged 6 months to 3 years with more salt, more soybeans, and less koji to yield a dark red or brown miso that is higher in protein, essential fatty acids, and salt. It is especially good in hearty soups and stews prepared during colder weather cooking. Varieties of long-term misos include mugi or barley miso; rice-based red, kome, genmai, or brown rice miso; soba or buckwheat miso; and hatcho or 100% soybean miso.

Natto miso is a chunky condiment made from soybeans, barley, barley malt, kombu (a sea vegetable), ginger, and sea salt. Use it as a relish or chutney on grains, beans, and vegetables, or in sandwich spreads. Try it in squash or sweet potato soup or add to your favorite barbeque sauce for sweet, salty, pungent zip.

Since miso is a concentrated food, use no more than 1/2 to 1 teaspoon of dark miso or 1-2 teaspoons of light miso per person. One tablespoon of light miso or a heaping 1 1/2 teaspoon of dark miso equals 1/4 teaspoon of sea salt.

GINGERY MISO SOUP

5 cups water
1 medium onion, thinly
    sliced
4" piece of wakame sea
    vegetable (opt.)
2 medium or 1 large
    carrots, cut in 1/2"
    diagonal slices
1/2" piece fresh ginger
    root, thinly sliced
2 tsp. rice or barley miso
2 green onions thinly
sliced or chopped parsley
    for garnish

Bring water to a boil. Add onion, reduce heat, and simmer 5 minutes, uncovered. If using wakame, quickly rinse under water and add to soup. Add carrots and ginger, cover pot, and continue to simmer soup for 15 minutes. Remove pot from the heat. Dilute miso with a small amount of the broth and return to soup, allowing flavors to mingle for 5 minutes before serving. For added color, garnish each bowl with sliced green onions or parsley.

Serves 4.
(Pyramid servings: 1 Veg. Group)

Nutrition Facts

Serving Size 1/4 recipe (367 g)
Servings Per Container 4

Amount Per Serving

Calories 35

	% Daily Value*
Total Fat 0g	0%
Sodium 120mg	5%
Total Carbohydrate 7g	2%
Dietary Fiber 2g	7%
Sugars 4g	
Protein 1g	

Vitamin A 200%	•	Vitamin C 10%
Calcium 2%	•	Iron 2%

Not a significant source of Calories from Fat, Saturated Fat and Cholesterol.
* Percent Daily Values are based on a 2,000 calorie diet.

Dissolve miso in a small amount of liquid before adding to soups, sauces, or other dishes to activate the beneficial enzymes in miso. Steep 3-5 minutes in the hot liquid at the end of cooking but do not boil. Miso used in spreads, dips, and salad dressings is primarily used for flavor, so the heat activation step is generally eliminated. However, many of the health benefits will still be present.

Unpasteurized miso is preferred since it leaves the beneficial lactobacillus bacteria and other enzymes intact, thus insuring the medicinal benefits and full flavors of miso. Previously, unpasteurized miso was available only in bulk, since, due to on-going fermentation, naturally occurring carbon dioxide expanded and burst packages of miso. Small refrigerated tubs of unpasteurized miso seem to have no problem. Furthermore, some brands of packaged miso have been heated at temperatures lower than pasteurization levels (they can still be called unpasteurized) to delay overzealous fermentation.

Previously, most miso was made in Japan. Now much is being made in the United States using traditional methods and often organically grown soybeans and grains.

Soy Sauce

The quality and purity of soy sauce vary tremendously.

Common soy sauce is made from defatted soy meal that is treated with hydrochloric acid, heated, then treated with sodium carbonate to neutralize the acid. It is unfermented and contains additives such as caramel color, corn syrup, and preservatives.

Traditional Japanese soy sauce is naturally fermented in wooden kegs for many months and then pressed. What we call "tamari," the product made from soybeans, wheat, water, and sea salt, is technically **shoyu**. Traditional **tamari** is wheat-free, originally the liquid which rose to the surface or settled on the bottom of miso kegs.

The confusion in names stems from a lecture George Ohsawa (the person responsible for introducing macrobiotic principles to the West) gave in Hamburg, Germany. A man in attendance was so enthralled with the shoyu that he sampled there that he registered the word "shoyu" as his own trademark and brand name, thereby giving himself exclusive rights to the name in Germany. Because of the problem, the Ohsawas renamed shoyu with the term "tamari" and "tamari" became a generic term for both shoyu and traditional tamari.

Attempts are now being made to return to the original names. Soy sauce containing soy, wheat, water, and sea salt is labeled as "tamari shoyu" or "shoyu" while the name "tamari" indicates the real wheat-free product.

Both shoyu and tamari develop a small amount of alcohol, about 11/4-11/2 %, during fermentation. To retain good flavor, some companies add another 1/2% or so of food-grade grain alcohol to stop fermentation and the growth of aerobic yeasts. In Japan, the adding of alcohol is considered an incidental additive and is not required on labels as it is in the United States.

Genuine traditionally made tamari made from soybean miso is in small supply since extracting too much of the tamari adversely affects the quality of the miso. Now most companies utilize a process developed specifically for making tamari. Because tamari has a stronger, deeper flavor which is retained in longer cooking and contains 36%

more glutamic acid (a natural flavor enhancer) than shoyu, commercial food processors always use tamari. Likewise, home cooking which benefits from a salty seasoning added early in cooking, such as soups, roasted veggies, and casseroles, is best seasoned with tamari.

In contrast, shoyu has a rich, savory aroma and sweeter flavor that is suitable for both cooking and condiment uses. Add tamari shoyu only during the last few minutes of cooking. Longer cooking robs it of its delicate flavors as its slight alcohol content evaporates.

Both shoyu and tamari contain about 1000 mg. of sodium per tablespoon. If on a salt-restricted diet for medical or personal reasons, consider a low sodium shoyu which, depending upon the brand, contains 133-560 mg. per tablespoon in comparison.

Good quality **low sodium shoyu** is made from a double fermentation process. After the normal 2 years incubation of regular shoyu, extra wheat and soybeans are added to the fermentation mash but without the salt, thus lowering the salt concentration. It is then fermented for an additional 11/2 to 2 years to yield a 9% salt content instead of the normal 16% of regular shoyu. The double fermentation process insures a full-bodied flavor similar to regular shoyu without tasting like some watered-down low-sodium soy sauces. Another technique used by some companies is to heat the soy sauce at lowered atmospheric pressure. The moisture content is reduced until the salt forms as a precipitate and the salt is then removed in a centrifuge.

Lower-quality low-sodium shoyu uses an ion exchange process which removes much of the salt from regular shoyu. The shoyu passes through a tank containing two electrically charged plates. The salt precipitates out onto the plates, resulting in a shoyu that is of questionable quality.

TEMPEH BOUQUET

1 Tbsp. sesame oil
1/4 lb. mushrooms, chopped
1 small onion, thinly sliced
8 oz. tempeh, cut in 1/2" squares
1 tsp. bouquet garni herbal seasoning mixture
1 Tbsp. tamari soy sauce
1 cup water or vegetable broth
1 carrot, cut in 1/2" slices

Preheat oven to 350° F. Heat oil in a skillet. Add mushrooms and onions and sauté 5 minutes. Add tempeh, sprinkle with bouquet garni and tamari and sauté another 5 minutes. Add 1 cup water or broth, cover skillet, and simmer for 10 minutes. Transfer contents and carrot slices into an 8" X 8" baking dish. Cover with foil and bake for 30 minutes. Remove foil and bake another 15 minutes. Serve over pasta or cooked grains.

Serves 3.
(Pyramid servings: 1/2 Veg. Group, 1 1/2 Meat/Protein Group, 11 grams Fat)

Nutrition Facts

Serving Size 1/3 recipe (250 g)
Servings Per Container 3

Amount Per Serving

Calories 220   Calories from Fat 100

	% Daily Value*
Total Fat 11g	16%
Saturated Fat 1.5g	8%
Sodium 330mg	14%
Total Carbohydrate 19g	6%
Dietary Fiber 2g	6%
Sugars 4g	
Protein 16g	

Vitamin A 150%	•	Vitamin C	8%
Calcium 8%	•	Iron	15%

Not a significant source of Cholesterol
* Percent Daily Values are based on a 2,000 calorie diet.

High-grade shoyus form a thick head of foam when shaken that may take as long as 15 minutes to dissipate. An inferior brand will form a weaker foam that dissolves quickly.

Another quality-control test involves placing a drop of shoyu in a glass of water. Good-quality, natural shoyu will sink to the bottom of the glass before dispersing, while an inferior shoyu disperses almost immediately near the surface.

High-grade, naturally aged shoyu enhances the flavor while aiding digestion of countless foods. Use in marinades, vegetable dishes, soups, stews, beans, salad dressings, and grains dishes instead of salt or miso for variety. To preserve the flavor and chemical structure of shoyu, store away from sunlight and heat, including the stove. Some even suggest refrigeration.

Tempeh

Tempeh is a traditional Indonesian soy food whose chewy texture and mild, mushroomy flavor make it a terrific meat substitute. Tempeh is made by culturing cooked, cracked soybeans with a starter called *Rhizopus oligosporus*, similar to the process involved in making blue cheese and similar types of cheeses. After an incubation period of 24 hours, the soybeans form into a cake bound by threads of white cottony mycelium. Grains such as rice, quinoa, and amaranth, as well as sesame seeds and peanuts are often combined with the soybeans before inoculation for increased flavor.

As a result of the fermentation process, proteins, fats, and especially the complex oligosaccharides (responsible for problems with intestinal gas) are broken down into simpler compounds, making tempeh easily digested and assimilated. Its protein is particularly high in quality and quantity, providing 17 grams protein per 4 oz. serving.

Tempeh has often been considered a significant source of B_{12}, but generally this is not true of tempeh that is processed in the United States. The source of B_{12} in tempeh is neither the soybeans nor the Rhizopus mold, but a bacterium of the genus Klebsiella which develops during prefermentation "accidental" inoculation. In traditional Indonesian preparation, the bacteria are also introduced via the mixed starter culture which is grown on hibiscus leaves. Since most U.S. shops use a pure Rhizopus oligosporus culture, any B_{12} that would be present would come from unreliable environmental sources.

While tempeh can be sold refrigerated, more often than not you'll find it in the frozen food department since the beneficial mold used to make tempeh continues to grow even when refrigerated. Although it may sound awful, black spore formation is perfectly safe, and yet tempeh's flavor is milder when the tempeh appears more white. Refrigerated, tempeh will keep 7 days and up to 6 months when frozen. Throw it away if it begins to have an ammonia-like smell or starts to grow patches of rainbow colors.

Preparation of tempeh is very easy. It can be marinated for hours or minutes with your favorite seasonings. Tamari soy sauce, ginger, garlic, and coriander are particularly delicious cooked with tempeh. Once seasoned, simmer in a small amount of water or broth with or without other vegetables, panfry, bake, broil, stir-fry, or deep-fry.

As a clue for what to do with tempeh, consider that when crumbled, it has a meat-like texture. Try it in chili, stews, and soups. Cut it into medium-size pieces and serve as a burger in a bun with all the trimmings. Cut it in strips, marinate in olive oil, lemon pepper, and tamari soy sauce, and serve fajita-like in a whole wheat tortilla. Simmer or bake in Italian seasonings and serve on pizza instead of pepperoni.

To make things even easier, preseasoned, precooked tempeh burgers and cutlets are also available, that require only warming in the oven or microwave.

Texturized Vegetable Protein

Texturized vegetable protein (TVP™) is a concentrated soy protein product used to extend or replace meat in burgers, casseroles, stews, chilis, meatballs, and loaves. TVP™ is a registered trademark of its developer, Archer Daniels Midland, Inc., the world's largest food processor of soy products.

Considered a second-generation soy product, TVP™ is made by removing 90% of the soluble sugars from defatted soy flour through a chemical-free aqueous extraction process. Comprising 70% protein, it is then extruded into granules and chunks. Once rehydrated, TVP™ has the appearance and texture of meat.

Although TVP™ and soy protein concentrates are primarily sold to manufacturers for use in prepared foods, you'll likely find TVP™ in natural food stores sold in bulk and as an ingredient in vegetarian chili and burger mixes. Avoid TVP™ products which contain artificial flavors or artificial colors. Instead, look for unflavored varieties or those seasoned only with herbs and spices or other natural flavors.

To use, pour 7/8 cup boiling water over 1 cup granules or 1 cup boiling water over 1 cup chunks. Stir, cover, and allow to soak for 5 minutes. Then add to your recipe as you would meat, simmering another 15-20 minutes.

One serving of granules is considered approximately 1/4 cup dry. It contributes 11 grams of protein, 7 grams of carbohydrates, 0.2 grams of fat, and 59 calories.

Related to TVP™ is **soy protein isolate.** Containing about 90% protein, it stands as the most highly processed soy ingredient, concentrated through the use of various acids and alkalis. In addition to its high protein content, soy protein isolate is used in many soy products and other foods for its binding and gelling properties.

Tofu

Tofu has gone from relative obscurity to being one of the most celebrated foods due to its versatility, nutritional attributes, and low price.

Admittedly, the flavor of plain tofu is quite bland, but this bland quality of tofu is partially what is responsible for its versatility. Rather than consumed plain, tofu depends and benefits from marinating, simmering, baking, sautéeing, or blending with other foods and seasonings. If any food could be considered a chameleon, tofu would be first on the list. Depending upon what it is cooked with and how it is cooked, every tofu dish you prepare can be unique.

Tofu can also be transformed to emulate the flavor and texture of dairy products such as cream cheese, sour cream, cottage cheese, ricotta, and whipped cream. For those who prefer to avoid eggs as a leavener in baked goods, 1/4 cup mashed tofu can be substituted for each egg. When crumbled and sautéed with onion, scrambled tofu makes a worthy stand-in for scrambled eggs, especially when a pinch of turmeric is added to give the dish its characteristic yellow hue.

Nutrition

Nutritionally, tofu is the most easily digested soy food due to the fact that the oligosaccharides, the hard-to-digest complex carbohydrates, are removed as a result of the manufacturing process. A four-ounce serving of firm tofu contains approximately 120 calories, 12 grams of high-quality protein and no cholesterol. This same serving size also contains 7 grams of fat, making 53% of tofu's calories from fat.

Although this may seem quite high, it is important to keep it in perspective of how much fat is found in equivalent protein sources. Four ounces of lean meat such as a round steak trimmed of fat contributes 11 grams of fat, roasted dark meat turkey provides 8 grams of fat, roasted turkey breast has 3.8 grams of fat, and braised pork shoulder trimmed of fat weighs in at 13 grams of fat. Tofu's 7 grams of fat wins over the beef and pork and comes in just under dark meat turkey. Most of tofu's fat is unsaturated, as well.

Considering the fact that tofu is generally consumed with other foods, the total percentage of calories from fat from a meal containing tofu will generally be well within reasonable guidelines suggested as optimum. However, since tofu is fairly high in fat, sauces or accompaniments to tofu such as nuts or nut butters are best kept to a minimum.

Some manufacturers are now producing a fat-reduced tofu, bringing the percentage of calories from fat down from 53% in regular tofu to 38%. In practical terms, that means a reduction from 7 grams of fat to 5 grams per 4 oz. serving. It's not that earth-shattering, but it's something. The reduction in fat is attributed to the use of dehulled, rolled soybeans that have had much of their soy oil removed. Expect to pay a bit more than the price of regular tofu.

Because they contain a higher percentage of water, some varieties of soft tofu and all silken tofu are lower in fat than regular firm tofu. Depending on the manufacturer, fat content in soft tofu can range from 2 -7 grams per 4 oz. serving. Silken tofu contains 2-3 grams per 4 oz.

Manufacturing the Varieties of Tofu

Regular tofu is made by washing, soaking, grinding, and boiling soybeans. The resulting soy milk is strained to remove the fiber and then reheated. A coagulant is added to curdle the soy milk. Finally, the curds are separated from the whey and put under pressure to harden.

Tofu is sold as either "soft," "hard," or "extra firm" depending upon how long the curds are pressed to expel the whey.

Soft tofu is like custard. It is the best type to use in dips, sauces, salad dressings, and for soft nondairy cheese substitutes for ricotta cheese and cottage cheese.

"Hard" or firm tofu holds its shape better. It is good to use in tofu salads, scrambled tofu, and cheesecakes. **"Extra firm"** is the preferred variety when using tofu in cubed or sliced form.

However, alterations can be made to make soft tofu harder and hard tofu softer. Soft tofu can be firmed by draining some of the liquid from the tofu. Place the tofu in a strainer or colander until the desired texture is reached. Another method is to lay the tofu in a cloth or between paper towels and on a hard surface. Place a plate or cutting board on top, weighted down with a heavy object (try a bottle of juice or a heavy book) for a couple of minutes to expel the liquid. Conversely, if your recipe calls for soft tofu and you have hard tofu on hand, simply mash with liquid before adding to your recipe or soak the tofu in water.

Silken tofu is a type of tofu popular in traditional Japanese cuisine that is much lighter, delicate, and sweeter-tasting than regular tofu, resembling a custard or thick cream. Due to its silken nature, it imparts a creamy texture to soups, shakes, dips, dressings, sauces, and dessert recipes.

Modern-day manufacturing of silken tofu depends on a thicker, richer soy milk that is neither strained nor pressed. After mixing the soy milk with a coagulant, it is poured directly into individual cartons that are then sealed in an aseptic, sterile atmosphere. Immersion in hot water activates the coagulant to form the tofu inside the carton. Since the curds and whey are not separated in the process as with regular tofu, silken tofu has a higher water content which accounts for its softer, smoother consistency.

Three varieties of silken tofu plus a low-fat version are generally available. **Silken soft tofu** is best when puréed to make fruit shakes, soups, puddings, and creamy sauce bases. With some experimentation, it can also be substituted for milk, cream, or eggs in your favorite recipes.

Silken firm tofu has a firmer texture and higher protein content as a result of added soy protein isolates. Use it in recipes that require steamed, cubed, or crumbled tofu. **Silken extra firm tofu** is best when stir-frying.

The type of coagulant used in manufacturing tofu affects its flavor, texture, and calcium content. Nigari, the most traditional coagulant, is derived from refining most of the sodium chloride from natural sea salt, leaving a combination of magnesium chloride and other trace minerals. While it produces the best flavor, smooth texture, and high protein, it creates a tofu very low in calcium, providing only 42 mg. per 3 1/2 oz. Pure magnesium chloride yields a tofu with even less calcium, about 36 mg. per 3 1/2 oz.

To boost calcium levels, manufacturers often use calcium chloride or calcium sulfate as coagulants for tofu. There are two sources of calcium chloride. It can be synthesized as the by-product of the manufacture of soda ash, involving a reaction between a calcium source and hydrochloric acid or chlorine gas. It can also be mined from underground deposits, a source used by more reputable tofu manufacturers. Calcium chloride makes excellent quality tofu and boosts calcium levels to 108 mg. per 3 1/2 oz.

Calcium sulfate, also known as gypsum, is a minimally refined mined product. When used alone as a coagulant, flavor, texture, and protein content of the resulting tofu leaves much to be desired. Therefore, manufacturers who use calcium sulfate generally combine it with other coagulants for better results. By itself, it would create a tofu with 139 mg. of calcium per 31/2 oz. Obviously, if combined with another coagulant, calcium levels will vary according to the proportion of particular coagulants.

Lactone or glucono-delta-lactone is an acid derived from cornstarch to make silken tofu. It curdles the soy milk similar to the way lactic acid from lactobacillus bacteria cultures reacts with milk to make yogurt. Because it incorporates more water into the tofu during the process, silken tofu will have less protein. When used alone, it provides only 14 mg. of calcium per 31/2 oz. However, labels of most varieties of silken tofu will indicate another calcium source has been added.

Buying and storage

Tofu is a very perishable product susceptible to several microbiological pathogens such as Clostridium botulinum, Staphylococcus aureus, Salmonella typhimurium, and Yersinia enterocolitica if manufactured or stored in unsanitary or too warm conditions. Look for packages that list suggested "use by" dates and buy accordingly for fresh-tasting tofu. Spoiled tofu is characterized by murky water, a discolored appearance, and a slimy film.

Oddly enough, tofu keeps fresh when stored in water. Once made and transferred to a container, it will keep fresh under refrigeration for 7 days if the holding water in the container is drained and replenished daily.

Tofu sealed in packages by the manufacturer has a longer shelf life until the package is opened. When packaged in **water-packed** tubs that are heat-sealed to keep the air out, tofu has an average refrigerator-life of 7-14 days.

Tofu that has been **pasteurized** before packaging may last up to 28 days. Once made, it is immersed in a tank filled with water heated to 145-165° for 20-60 minutes, followed by rapid chilling. In exchange for the extended refrigerator-life, flavor is only slightly impaired.

Vacuum-packed tofu can potentially last 21-35 days. In this method, the tofu is heat-sealed without water in a multi-laminant plastic bag in which all the air has previously been extracted.

Silken tofu is sold in **aseptic packages** sealed under extremely sterile conditions. They can be sold and stored without refrigeration for about 9 months.

Despite the fact that it appears more environmentally friendly since it eliminates excess packaging materials, avoid buying tofu in bulk. Without the benefit of a seal to keep bacteria or air out, tofu should be rinsed daily and stored in fresh water—a practice not common when stores are dealing with 20 lb. water-filled buckets of tofu. When you add in the increased likelihood of bacteria from utensils (or hands!) used to scoop out the tofu, it's just not worth the chance. On the other hand, if the store where you buy bulk tofu changes the water religiously and only allows an immaculate employee whose primary job is the privilege of waiting on tofu

SAVORY BAKED TOFU

1 tsp. olive or sesame oil
1 lb. fresh firm tofu, cut in
    1/2" slices
1 tsp. pizza seasoning or
    curry powder
1 Tbsp. tamari soy sauce

Preheat oven to 350° F. Oil a 9" X 13" baking dish. Place tofu slices in a single layer. Sprinkle with seasoning and tamari. Cover with foil and bake for 30 minutes.

Variation: For a more meaty texture, thawed frozen tofu slices may also be used instead of the fresh tofu.

Serves 4.
(Pyramid servings: 1 1/2 Meat/Protein Group, 11 grams Fat)

Nutrition Facts

Serving Size 1/4 recipe (119 g)
Servings Per Container 4

Amount Per Serving

Calories 180   Calories from Fat 100

	% Daily Value*
Total Fat 11g	**17%**
Saturated Fat 1.5g	**8%**
Sodium 250mg	**10%**
Total Carbohydrate 5g	**2%**
Protein 18g	

Vitamin A 4%	•	Calcium 25%
Iron 70%		

Not a significant source of Cholesterol, Dietary Fiber, Sugars and Vitamin C.
* Percent Daily Values are based on a 2,000 calorie diet.

---

customers, then perhaps the relative safety of dispensing bulk tofu could be argued.

Also avoid tofu sold in produce sections of your local grocery or natural food store. The average temperature in these departments is above 50°. Tofu needs temperatures of 41° or less to avoid spoiling.

Cooking with tofu

All tofu, with the exception of silken and just-made tofu, should be cooked briefly to protect against potential bacteria that may have formed during storage and to give it a freshness boost for improved flavor. If planning to use tofu for dips and other recipes in which it won't be subjected to any further cooking, immerse in boiling water and cook briefly for 5 minutes. Remove the tofu, allow it to cool, and then proceed with your recipe. Tofu that will be simmered, baked, fried, or grilled needs no prior simmering.

If you're new to tofu, one of the easiest ways to get acquainted with its possibilities is to try some of the prepared tofu products sold in the dairy case and frozen food areas in your favorite food store such as tofu "no egg" salad, cottage tofu, dips, frozen dinners, tofu burgers, tofu "hot dogs," tofu "bologna," and tofu mayonnaise and tofu salad dressings. Many "tofu-helper" type mixes are also available to make burgers, stir-fries, and casseroles with tofu. Once you understand that there are no restrictions on your creativity, you're ready to give tofu a whirl.

Start out traditionally and stir-fry it Chinese-style with lots of veggies.

Mash it and add just a bit of salad dressing, nut butter, avocado, lemon juice, vinegar, fresh herbs, hot sauce, spaghetti sauce, chutney, soy sauce, or any other condiment you enjoy. The point is to give the tofu a subtle flavor boost, not overwhelm it. Serve as a dip, sandwich filling, or use it instead of ricotta in pasta dishes.

Then move on to simmering. Add to stews, soups, chilis, and vegetable medleys. The tofu will contribute its soft texture while absorbing the flavors in which it is immersed.

Baking is easy. Slice or cube, sprinkle with herbs and soy sauce, place on a baking pan, and bake at 350° for 20-30 minutes, covered or not, as you please.

Once you've spent some time experimenting with tofu in its fresh state, place a block of tofu in a container or plastic bag without water and put it in the freezer for about a week. (Unless the thought of tofu slush sounds appealing, don't freeze silken tofu.) Tofu's naturally white color will turn yellow while in its frozen state but, once thawed, it will return to its original color.

Thawed **frozen tofu** has a chewy, meaty texture which, when crumbled, is perfect as a substitute for ground beef in casseroles, pizza, stews, or spaghetti sauces. Sliced or cubed frozen tofu has a texture similar to chicken, great for mock chicken salads and cutlets. Freezing tofu also increases its ability to absorb flavors. Use frozen tofu within 6 months.

Freeze-dried tofu is a further expansion on the frozen tofu theme. It has a finer, firm-grained texture and is more absorbant and soft when reconstituted. When available, it can be found in the Oriental foods section of a natural foods or specialty food store. Unusual in appearance, it looks like a pack of beige-colored 2 x 21/2" sponges wrapped in cellophane.

The traditional manufacture of freeze-dried tofu is just as intriguing. In the mountains of Japan, the tofu is suspended on wooden racks where it is allowed to freeze during the night and thaw during the day, allowing for evaporation of its moisture content. After about 20 days, the tofu is extremely dry, light in weight, and finely textured.

Freeze-dried tofu needs no refrigeration. However, once the package is open, it should be stored in an airtight plastic bag or container and used within 4 months. To reconstitute, soak the cakes in warm water for 3-5 minutes. Since freeze-dried tofu is such a concentrated energy source, containing up to 7 times more nutrients than an equal weight of fresh tofu, one cake is usually enough per person.

Press between towels or the palms of your hands to squeeze out excess liquid. Then cook with soups, stews, vegetables, or alone with your choice of seasonings to absorb flavors.

Eggs

WHEN IT comes to value, convenience, and nutrition, eggs provide a package deal. No other concentrated protein food is as inexpensive and quick to prepare. Its protein content and riboflavin (B_2) are equally divided between the yolk and the white. Most of the egg's other major nutrients: iron, vitamins A, D, and B_{12} are found in the yolk. However, the yolk also provides all the fat and cholesterol that is found in the egg, a fact that has put the yolk on shaky nutritional ground.

NUTRITION

By virtue of being the most concentrated source of cholesterol found in our diets, eggs were first singled out as a major contributor to heart disease by the American Heart Association in 1964. Considering the Association's suggested limit of 300 mg. of cholesterol intake per day, eating a single egg with its 274 mg. of cholesterol left little room for the daily consumption of other commonly consumed cholesterol-containing animal proteins. Accordingly, they recommended the average person eat no more than 3 whole eggs per week, including those used in baking. No restrictions were placed on egg whites.

Much has been learned about both cholesterol and eggs since then. New research has disproved the theory linking dietary cholesterol directly to blood cholesterol. Instead, the body has an internal self-adjusting system that regulates the amount of cholesterol absorbed and recycled depending on dietary intake. How well this system actually works can vary considerably among the population, a fate determined by the genetic luck of the draw.

While some of us may be genetically hypersensitive to dietary cholesterol, what's more important for everyone is to limit saturated fat intake. Saturated fats in foods are the primary contributors to elevating blood cholesterol. Therefore, even if a low-cholesterol diet is maintained, one high in saturated fats can still mean trouble.

Eggs present the opposite situation. Although they are undoubtedly high in cholesterol, their fat is primarily unsaturated, underscoring the fact that eggs may, after all, be an acceptable adjunct within a healthy diet. However, since it is hard to determine who is hypersensitive to cholesterol and who is not, moderate consumption of eggs is still advised.

It has also been discovered that eggs have less cholesterol than we've all been led to believe. Attributed largely to changes in analytical methods, in 1989 it was announced that eggs actually contained 213 mg. of cholesterol per egg rather than the 274 mg. as previously believed.

Consequently, the American Heart Association slightly modified their former position to allow the addition of another egg to its suggested weekly egg allotment per person, making 4 whole eggs per week as the new standard. As before, the consumption of egg whites remains unrestricted.

FOOD SAFETY CONCERNS

As if cholesterol wasn't enough of a public relations problem for eggs, thanks to a new strain of salmonella bacteria, in 1990 the FDA designated fresh eggs as a "potentially hazardous food."

Unlike its predecessors which could be transmitted only through cracked or thin-shelled eggs, Salmonella enterititis can spread directly from infected hens into their eggs. When contaminated eggs are consumed, severe intestinal illness can occur within 12-14 hours and last 1-4 days. Even worse, it can be fatal to cancer or heart patients, the very young and old, and individuals with immune-system disorders.

While the risk of eating a contaminated egg is less than 1 in 10,000, it still makes sense to use any precautions possible to avert a potentially serious problem.

Most cases of egg-related Salmonella enterititis food poisoning have occurred from eating raw or undercooked eggs. Therefore, it's best to avoid beverages and foods made with raw eggs that do not undergo any further cooking, such as eggnog, some health drinks, Caesar salad, hollandaise sauce, egg-based homemade ice cream, and homemade mayonnaise. Snitching batter from bowls of cookie or cake mixes that contain raw egg should definitely become a thing of the past.

Most restaurants and manufacturers have switched to using pre-shelled eggs that have been ultra-pasteurized to destroy harmful bacteria in most of their egg-containing drinks and foods. Other sterilization techniques are still being explored, including high-pressure injections of pure oxygen and ozone into the egg to provide salmonella-free raw eggs, still in the shell.

But sterilized or ultra-pasteurized eggs aren't the only answers to beating Salmonella enterititis. Proper storage combined with thorough cooking can virtually make any egg safe to eat.

Cooking Eggs Safely

Thoroughly cooked, properly stored eggs can effectively destroy Salmonella enterititis. Just make sure to cook eggs until both the white and yolk are firm in a skillet over medium heat, in boiling water, or in a moderate oven. Refer to the table below for approximate timing required for thorough cooking.

Cooking Method	Suggested Safe Cooking Timing
scrambled	at least 1 minute
sunnyside up	5 minutes
fried over easy	3 minutes on the first side and 2 minutes on second
poached	5 minutes
boiled eggs	7 minutes
meringue-topped pies baked in 326° F. oven	25-27 minutes

BUYING AND STORING

Several factors influence the size and quality of eggs: the age, weight, and breed of the hen, environmental temperatures, the quality of feed, and living conditions.

Young hens lay small eggs while older hens produce large to jumbo-sized eggs. The occasional double yolk results from a young hen whose laying cycle needs some fine-tuning.

The color of the shell indicates only the breed of hen that laid the eggs, not nutrient value. White leghorn chickens lay white eggs, Plymouth Rock hens and Rhode Island Reds lay brown eggs, and other breeds are responsible for the many varying colors of eggs that are available.

Fertile vs. Nonfertile Eggs

A hen will routinely produce eggs whether or not she has mated with a rooster. While still fit to eat, these non-fertile or sterile eggs will never mature into chicks, even after proper incubation. Living conditions for the laying hens account for the main differences between fertile and non-fertile eggs.

Most eggs sold in grocery stores and served in restaurants are produced from caged hens. The poultry industry has conducted considerable research to discover the most efficient and cost-effective, but not necessarily humane, way to produce eggs. Accordingly, most laying hens are stuffed, three to five into a small wire cage, where they will live for up to 2 years cranking out eggs in an uncomfortable, restricted, stressful environment.

By nature, during the day chickens like to run, fly, explore, as well as scratch and peck at the ground looking for food, even if given access to plenty of feed. At night, they like to roost above the ground. As social animals, they like to eat and dust-bathe together in groups. Laying hens also like to nest, spending considerable time looking for just the right place and getting it just so.

But none of these natural behaviors are being satisfied with the "battery" cage confinement system for laying hens. As a result, the stress can drive them to peck each other in the small cages. The poultry industry took care of this problem by removing a part of the hen's beak (debeaking), thus depriving the hens normal preening, exploring, and eating. Since hens are very sensitive to touch, temperature and pain, such a procedure is very cruel. Lack of exercise and the demands of high egg production cause hens to have very brittle bones.

Although hens naturally produce eggs according to day/night and seasonal cycles, overhead lights may be left on 24 hours per day to confuse the birds and encourage maximum production. Some producers routinely add antibiotics to the feed to help counter disease which can run rampant when hens are confined in small quarters. For collecting ease, the average producer has an egg collection system connected to a conveyer belt or trough.

Many "battery" eggs may have deep, yellow yolks, reminiscent of eggs laid by hens who have access to sunlight and vegetation. But it is the addition of yellow corn, green grass, alfalfa, or marigold petals to their feed that enhances the color of the yolk.

In contrast, hens raised in floor houses have at least 2 square feet allotted per bird, often with open access to the outside. In addition to their feed ration, hens that are raised in a chicken house also have access to eat whatever they find such as grubs and bugs. Not only does this give them access to cafeteria-style dining, it also allows them the opportunity to try to find something that could fill in the nutritional gap they may inherently find missing, as well as having access to vitamin A-rich vegetation to produce deep, yellow yolks.

Exposed to natural light and, in many cases, temperatures, hens are also allowed the opportunity to live and breed according to the cycles of nature, thus allowing them the dignity of their species rather than living their lives simply as egg machines.

A **fertile egg** is one that has been produced by a hen who has mated with a rooster. Since a rooster in every cage would be too expensive (they eat a lot) and very noisy, hens who have access to a rooster will always be quartered within a house instead of a cage. Therefore, buying fertile eggs is a guarantee that the eggs come from hens allowed to freely roam within a chicken house and possibly in a yard.

In flocks where hens and roosters are kept together, 80-95% of the eggs will be fertile. Since the embryo remains microscopic, it is very difficult to tell whether or not an egg is fertile. Contrary to popular belief, a small blood spot on the yolk is not a sure sign of a fertile egg.

And there's no need to worry that your carton of fertile eggs will hatch into chicks on the way home from the store. The eggs are chilled shortly after they are laid to prevent the natural hatching progression from initiating.

When it comes down to it, there is little, if any nutritional difference between a fertile egg and a sterile egg. However, in addition to feeling good about supporting a more humane existence for the laying hens, many people find fertile eggs are richer in flavor than typical sterile eggs. The yolks and whites from eggs laid by uncaged hens are also denser than those laid by hens stuffed into a small cage.

Sometimes laying hens are raised in floor houses without the companionship of a rooster. Free-range hens in this situation will lay sterile eggs, much like their caged cousins.

Switzerland and Sweden have both passed legislation banning the wire caging system for laying hens. As a result, more humane housing systems have been developed that allow freedom of movement and the expression of natural behaviors, including dust bathing, perching, and private nesting.

In this country, the plight of laying hens has largely been ignored. Current conditions will likely stay the same unless consumers demand a change. Make a conscious choice when choosing eggs at the grocery store. Buy only eggs laid by humanely treated hens, commonly referred to as "free-roaming," "free-range," "free-running," or "uncaged." Urge your favorite restaurants and bakeries to do the same.

Egg Grading

Grading for quality depends upon the interior quality of the egg and on the condition and appearance of the shell. USDA inspection is required only if the distributor/producer sells eggs produced at other farms or if his/her flock numbers more than 3000 hens.

Eggs can be sized and graded by the producer without USDA supervision but "U.S.D.A." may not appear on the label. Small producers can also market eggs as "ungraded."

GRADE AA eggs represent the best in quality and freshness. The height of the egg as well as the firm centering of the yolk gives the egg a superior appearance. The clear, firm, thick egg white is best for poaching, frying, and cooking in the shell when the appearance of the egg is important.

GRADE A are not as satisfactory for poaching but still excellent for frying and cooking purposes. After 10 days a Grade AA egg will become a Grade A. Most egg packers list their eggs as Grade A to give themselves flexibility in the length of time they can sell their eggs, even though it may have been Grade AA at the time of packing. Grade A eggs will keep up to 30 days under proper conditions.

GRADE B eggs can be used when the appearance of the egg doesn't matter, i.e., scrambled eggs or blended cooked foods. Its shell is unbroken, slightly abnormal, and ranges from clean to very slightly stained. The egg white is clear but may be slightly weak.

SCRAMBLED EGG WHITES

8 egg whites
1/8 tsp. turmeric
2 tsp. canola oil
2 Tbsp. nonfat dry milk powder

Whisk ingredients together. Heat skillet over low heat and brush lightly with oil. Add egg white mixture and scramble as usual.

Serves 2.
(Pyramid servings: 2 Meat/Protein Group, 41/2 grams Fat)

Nutrition Facts
Serving Size 1/2 recipe (144 g)
Servings Per Container 2

Amount Per Serving

Calories 130   Calories from Fat 40

	% Daily Value*
Total Fat 4.5g	7%
Sodium 260mg	11%
Total Carbohydrate 5g	2%
Sugars 5g	
Protein 17g	

Calcium 10%

Not a significant source of Saturated Fat, Cholesterol, Dietary Fiber, Vitamin A, Vitamin C and Iron.

* Percent Daily Values are based on a 2,000 calorie diet.

Storing Eggs

Salmonella enterititis multiplies at room temperature, so keep both raw and cooked eggs refrigerated at temperatures under 40° F. To avoid odors and flavors of other foods also stored in the refrigerator, refrigerate eggs in their carton rather than the egg compartments provided in the door of many refrigerators. Eggs will remain fresher and the yolk more centered if they are stored round side up to prevent movement of the egg cell toward the yolk.

Fresh eggs should be used within 5 weeks. Use leftover egg yolks and egg whites as well as hard-boiled eggs, whether in or out of shell, within 4 days. Freshly cooked eggs or foods containing eggs should be served immediately after cooking or, if intended to be served later, refrigerated quickly.

When dyeing hard-boiled eggs for holiday decorations or Easter egg hunts, consider making separate batches for eating and displaying or hiding. Under no circumstances should eggs be consumed after being left unrefrigerated for more than 2 hours.

EGG-BASED SUBSTITUTES

Many people find that they can still enjoy eggs and eliminate the usual amount of cholesterol by using more egg whites than yolks in their cooking. Substitute 2 egg whites to replace each whole egg when scrambling eggs or in recipes that don't depend on the yolk for flavor and texture. Or compromise with a combination of egg yolks and egg whites, substituting 1 whole egg and 2 egg whites for 3 whole eggs.

Commercially prepared egg substitutes are available in two basic models. Most familiar are the liquid substitutes based primarily on pasteurized (salmonella-free) egg whites with oil, cornstarch, emulsifiers, and, depending on the brand, artificial coloring.

SCRAMBLED TOFU

Tofu can be mashed and sautéed with 1/4 teaspoon turmeric (a spice) to imitate the soft texture and characteristic yellow color of scrambled eggs. Try this recipe for starters and then experiment with your own special seasonings.

1 Tbsp. sesame or olive oil
1/4 tsp. turmeric
1 small red onion, minced
2 cloves garlic, minced
2 ribs celery, finely diced
3 medium-sized mushrooms, sliced (optional)
1 lb. tofu, soft or firm
1 Tbsp. tamari shoyu or 1/4 tsp. sea salt
1/4 tsp. dillweed (optional)

In an large oiled skillet over medium heat, sauté tumeric for 30 seconds. Add onion and garlic and sauté 3 minutes or until onion becomes translucent. Add celery and mushrooms and continue to sauté for another 2 minutes. Crumble tofu and add to vegetables. Season with shoyu or salt and dillweed. Cover, reduce heat to medium-low and cook for 10 minutes, stirring occasionally. Serve with toast, bagels, or tortillas.

Serves 4.
(Pyramid servings: 1/2 Veg. Group, 1 1/2 Meat/Protein Group, 13 grams Fat)

Nutrition Facts

Serving Size 1/4 recipe (184 g)
Servings Per Container 4

Amount Per Serving

Calories 220   Calories from Fat 120

	% Daily Value*
Total Fat 13g	21%
Saturated Fat 2g	10%
Sodium 270mg	11%
Total Carbohydrate 9g	3%
Dietary Fiber 1g	5%
Sugars 2g	
Protein 19g	

Vitamin A 4%	•	Vitamin C	8%
Calcium 25%	•	Iron	70%

Not a significant source of Cholesterol
* Percent Daily Values are based on a 2,000 calorie diet.

Like the home-separated egg whites, these egg substitutes can be used in cakes, cookies, muffins, quiches, and omelets. However, they are not suitable for making meringues, in recipes that call for more than 3 eggs, or in recipes that require both separated yolks and whites. A teaspoon of oil may be needed to improve texture in baked goods that are already low in fat.

Another type of egg substitute is made by first treating the egg yolk to remove 80% of the cholesterol and recombining it with the egg white to make a pasteurized (salmo-nella-free) liquid whole egg product called "Simply Eggs"™. The cholesterol is reduced by centrifuging the egg yolk with modified cornstarch which causes much of the cholesterol to stick to the cornstarch. Except for a small amount of sodium and only 45 mg. of cholesterol per equivalent egg, "Simply Eggs"™ contains the same nutrients as found in a regular egg. It is packaged in half-pint containers, the equivalent of 4 whole eggs. Refrigerated and unopened it will last 9 weeks but, once the package is opened, it must be used within 3 days. "Simply Eggs"™

can be used in any recipe requiring whole, unseparated eggs, including egg dishes, baked goods, and beverages.

"NON-EGG"-BASED SUBSTITUTES

Various "non-egg"-based substitutes are available that, to a limited degree, can emulate an egg's intended function in some recipes.

Leavening: to lighten and increase volume in baked goods.

Baking powder: In cake and cookie recipes that require only 1 egg, substitute 2 tablespoons water and 1/2 teaspoon baking powder.

Buttermilk/thinned yogurt: Replace the liquid in the recipe with buttermilk or thinned yogurt. You must also replace the baking powder with an equivalent amount of baking soda to a maximum of 1 teaspoon per cup of flour used.

Ener-G Egg Replacer™: This is a dry product found in most natural food stores made from potato starch, tapioca flour, leavening agents (calcium lactate, calcium carbonate, citric acid), and a vegetable-derived gum. For each egg, mix 11/2 teaspoon of the powder with 2 tablespoons of water and add to your recipe. It works best in recipes made from scratch.

Flaxseeds: For the equivalent of 3 eggs, combine 1/4 cup flax-seeds and 3/4 cup water. Process 5-10 minutes in a blender to make a gluey slurry. Add an equivalent amount to baked goods instead of the required eggs.

Binding Substitutes: to hold ingredients together or to provide body

Apple butter, fruit puree, cooked starchy vegetable puree: use 3 tablespoons to replace each egg. Various commercially prepared fruit purees based on plum puree (prunes) and advertised as fat replacers can also be used instead of eggs to provide body.

Ener-G Egg Replacer™: See above, under "leavening."

Flaxseeds: See above, under "leavening."

Tofu: substitute 1/4 cup regular or firm mashed tofu to replace each egg.

Miscellaneous: mashed beans or potatoes, nut butters, cooked oatmeal can all be added to provide body when making casseroles or grain or bean-based "burgers."

Nuts and Seeds

NUTRITION

Nuts and seeds provide rich flavor and crisp texture when added as an ingredient or a garnish to fruit and vegetable salads, breakfast cereals, whole grains, and pasta. It's also no secret that they are terrific eaten out of hand as a snack, served alone or combined with dried fruits.

What may not be so obvious is that nuts and seeds are classified as proteins instead of fats on the Food Guide Pyamid. While there is no doubt that nuts and seeds are high in fat, like other protein foods, they also supply B vitamins and minerals, particularly iron, zinc, and potassium. Unlike meats, fish, and poultry, nuts and seeds supply fiber. One-third cup nuts and seeds or 2 tablespoons of nut butter are equivalent to 1 oz. of lean meat.

In general, seeds are higher in protein than nuts. Using the classic protein complementary system, the protein quality of both nuts and seeds can be enhanced when combined with beans or dairy products to provide amino acids (lysine and isoleucine) that are deficient in nuts and seeds. Since peanuts and soynuts are beans, their protein can be complemented with grains and dairy to make up for the amino acids (tryptophan and methionine) deficient in beans. Even though it is not necessary to eat complementary proteins at the same meal, you probably already combine them as a matter of taste. Examples include hummus (garbanzo beans plus sesame seeds) and peanut butter sandwiches (peanuts plus grains).

Depending on the particular nut or seed, its fat is primarily monounsaturated or polyunsaturated. Unlike saturated fat, the type of fat considered the primary culprit in the American diet for elevating blood cholesterol, both monounsaturated and polyunsaturated fats can help lower total cholesterol when substituted in the diet for saturated fats. Monounsaturated fats go one step further than polyunsaturated fats. Instead of lowering the "good" cholesterol (HDL or high density lipoproteins) along with the "bad" cholesterol (LDL or low density lipoproteins), monounsaturated fats spare the HDL to allow them to continue their work of reprocessing and removal of cholesterol from the body. Some nuts and seeds are also good sources of essential fatty acids. Just the same, even though nuts and seeds supply the right kinds of fat, they are best eaten in moderation.

BUYING AND STORING

Fresh Nuts

Nuts should be stored carefully in warehouses, grocery stores, and at home to retard rancidity (oxidation of fat). Not only does rancidity damage cells within the body, it also destroys the flavor of the otherwise delicious nut or seed. Since dark patches indicate that rancidity is starting to occur, make sure the inside portions of the nuts or seeds you buy are of uniform color.

When possible, taste bulk nuts and seeds before purchasing. Upon inquiry, most stores will gladly give you a sample to test for freshness. If they refuse, buy nuts and seeds elsewhere. For optimum freshness and quality, choose varieties packaged in nitrogen-flushed packages.

Make sure to avoid any nuts that are moldy, discolored, or shriveled. Almonds, brazil nuts, pecans, pistachios, walnuts, and, especially peanuts are vulnerable to aflatoxin, a carcinogenic mold produced by a fungus called Aspergillus flavus that grows on plants weakened by insects or drought conditions.

Organically grown nuts and peanuts, raised according to a system that enhances the natural ecological balance within the soil, are generally less likely to be affected by aflatoxin.

Nuts in the shell keep the longest, up to 1 year if stored in a cool, dry place. Shelled nuts are best refrigerated in tightly sealed glass or plastic containers to compensate for the removal of their natural protective covering.

Depending on the particular nut or seed, shelled nuts can retain their quality 3-9 months in the refrigerator and up to 1 year in the freezer. When traveling or stashing nuts and seeds in your desk or locker at work or school, buy small amounts at a time and replenish with a fresh batch frequently.

Nuts and seeds vary in weight, but a good rule of thumb is to buy twice the quantity of nuts in the shell for the amount needed *shelled*.

Broken nuts are very susceptible to rancidity, so it's best to buy whole nuts instead of prechopped or ground nuts. Process your own at home in a blender, food processor, or electric nut and coffee mill just prior to use.

Raw nuts can be pan- or oven-roasted at home. To pan roast, put a thin layer of nuts in a skillet over low heat and stir frequently. Check for doneness after 5 minutes and every couple of minutes thereafter to prevent burning. To oven roast, spread nuts or seeds on a baking sheet and place in a preheated 325° oven, stirring occasionally. Like pan-roasting, check nuts frequently. Since nuts and seeds will continue to roast while cooling, remove them from the heat as soon as the roasting aroma permeates the room.

For a special treat, towards the end of roasting, sprinkle nuts with tamari shoyu (natural soy sauce), stir to coat, and place back in the oven to dry for about 2 minutes. Tamari roasted nuts are terrific as a snack (especially when combined with raisins) or as a condiment on foods.

Because roasting brings oils to the surface, roasted nuts tend to turn rancid more quickly. For best flavor, roast no more than you can use within a month. Avoid commercially roasted nuts that are laden with preservatives, sugar, monosodium glutamate (MSG), vegetable gums, salt, and seasonings to mask any "off" rancid flavors. Fresh, high-quality roasted nuts have no need for such additives.

Nut Butters

Nut butters are another way to enjoy the flavors and nutrition of nuts. Typically used as spreads for bread and crackers, nut butters can also be used as the basis for sauces, gravies, dips, and cookies.

Thanks to the force of gravity, the oils and solids of natural nut butters tend to separate. However, once the oils are stirred in with the solids and subsequently refrigerated, the oils and solids remain suspended. Another trick is to store unopened jars of nut

BASIC NUT MILK

1/4-1/3 cup nuts
3 1/2 cups hot water or
    juice
1 Tbsp. flaxseeds or 1 tsp.
    lecithin granules
    (optional)
1-2 Tbsp. rice syrup,
    honey, or maple syrup
dash of flavor extract
    (optional)
2 Tbsp. carob powder
    (optional)

Grind nuts (and flax seeds if used) in a blender to the consistency of flour. Gradually add hot water (and lecithin, if used) until creamy. Then blend in 1-2 tablespoons of sweetener (and flavor extract and/or carob, if used). Pour the nut milk through a fine strainer into a bowl or large measuring cup. Use the nut milk immediately or pour into a jar or pitcher, cover tightly, and refrigerate.

Makes 1 quart.
(Pyramid servings: 1/4 Meat/ Protein, 6 grams Fat, 3 grams Sweets)

Nutrition Facts

Serving Size 1 cup almond milk (226 g)
Servings Per Container 4

Amount Per Serving

Calories 90	Calories from Fat 60

	% Daily Value*
Total Fat 6g	10%
Saturated Fat 0.5g	3%
Sodium 10mg	0%
Total Carbohydrate 7g	2%
Dietary Fiber 1g	6%
Sugars 5g	
Protein 3g	

Calcium 4%	●	Iron 8%

Not a significant source of Cholesterol, Vitamin A and Vitamin C.
* Percent Daily Values are based on a 2,000 calorie diet.

---

butters upside down at room temperature to help distribute the oils. You'll still have some stirring to do, but it will be much easier.

To prevent separation both before and after the jar is opened, some nut butters are hydrogenated to harden the oils into a semi-solid. While it may save a minute's worth of initial stirring, the process of hydrogenation transforms the chemical structure of many unsaturated fatty acids. Referred to as trans-fatty acids, these altered fats have been shown to raise "bad" cholesterol almost as much as saturated fats. All in all, your best bet is to buy unhydrogenated nut butters or one of the new peanut butters whose solids are naturally suspended using a new process involving lecithin.

You can also make your own nut butters at home. First roast the nuts and process in a blender or food processor until creamy. A teaspoon or tablespoon of oil per 2 cups of nuts or peanuts may facilitate the grinding and yield a better consistency. Some juicers have attachments specifically for making nut butters.

According to the Food Guide Pyramid, consider 2 Tbsp. of peanut butter equivalent to 1 oz. of lean meat. Like whole nuts, this protein contains a significant amount of fat and should be eaten judiciously.

Nut Milks

Nuts and seeds can also be transformed into a nondairy milk substitute that can be used like milk in almost any application: as a delicious beverage, to moisten hot and cold cereals, as a base for sauces and gravies, and for baking. Preparation is minimal. Similar to dairy milk, nut milk will keep up to 5-7 days in the refrigerator.

Keep in mind that nut milks provide minimal calcium compared to dairy milk. Be sure to include other sources of calcium such as collard greens, kale, mustard greens, broccoli, or even calcium supplements to provide your daily calcium requirement.

The composition and texture of blanched almonds, cashews, and sesame seeds make them the best candidates for nut milks. A tablespoon of flaxseeds ground with the nuts or a teaspoon of lecithin granules blended with the hot water will help emulsify the mixture to keep the fats and liquid in suspension. Pouring the "milk" through a fine strainer will remove any coarse pieces of nuts or hulls that could make the final product gritty.

Exploring Your Options

ALMONDS

Facts and Features

Grown extensively in California, almonds are related to peaches, nectarines, and other members of the rose family. Sweet almonds are the edible variety while bitter almonds are used as an ingredient in cosmetics and to make almond extract.

Almonds are a fairly good source of calcium, supplying as much calcium in 3 tablespoons as in 1/4 cup milk. Eighty-one percent of their calories are from fat, predominantly monounsaturated.

One pound of almonds in the shell will yield 11/4 cups shelled whole almonds. Store shelled almonds in the refrigerator for up to 9 months and in the freezer for up to 1 year. Thanks to their edible but tough brown skin that is retained after shelling, almonds resist rancidity better than any other nut.

Varieties and Preparation Guidelines

Since the skin also adds fiber and a slightly assertive flavor some recipes call for blanched almonds. For best flavor, blanch your own at home. Simply pour boiling water over the almonds, allow them to set for 3 minutes, and drain. Then put the almonds into cold water for 1 minute. The skins will slip off easily when the nut is gently rubbed between your thumb and fingers. Blanched almonds are also a favorite for making nut milks.

Almond butter, available in both smooth and crunchy versions, can be used similarly to peanut butter to make sandwiches, cookies, and spreads with a rich, gourmet flair. For a real treat, spread almond butter on bananas, apple slices, or cooked and sliced sweet potatoes.

BRAZIL NUTS

Facts and Features

Brazil nuts are harvested from the wild in Venezuela and, of course, in Brazil. A good source of dietary fiber, they also contain a significant amount of fat. Ninety-two percent of their calories are from fat, predominantly polyunsaturated.

Store in the refrigerator or freezer up to 9 months.

Varieties and Preparation Guidelines

Brazil nuts make delicious snacks, especially when eaten with fresh or dried fruit, including apples, pears, raisins, dates and figs. They contribute a special creamy texture when added to smoothies. Try a few chopped brazil nuts in poultry stuffings for extra texture and flavor.

CASHEWS

Facts and Features

Cashews are imported from India and Brazil only in their shelled form due to a toxic oil that lies between the outer shell and an inner shell that surrounds the nut itself. Exposing the cashew to heat causes the outer shell to burst and release the toxic oil. Although generally marketed as "raw," once the outer shell is removed, all cashews are roasted to remove the inner shell. In their "raw" state, cashews taste sweet. Further roasting adds more depth in flavor.

Cashews are lower in fat than many nuts, with 72% of their calories from fat, predominantly monounsaturated.

Store in the refrigerator for up to 6 months or in the freezer for 9 months.

Varieties and Preparation Guidelines

Because of their sweet flavor and creamy texture, cashews are perfect when ground for making nondairy sauces and nut milks. When left whole, cashews are especially good in stir-fries and East Indian dishes. Since they become unpleasantly soggy when cooked too long, add cashews at the end of cooking to maintain crispness. Nothing seems to correct the tendency for cashews to become limp in baked goods. Therefore, if you're really hankering for the flavor of cashews in muffins or breads, wait until after baking and spread on the cashew butter.

To compensate for its lower fat content, both raw and roasted **cashew butter** are commonly made with the addition of an oil to facilitate grinding. Higher-quality cashew butters use unrefined, expeller-pressed safflower oil.

Besides spreading it on bread, use cashew butter instead of cream to thicken soups. First whisk it into a small amount of broth before mixing it with the rest of the soup. Or dilute it with vegetable broth and thicken with arrowroot for a luscious sauce.

CHESTNUTS

Facts and Features

Once prolific throughout the United States, a devastating blight in the early 1900s nearly wiped out our own native North American species of chestnut tree. Accordingly, most chestnuts available now are imported from Europe, making what was once a common ingredient collected from the tree in one's backyard a gourmet treat.

Now a new generation of cooks are discovering chestnuts' amazing nutritional profile and delicious flavor. High in complex carbohydrates, only 13% of chestnuts' calories are from fat, creating a nut that is decidely more starchy than crunchy and oily. The fat in chestnuts is predominantly monounsaturated.

Plan on buying 1 pound of chestnuts in the shell to yield 2 1/2 cups shelled chestnuts. Chestnuts in the shell will keep 4-6 months when stored in a perforated bag in the refrigerator. Shelled and blanched chestnuts can be frozen 9-12 months.

Varieties and Preparation Guidelines

You won't see chestnuts in trail mixes or as an ingredient in nut milks. Instead, use them to add flavor and texture to soups, stuffings, pastas, stir-fries, and desserts.

Chestnuts can be roasted, steamed, or boiled to remove the outer shell that envelopes its richly flavored meat. Before roasting or cooking, the outer shell must be slit to keep it from exploding as the moisture within turns to steam when heated. Cutting the shell in the form of a cross will help make removal of the shell even easier after cooking.

To prepare, roast in a 400° F. oven or steam/boil for 15-20 minutes until the edges of the slit curl back and the chestnut meat becomes soft. While still warm, peel off the shell. Once it cools, the task becomes very difficult and frustrating.

Dried chestnuts are also available as convenient substitutes for shelled fresh chestnuts. Reconstitute them in water for 6-8 hours. Then simmer them until tender and add to recipes. You can also cook dried chestnuts with rice in a pressure cooker for a special richly flavored rice dish.

COCONUT

Facts and Features

A coconut comes to us from the coconut palm tree that grows in Hawaii and other countries with tropical climates. Actually the seed of the tree's fruit, the coconut meat comprises the seed's endosperm. When in its fresh form, coconut is often considered as a fruit. In its dried form, it is treated as the equivalent of a nut.

Eighty-eight percent of the calories from coconut are derived from fat. Unlike other nuts whose fats are predominantly monosaturated and polyunsaturated, coconut's fat is primarily saturated. Therefore, as delicious as it is, coconut is best used sparingly.

Refrigerate dried coconut after purchase and use within 1 month or 6 months in the freezer.

Varieties and Preparation Guidelines

Choose unsweetened dried coconut flakes or ribbons over the presweetened alternatives. If you haven't tried the unsweetened variety before, you'll be surprised at its nutty and subtly sweet flavor—perfect as is for baking, cooking, and mixing into fruit salads.

FLAXSEEDS

Facts and Features

Flaxseeds (linseeds) are tiny, oval-shaped, brown seeds. Bland in flavor, they are acclaimed as the richest food source of Omega-3 fatty acids (alpha-linolenic acid). Studies have shown that essential fatty acids stimulate the production of prostaglandins, hormone-like compounds which regulate many of the body's functions. Of particular interest, the Omega-3 fatty acids found in flaxseeds helps reduce the rate of blood clot formation, thus helping to reduce the risk of strokes and heart attacks.

Flaxseeds are also very high in fiber, swelling and increasing in bulk when moistened and during digestion. Only 64% of flaxseeds' calories are from fat.

Varieties and Preparation Guidelines

In their whole form, add flaxseeds to baked goods for crunch and extra fiber. When ground, they can be sprinkled over cereal or blended with juice. Be careful—a little goes a long way.

Flaxseeds can also be blended with water and transformed into an egg replacer for baking. For the equivalent of 3 eggs, combine 1/4 cup flax seeds and 3/4 cup water. Process 5-10 minutes in a blender to make a gluey slurry. Add an equivalent amount to baked goods instead of the required eggs. The flaxseed egg substitute is neutral in flavor and contributes a moist texture to the finished product.

HAZELNUTS

Facts and Features

Hazelnuts sold in the United States usually come from Oregon and Washington state. While the names hazelnuts and filberts are often used interchangeably, originally the American variety was referred to as hazelnut and the European version as filbert.

With 92% of their calories from fat, hazelnuts rank as one of the nuts highest in fat. Fortunately, most of the fat is monounsaturated.

Varieties and Preparation Guidelines

Hazelnuts' flavor is unique and delicious, especially when the nuts are roasted. Serve them as a snack or chop and use in cookies, breads, and mixed with vegetable medleys.

Like almonds, many cooks like to blanch hazelnuts to get rid of the fibrous brown skin that surrounds the meat. To blanch, pour boiling water over the hazelnuts, allow them to set for 3 minutes, and drain. Then put the hazelnuts into cold water for 1 minute.

Transfer the nuts to a towel and rub the nuts vigorously to remove the skins.

One pound of hazelnuts in the shell will yield 11/2 cups of whole nuts. Refrigerate shelled hazelnuts up to 9 months in the refrigerator or 12 months in the freezer.

Hazelnut butter is all the rage in Europe for cookies and baked goods. It can also be served with jam on breakfast breads or thinned with fruit juice for a terrific sauce over sliced bananas, apples, and pears.

MACADAMIA NUTS

Facts and Features

Macadamia nuts are grown on evergreen trees indigenous to Australia but now found in Hawaii and California. Since their shells are very hard to crack, macadamia nuts are always sold shelled.

Sweet and buttery, macadamia nuts also take the prize for being the nut with the highest percentage of calories from fat. Although 95% of their calories are from fat, most of it is monounsaturated.

Store in the refrigerator up to 6 months or in the freezer for 9 months.

Varieties and Preparation Guidelines

Serve as a snack, toss in salads, or chop and add to your favorite cookie recipe.

PEANUTS

Facts and Features

While commonly referred to as nuts, peanuts actually belong to the legume family. In the United States, peanuts are grown in the southern states.

Since the peanut is susceptible to a potent carcinogenic mold called aflatoxin, it is very important to buy peanuts from reputable growers who take special precautions during the growing process and in storing whole, undamaged peanuts in a dry, temperature-controlled environment. Strong, healthy plants, irrigated when necessary, naturally resist the mold which produces aflatoxin.

In 1969, the FDA set an upper limit of 20 parts per billion for aflatoxin in peanuts and peanut products, reportedly based on economic considerations rather than negligible risk. Peanuts grown in the dry arid climate of New Mexico and other parts of the Southwest are less susceptible to the aflatoxin mold.

Even though peanuts are very high in fat relative to other legumes, when compared with nuts they rank among the lower fat varieties with 77% calories from fat, predominantly monounsaturated. Lower-calorie peanuts with 20% of their calories removed through supercritical extraction are now being marketed. A chemical-free process, supercritical extraction involves exposing peanuts to carbon dioxide at warm temperatures and high pressure. Under these conditions, the carbon dioxide acts as a fluid and develops the ability to dissolve the oil.

Peanuts salted in the shell are seasoned by soaking them in a brine solution before roasting. Since a cup of shelled salted peanuts can contain up to 1000 mg. of sodium, it's a good idea to choose unsalted varieties more frequently. Fresh, high-quality peanuts are so flavorful that you'll discover they don't require salt to perk them up.

Buy 11/2 pounds of peanuts in the shell to yield 1 pound or 31/2 cups of shelled peanuts. Peanuts tend to go rancid quickly, so store peanuts in the shell in a cool, dry place for up to 2 months or in the refrigerator for 6 months. Shelled peanuts should be refrigerated and used within 3 months or frozen for up to 6 months.

Varieties and Preparation Guidelines

Besides eating them for snacks, peanuts are a natural in East Indian and Thai dishes. When chopped, they are equally delicious baked in cookies, breads, and muffins or as an ingredient in candies and even soups.

There are three main varieties of peanuts. Long, oval Virginia peanuts have a strong flavor. Spanish peanuts, the preferable peanut for peanut brittle, are mild-tasting and small and round. Valencia peanuts are richly flavored and medium-sized with an oval shape.

Most people prefer the flavor of roasted peanuts over raw. When buying preroasted peanuts, look for dry-roasted varieties free of unnecessary additives. To roast your own, place in a shallow baking pan in an oven preheated to 325°F. Roast peanuts in the shell for about 20 minutes and shelled peanuts for about 15 minutes. Check them frequently to prevent burning, removing from the oven as they begin to brown.

Peanut Butter

Fifty percent of the peanut crop is ground into peanut butter. By federal law, peanut butters must contain at least 90% peanuts with the option of adding sweeteners and stabilizers for the remaining 10%. Artificial sweeteners, colors, flavors, preservatives, and vitamin fortifiers are not allowed. New reduced-fat peanut butters made by substituting some of the peanuts with soy protein and sugar must be labeled as "peanut spread."

Several mass-market peanut butter manufacturers add hydrogenated vegetable oils and mono- and diglycerides to prevent the separation of peanut butter's heavy solids from its natural oils. This practice was pioneered by the makers of Peter Pan™ peanut butter in 1930, a time when reliable refrigerators weren't as commonplace in homes as they are today. Considering that any temperature below 50° F. will keep the oil in its proper place, an initial stirring to blend the solids and oils make stabilizers in peanut butter an unnecessary addition of extra calories as well as hard-to-metabolize trans-fatty acids.

Some of the oil can be removed, but be sure to retain enough to ensure spreadability. Approximately 1 Tbsp. of oil removed from peanut butter before the initial stirring will eliminate about 1/2 gram of fat per tablespoon. It's not much but if you're concerned that you are getting too much fat in your diet, every little bit helps. Of course, you could spread the peanut butter a bit thinner.

Sugar and salt have been added to peanut butters since 1910 to mask bland flavors. The fact remains, however, that brands made with fresh, high quality peanuts need no flavor enhancement. Be sure to read the ingredient label carefully to make sure what you're buying is 100% peanuts.

Also look to see if the peanuts were unblanched or blanched. Peanut butters made from unblanched peanuts offer more full-bodied flavor, aroma, and nutrients. While some manufacturers may claim the skin can make the peanut butter taste bitter, in reality the blanching process is largely used as a roundabout way to lengthen shelf life. During the process of removing the reddish skins loosened from blanching, mechanical rollers also remove the nutrient-dense peanut germ. Since the germ contains many natural oils, its removal creates a peanut butter that may not go rancid as quickly *when unrefrigerated* as an unblanched peanut butter under the same conditions.

Go for the flavor and nutrition of unblanched peanut butter. If refrigerated after opening and used within 3-4 months, there's no reason to worry about your peanut butter going rancid.

When you consider that a jar of peanut butter rarely lasts long in any household and that almost everyone has access to a refrigerator to keep their peanut butter fresh, sugar-free and stabilizer-free peanut butter made from unblanched peanuts is your best bet for flavor and nutrition.

Little needs to be said about how to use peanut butter. Just bring to room temperature for ease in spreadability and use it to top bread, crackers, carrots, and celery, as an ingredient in cookies and muffins, and when no one's looking.....

PECANS

Facts and Features

Pecans, one of the few truly native American nuts, are grown primarily in the southern states. Its name is derived from an American Indian word "pegan" meaning bone shell, an apt description of what faces anyone who has ever shelled a pecan.

Rich in flavor, eighty-seven percent of the calories in pecans are from fat, predominantly monounsaturated.

Two pounds of pecans in the shell will yield 1 pound or 4 cups shelled. Look for clean shells that are free from scars, cracks, or holes. If the nuts inside the shell rattle when shaken, they are past their prime. Good-quality pecans both in and out of the shell will keep up to 6 months in the refrigerator or up to 1 year in the freezer.

Shelled pecans should be crisp, golden brown, and relatively plump. Since they can easily go rancid, pecans should be purchased whole instead of ground or broken. Their soft texture enables them to be very easily processed at home using a blender or food processor. Refrigerate pecans up to 6 months. When frozen, they will keep 1 year. Store in a tightly closed container to prevent pecans from absorbing odors from other foods.

Varieties and Preparation Guidelines

Use pecans in both sweet and savory foods, in baked goods, or as a garnish. They can also be used interchangeably with walnuts in recipes.

PINE NUTS

Facts and Features

Pine nuts (pignolias) are harvested from pine cones of trees grown around the Mediterranean although a similar variety is grown on a limited scale in the United States. Slender, creamy white pine nuts from the European stone pine are the variety most commonly sold in stores. The smaller, darker pine nuts gathered in the wild from the pinon pine found in the southwestern parts of the United States have too small a yield for widespread commercial use.

Eighty-six percent of their calories are from fat, primarily polyunsaturated. Pine nuts are higher in protein than most nuts. One ounce or 3 tablespoons provides about 6 grams of protein and 17 grams of fat.

Even if refrigerated, pine nuts go rancid quicker than other nuts and seeds. Store up to 1 month in the refrigerator and up to 6 months in the freezer.

Varieties and Preparation Guidelines

Their aromatic flavor and crisp texture make them a favorite in pesto, dolmas, poultry stuffings, or as a garnish for vegetables and pasta dishes.

PISTACHIOS

Facts and Features

Pistachios are the seed of an evergreen grown in California and in the Middle East. This delicately flavored, pale-green nutmeat is naturally (and preferably) encased in a greyish-beige shell. Pistachios have been traditionally dyed red to hide blemishes and discolorations that can show up on the shell if not hulled quickly after harvesting. Modern harvesting and processing techniques make dyeing even more unnecessary.

With 78% of its calories from fat, most of it monounsaturated, pistachios are somewhat lower in fat than many nuts. Even though salted pistachios are more common, they are readily available unsalted.

One pound of pistachios in the shell will yield about 9 oz. or 4 cups of nutmeats. Refrigerate up to 3 months and freeze up to 1 year.

Varieties and Preparation Guidelines

Besides being a popular ingredient in ice cream, pistachios are delicious eaten as a snack and in stuffings, candies, and desserts.

Pistachio butter is the best way to enjoy pistachios without having to deal with the shells. Extremely rich, it is best served with fruit. Dip in apple slices, bananas, or pears for a simple, utterly satisfying dessert or snack. Or, even better, cut a medjool date in half, remove the pit, and stuff each date half with pistachio butter.

PUMPKIN SEEDS

Facts and Features

Pumpkin seeds that are sold commercially come from a special type of pumpkin grown in Mexico that yields long, flat, dark green seeds instead of the pale, fibrous seeds found in jack-o'-lantern pumpkins or pie pumpkins. Also called "pepitas," these seeds are known for their high concentrations of protein (1 oz.= 7 grams protein) and zinc.

Seventy-six percent of pumpkin seeds'

calories are from fat, much of it polyunsaturated. They also are a good source of Omega-3 fatty acid, supplying alpha-linolenic acid, one of the essential fatty acids that must be obtained from foods.

When stored in the refrigerator or freezer pumpkin seeds will last up to 1 year. On the shelf, they can remain relatively fresh for about 2 months, assuming that they were purchased in top condition.

Varieties and Preparation Guidelines

True to their origin, pumpkin seeds are terrific in Mexican cuisine and Southwestern cuisine. Roast and mix in with rice or veggies. Garnish enchiladas just before serving. For deeper, richer-flavored sauces, mix in a tablespoon of finely ground roasted pumpkin seeds.

SESAME SEEDS

Facts and Features

After enduring years of being sold in the spice section of grocery stores as an adornment for hamburger buns, the many forms of sesame seeds are finally finding their way into the new American cuisine.

Grown throughout the world, sesame seeds are sold both whole and hulled. While most nuts and seeds have their shells removed by machine, until recently sesame seed hulls were commonly removed using a chemical bath containing lye, acids, and enzyme solutions in which the seeds were soaked until they burst. Sesame seeds hulled in this manner have a white, glossy sheen, a bitter, slightly soapy and salty flavor. Even though the seeds are washed after treatment, traces of these solvents may remain. Sesame seeds can also be hulled using a salt brine instead of the chemical solvent.

Companies concerned with quality are now using a chemical-free mechanical hulling process. The seeds are first steam-heated to loosen the hulls and then mechanically rolled to remove them. Mechanically hulled sesame seeds have a dull, off-white appearance with some color variation.

Besides color and appearance, another telltale way to determine the hulling method is to look at the sodium content. Those processed with chemicals or saltbrine will be quite high in sodium. Mechanically hulled seeds will have negligible sodium levels.

Sesame seeds provide good-quality protein when combined with beans or dairy. Calcium content is another story. While a nutritional analysis may indicate that whole sesame seeds are high in calcium, oxalic acid from the hull binds up the calcium, a substance which prevents the mineral's absorption.

Seventy-six percent of sesame's calories are derived from fat. Much of it is polyunsaturated.

When stored in the refrigerator or freezer sesame seeds will last up to 1 year. On the shelf, they can remain relatively fresh for about 2 months, assuming that they were purchased in top condition.

Varieties and Preparation Guidelines

To toast seeds, place in a dry skillet over medium-low heat for 5-6 minutes or until golden brown. Stir constantly to prevent burning.

Sesame seeds add terrific flavor and texture when sprinkled in stir-fries or added to cookies and breads. For a flavorful switch from the usual butter and syrup routine, try topping your pancakes with a mixture of ground sesame seeds and applesauce or maple syrup .

Sesame seeds are also the main ingredient in gomasio, a delicious low-sodium condiment made by roasting and grinding sesame seeds with salt in a proportion of about 14 to 1.

Strong, earthy-flavored **black sesame seeds** are imported from China and Japan. Traditional use of black sesame seeds is as an ingredient in dessert recipes. Sprinkle some over steamed or baked carrots, sweet potatoes, or squash for a striking color accent.

Gomasio or sesame salt is a combination of ground roasted sesame seeds and sea salt. It is used as a low-sodium alternative to salt and as an additional source of protein and calcium. As a natural home remedy, a teaspoon of gomasio is a good antidote to the unfocused, queasy feeling from overconsumption of fruit or sweets.

The proportions of sesame seeds to sea salt in prepared, moderately salty gomasio ranges from 8:1 to 14:1 depending on the brand. A gomasio with 20:1 proportion can easily be made at home if a less salty condiment is preferred. Sprinkle on grains and vegetables as you would salt.

As peanuts are to peanut butter, sesame seeds are to **sesame tahini**. A delicious, creamy spread popular in Middle Eastern, African, and Oriental cuisines, tahini is made from hulled sesame seeds, available both raw and roasted. Raw tahini has a nutty, subtly sweet flavor and thin consistency. Tahini made from roasted sesame seeds has a deeper, richer flavor, making it more appropriate as a spread or combined with miso and vegetable broth for a distinctive sauce.

Tahini is very versatile and suitable at any meal. At breakfast, spread some on your toast instead of butter, add a tablespoon to smoothies, or thin with a small amount of juice as a sauce for fruit salads. At lunch or dinner, tahini can be a both binder and flavor component for garbanzo bean-based hummus or combined with other beans for

sandwich spreads, fillings, or dips. Or use it to make salad dressings or nondairy "cream of" soups. The possibilities are endless.

A simple nondairy milk substitute can be made by blending 1 tablespoon of tahini with 1 cup of water and a dab of sweetener. Use as you would milk as a beverage or in cooking and baking.

Sesame butter, made from whole ground sesame seeds, is darker in color and stronger in flavor. It is used primarily as a spread rather than as an ingredient in cooking.

SUNFLOWER SEEDS

Facts and Features

Sunflower seeds have their roots in the United States but are used extensively throughout the world as a concentrated energy source. Collected from the dried heads of huge flowers, sunflower seeds are easily obtained from a crop of sunflowers grown in your own backyard.

Sunflower seeds are particularly high in protein, providing 8 grams per quarter cup. Seventy-eight percent of their calories are from fat, predominantly polyunsaturated.

For best nutrition, choose unsalted, raw or dry roasted seeds. Avoid broken or discolored seeds, significant indications that the seeds may be rancid.

When stored in the refrigerator or freezer sunflower seeds will last up to 1 year. On the shelf, they can remain relatively fresh for about 2 months, assuming that they were purchased in top condition.

Varieties and Preparation Guidelines

Besides being consumed as a nutritious snack, sunflower seeds' flavor and texture make them a good addition to baked goods and as a crunchy substitute for bacon bits

PECANOA PILAF

1/3 cup pecans
1 Tbsp. safflower oil
1 small onion, diced
1/2 bunch parsley,
    chopped
1/2 tsp. each: ground
    cumin, coriander,
    curry powder
1 1/3 cup quinoa,
    thoroughly rinsed
3 cups water
1/4 tsp. salt

Preheat oven to 300°. Dry-roast pecans for 10-15 minutes while preparing pilaf. Stir occasionally to prevent burning.

Heat oil in a saucepan and add onions. Sauté 3 minutes and add parsley and spices. Sauté an additional 3 minutes and then add quinoa, water, and salt. Bring to a boil and cover.

Reduce heat and simmer 15 minutes. Remove the saucepan from the heat and stir in coarsely chopped pecans. Let sit about 5 minutes before serving.

Serves 4.
(Pyramid servings: 3 Bread/Grain Group, 1/4 Veg. Group, 14 grams Fat)

Nutrition Facts

Serving Size 1/4 recipe (270 g)
Servings Per Container 4

Amount Per Serving

Calories 320   Calories from Fat 120

	% Daily Value*
Total Fat 14g	**21%**
Saturated Fat 1g	**6%**
Sodium 90mg	**4%**
Total Carbohydrate 43g	**14%**
Dietary Fiber 5g	**19%**
Sugars 2g	
Protein 9g	

Vitamin A 4%	•	Vitamin C	10%
Calcium 6%	•	Iron	35%

Not a significant source of Cholesterol
* Percent Daily Values are based on a 2,000 calorie diet.

and croutons on cooked vegetables and salads. Roast for best flavor.

Unhulled, raw sunflower seeds can be sprouted. Crisp in texture and slightly bitter, sunsprouts are a great addition to salads and sandwiches.

WALNUTS

Facts and Features

Originating in ancient Persia, walnuts have been grown in California since the late 1700s. No other nut has been so revered in cooking and baking

Eighty-nine percent of walnuts' calories are from fat, much of it polyunsaturated. They also contribute Omega-3 fatty acids, a type of essential fatty acid not often found in the diet.

Like pecans, they tend to go rancid quickly, especially when shelled. Of all the nuts, it is most critical to sample walnuts before purchasing. Buy walnut halves instead of walnut pieces. They can be easily chopped or crushed at home.

One pound of English walnuts in the shell will yield 2 cups shelled nuts. For best flavor and texture, avoid walnuts that rattle within their shell. Unfortunately, the shells of whole walnuts are often bleached for cosmetic purposes. The shells of walnuts that are commercially cracked are not bleached.

Store walnuts in the shell at room temperature for 2-3 months. Both in- and out-of-shell walnuts store up to 1 year in either the refrigerator or freezer.

Varieties and Preparation Guidelines

Use walnuts in cookies and other desserts, breads, stuffings, salads, vegetable, grain, and chicken dishes, and cereals.

The thin skin covering the walnut meat is both a blessing and a curse. It provides much of walnuts' flavor and yet, in some cases, it can taste too bitter and astringent. Some recipes specify to remove the skin. The easiest way to do this is to lightly roast the walnuts, just enough so that the skin loosens, but not so much that the nuts taste too toasted. Then place the walnuts in a towel and rub vigorously to remove the skins.

There are two main varieties of walnuts. Most commonly sold are **English walnuts**, named as such in reference to the English merchant marines who transported the nut throughout the world.

The **black walnut**, native to the United States, is slightly higher in protein and stronger in flavor. Since it is an extremely hard nut to crack, it is usually sold shelled as bits and pieces

MILK, YOGURT & CHEESE GROUP

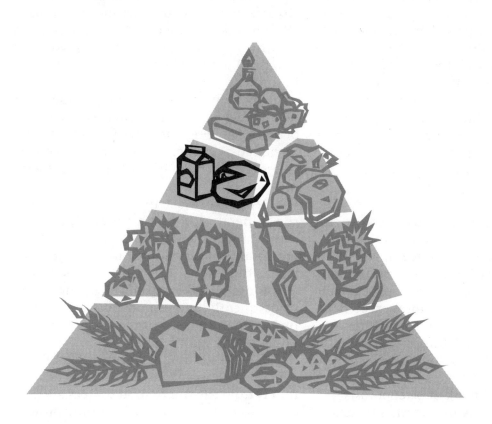

Dairy Products

IN THE United States alone, milk is an $18 billion industry. According to government statistics, in 1991 there were about 182,000 dairy farms in the United States, representing 10 million dairy cows that produce about 17 billion gallons of milk. Over 700 dairy plants process milk and milk products.

Through advertisements on television and in magazines and throughout basic nutrition classes interspersed throughout one's school career, we're constantly reminded that milk is good—and necessary—food. A source of high-quality protein, milk and products made with it also contain vitamin A, riboflavin and other B vitamins, phosphorus, magnesium, potassium, sodium, chloride, sulfur, and a significant amount of easily absorbed calcium.

NUTRITION

Dairy products are most noted for their calcium content, a critical mineral for density and strength of bones and teeth, as well as normal muscle contraction, transmission and interpretation of nerve impulses, and maintenance of cell membranes. A deficiency of calcium, either from too little supplied in the diet or malabsorption, can cause skeletal abnormalities such as misshapen bones, retarded growth, or reduced density in bones—the hallmark of osteoporosis.

One cup of milk or yogurt, 11/2 oz. of natural cheese, or 2 oz. of processed cheese constitute a serving. The Food Guide Pyramid suggests 3 servings daily for children, teenagers, and young adults up to 24 years of age. Calcium intake is especially important during these years when bones grow larger and heavier. Accordingly, pregnant and lactating women must also ingest adequate amounts of the mineral to help calcify fetal bones and produce mother's milk— all while keeping their own bones strong and healthy. A good basis of calcium in younger years will help maintain bone density later in life.

To help maintain strong bones and teeth, older adults require at least 2 servings of dairy. Some researchers suggest that postmenopausal women not taking estrogen increase their calcium intake back up to 3 servings a day.

Several factors help in the absorption of the mineral. Too much protein produces excess nitrogen and sulfur in the blood, leading to an acid condition. In order to neutralize the acidity, calcium is leached from the bones and then excreted in the urine. Consequently, more moderate amounts of protein in the diet may make it easier to keep bones strong with less calcium.

Besides keeping your protein intake to a moderate level, adequate amounts of Vitamin D from the sun or food sources are necessary to make the calcium-binding protein that helps regulate absorption for both

PERCENTAGE OF CALORIES FROM FAT

TYPE	FAT	CHOLESTEROL	% OF CALORIES/FAT
whole milk	8 grams	33 mg	48%
2% milk	5 grams	22 mg.	37%
skim milk	trace	4 mg.	5%
goat milk	10 grams	28 mg.	54%
buttermilk	2 grams	9 mg.	2%
whole yogurt	7.4 grams	29 mg.	48%
lowfat yogurt	3.5 grams	14 mg	21%
nonfat yogurt	trace	4 mg.	3%
cheddar cheese	14 grams	45 mg.	74.2%
part skim mozzarella	7 grams	40mg	52.7%

proper maintenance of blood calcium levels and mineralization of the bones.

Calcium is also best absorbed with phosphorus in a 1:1 ratio, a proportion that can easily get out of balance in diets heavy in high phosphorus foods and drinks, including consuming too many animal proteins, foods processed with sodium phosphates, and soft drinks throughout the day. And, even though your diet should be high in fiber, supplying at least 25 grams per 2000 calories a day, an overabundance will bind up calcium, thus decreasing its absorption.

High in Fat

Although dairy is a significant source of easily absorbed nutrients, it also contains cholesterol and high amounts of total fat, especially saturated fat. This fact is most apparent when you compare labels of whole milk dairy products with those reduced in fat. But what you don't see is the actual **percentage of calories from fat**, a statistic that shows the grams of fat contained in a product in more realistic terms. The above chart shows what you'll get from various dairy selections, all based on the standard serving sizes, i.e.,

8 oz. serving of milk or yogurt or 11/2 oz. serving of cheese.

Even if you were to drastically cut back on meats in order to lower total fat and cholesterol, as long as dairy is still a main part of the menu, the percentage of calories from fat will still hover too high. Fortunately, many lower-fat versions of fluid milk, yogurt and cheese are readily available.

LABELING

The calcium information included on the Nutrition Facts label is another guide to monitoring your calcium intake. Rather than listing its actual amount in milligrams, the calcium content of a food is noted by its percentage of the Daily Value of calcium, 1000 mg. To get the optimal amount, just add up the percentages listed on the labels of the foods you consumed during the day, shooting for a daily total of 100%.

A food whose label carries the "calcium helps osteoporosis" health claim, thus implying the product is a good source of calcium, must contain 20% (200 mg.) or more of the Daily Value for calcium per serving. Regulations also stipulate the calcium must be a source that is easily absorbed and the food's phosphorus content must be less than the amount of calcium found in the food per serving.

Foods that claim to be non-dairy such as coffee whiteners and soy cheese but include caseinate (milk protein) as an ingredient must now indicate that caseinate is derived from milk.

Curiously, a glance at the sugar content of Total Carbohydrate listed on the Nutrition Facts label makes dairy products look like they contribute a lot of sugar and little, if any, complex carbohydrates. If it is a label for plain milk, yogurt, or cheese, the grams of carbohydrates listed under "Sugars" merely indicates the product's lactose content. A simple sugar naturally present in milk, lactose is a unique type of sugar in that it helps increase the absorption of calcium, phosphorus, magnesium, and zinc and also helps promote the growth of "friendly bacteria" in the intestines.

As long as your digestive system can easily metabolize the lactose, you don't have to give the high percentage of sugars in the milk product a second thought.

In contrast, the "Sugars" content of flavored milk products will also include more simple sugars than naturally occurs in the milk. It's these added sugars that are most important to curtail.

FOOD SAFETY CONCERNS

MILK PROCESSING

Milk is a perishable food, very susceptible to bacterial contamination. Subsequently, most states require that milk be pasteurized before sale.

During **pasteurization**, milk is heated to 161° F. for 15 seconds to kill yeasts, molds, pathogenic microorganisms, and most of the less harmful strains of bacteria. The process causes slightly decreased levels of vitamins B_1, B_{12}, and C. About 6% of the calcium be-

comes insoluble and about 1% of the proteins coagulate and some of the milk's fat globules also become more dispersed.

Advocates of raw milk believe that unpasteurized milk tastes better and protects the natural enzymes present in the milk. Serious cheese-ophiles insist that cheese made from raw milk has more depth of flavor than cheese made from pasteurized milk.

What made the arguments for raw milk harder for state health officials to accept was the June 1985 tainted cheese incident in Los Angeles which caused 29 deaths or stillbirths and 60 illnesses. The culprit in the freshly made, unaged cheese was Listeria monocytogenes, a bacterium that can be effectively killed by pasteurization.

As a result, current FDA regulations stipulate that all cheese must be made from pasteurized milk or aged at least 60 days before sale to ensure that any problems from harmful bacteria are eliminated by the naturally occurring acidity of the cheese.

Access to raw fluid milk remains at each state's discretion. A few states allow milk to be sold as raw, as long as it passes very rigorous certification testing, including the fulfillment of higher than normal sanitation standards at the dairy.

Ultrapasteurization, the process of heating milk to 280° F. for 2-4 seconds, kills off more bacteria. Milk destined for aseptic packaging is ultrapasteurized and then cooled rapidly to 45° F. before it is sealed in sterile containers under sterile conditions.

Most whipping cream and half-and-half products are also ultrapasteurized since the process significantly extends shelf life, an outcome manufacturers adore since fresh cream products sell much slower than milk.

But many cooks claim ultrapasteurized cream doesn't whip as easily as varieties which have been pasteurized at lower temperatures like other dairy products. To compensate, many manufacturers add **polysorbate 80** as an emulsifier to improve the cream's whipping quality and to produce a smoother body and texture.

Polysorbate 80 (polyoxyethylene sorbitan monooleate) is made by reacting oleic acid (one of the fatty acids found in oil) with sorbitol (a sugar alcohol which acts as a humectant) to yield a compound which is then reacted with ethylene oxide. While its name sounds like it should be unbelievably bad, in reality it is relatively safe, digested in the same manner as its components, fats and sorbitol, would be metabolized.

That being said, whipping creams and half-and-half that contain polysorbate 80 are no match for real fresh cream that is merely pasteurized. Therefore, first look for brands that contain cream and little else. Choose those with polysorbate 80 as a last resort.

The same advice goes for the other additives commonly found in whipping cream: mono- and diglycerides, another emulsifier also made from fats, as well as thickening agents such as guar gum, cellulose gum, and carrageenan (derived from a sea vegetable). If you can avoid them, all the better for real taste. If all the brands you have available to you contain emulsifiers and thickeners, they're safe to use but certainly not the optimum choice.

Homogenization distributes the fat particles evenly throughout the milk so there is no separation of the cream from the rest of the milk. In the process, milk is sprayed at high pressure through a small nozzle onto a hard surface to break the fat particles into very small particles.

Undoubtedly, homogenization has its drawbacks. The milk is more bland in flavor, more sensitive to spoilage from light, and, when heated, more likely to curdle. Since the fat globules have been decreased in size, homogenized cream doesn't whip as well.

Fortunately, pasteurized, unhomogenized milk is occasionally available, especially from smaller dairies. Besides having access to better flavor and cooking properties, many people enjoy unhomogenized milk for the cream that floats to the top. Gently skimmed from the milk, the cream can be used as a topping for fruit, desserts, and cereals or whipped. Whirled in a blender or food processor, the cream can be transformed into homemade butter. It can also be stirred to disperse cream throughout the milk without disturbing the nature of the fat globules. If you prefer not to use the cream, it can also simply be discarded.

Drug Residues in Milk

Although pasteurization removes bacteria in milk which could be harmful, it does not remove residues from the many drugs used to treat dairy cows.

The FDA is responsible for approving new animal drugs before they can be legally marketed in the United States. It is up to them to determine residue tolerances, the amount that the FDA believes can legally be present in milk safe to drink, as well as withdrawal periods, the time required from cessation of the drug until the milk from the cow can be sold for consumption. As of May 1992, 60 drugs, including those used for topical application, have been allowed for use on dairy cows.

It is also the FDA's duty to monitor the purity of milk by coordinating with the states the testing of milk for not only bacteria and somatic cell counts (indicative of infection in the cow) but also for illegal residues of drugs.

Even low levels of drug residues are dangerous. They can cause: 1) allergic reactions in persons sensitive to antibiotics that may have been used to treat a cow, 2) the development of bacteria resistant to antibiotics,

3) the suppression of the human immune system through constant exposure to low levels of antibiotics, 4) the emergence of antimicrobial-resistant bacteria linked to the use of antibiotics in dairy cows, which could lead to increased risk of human infection, and 5) a slightly increased risk of adverse chronic effects, such as cancer.

In December 1989 an article that appeared in the Wall Street Journal shattered milk's pure image when it outlined the results of two surveys conducted on animal drug residues in milk. One study sponsored by the Wall Street Journal indicated that 20% of retail milk was contaminated with animal drug residues, possibly including sulfamethazine, a suspected carcinogen not approved by the FDA for use in dairy cows. The other study, sponsored by the Center for Science in the Public Interest, a consumer food safety and nutrition activist organization, claimed that 38% of retail milk contained drug residues.

Critics, including the FDA, claimed that the testing methodology may have been oversensitive to some drugs and that further testing was needed using more sophisticated methodology to confirm the results. As a response to the country's concern about the real story on the milk purity, the FDA conducted their own survey in 1990 to determine whether residues of certain animal drugs could be found in milk. After tabulating the results of their survey, later on that year the FDA declared milk to be safe.

However, in November 1990, a disturbing report from the General Accounting Office, an independent investigating arm of Congress, contradicted the FDA's milk safety claim. They revealed that testing methodology used by the FDA and states only detect four animal drugs—ampicillin, cephaparin, hetacillin, and penicillin—at tolerance levels. Furthermore, sulfa drugs and tetracyclines that were believed to be used on dairy

cows could only be detected at levels of 15 parts per million, despite that the safe level set by the FDA was much lower—at levels of 10 parts per billion.

Presented with the facts, the FDA made renewed efforts to increase testing frequency and implement new methodologies to detect more animal drugs. However, a subsequent review by the General Accounting Office in August 1992 found little progress had been made since 1990 on insuring the public that milk is safe. According to their investigations, 82 drugs are commonly being used on dairy cattle, far more than the FDA's tests can detect. Of that number, 42 are not even approved for use in any food-producing animal, much less dairy cows.

Connected with these findings is the loophole created in 1984, the extra-label drug use policy, under which veterinarians can treat food animals under emergency circumstances with drugs not approved for use for the specific animal in question. The GAO found that, rather than being used only in emergencies as the regulation allows, unapproved drugs were being used routinely. In response, several veterinarians claimed that common usage of unapproved drugs was necessary because the drugs currently approved for use on dairy cows are less effective, less potent, and more expensive than other drugs. And it's not just the veterinarians. Many animal drugs are available over-the-counter, giving any milk producer a virtual smorgasbord of drugs from which to choose, whether approved for dairy cows or not.

The bottom line is that the milk and, consequently milk products that we buy may potentially contain residues from the several drugs given to dairy cows. Thanks to irresponsible actions by some producers and their veterinarians, milk's purity image has been severely tarnished.

Growth Hormones in Dairy Cows

Another issue related to the uncertainty of the presence of drug residues in milk is the use of genetically engineered bovine growth hormones in dairy cows. Commonly referred to as BST (bovine somatotropin) or rBGH (recombinant bovine growth hormone), it is injected into dairy cows every 14 days to increase milk production 5-10%.

Several dairies and consumers vehemently object to its use for several reasons.

There is a glut of milk already in the United States, so any drug used to increase milk production is unnecessary and irresponsible. Elevated milk surpluses can make the price for milk on the open market extremely low, requiring more of our tax money to pay the difference between actual market prices and the price the government guarantees to the dairy industry.

Cows treated with BST have higher levels of clinical mastitis, an infection of the udder. It's a fact even admitted in the list of warnings printed on the package insert of the product. Hand in hand with more infections comes the increased use of drugs, particularly antibiotics, to quickly get the cows well so their milk can be sold. As discussed above, the FDA's system for policing drug residues in milk is no assurance that the increased use of medication with the administration of BST will not interfere with milk's presumed purity.

Unfortunately, it is impossible to test whether the presence of BST in milk or dairy products is naturally occurring or the result of injections with the bioengineered form. Therefore, no retail store can unequivocally claim that all their dairy products are free of the genetically engineered growth hormone. Dairy products made from milk supplied by dairy cooperatives are most difficult to guarantee as BST-free since hundreds of farmers can collectively contribute to the milk pool.

Retailers can, however, let you know the names of the companies they believe can guarantee the source of their milk is free of administered BST, based on the fact that the milk comes only from the manufacturer's own herds or from other dairies with whom they have specific contracts which preclude the use of BST. When it comes down to it, your best bet is milk from certified organic dairies which have systems in place to substantiate their "no BST" claim.

But don't expect to find much labeling on dairy products claiming no BST was used to produce the milk. Unbelievably, several producers who labeled their products as such were sued by the manufacturer and warned by the FDA that such statements were false and misleading. The FDA claims that milk produced with the synthetic hormone is virtually the same as milk produced without it.

They even went so far as to say that dairies, food companies, distributors, and supermarkets who have made public pledges not to use, buy, or sell milk or milk products from cows treated with the hormone might gain an unfair competitive advantage because of a stigma they fear can be attached to milk from treated cows. To prove their point and to show their support for BST, the FDA decreed that any producer labeling their product as BST- or rBGH-free must include a footnote stating that "no significant difference has been shown between milk derived from" cows that were given the drug and those that were not. So much for consumer choice.

HUMANE TREATMENT OF FARM ANIMALS

Ironically, dairy cows, the major players in the issues of drug residues and the use of BST, are rarely considered for the effect drugs have on them physically and, let's admit it, emotionally.

Milk production per cow has increased significantly over the last 40 years due to what the dairy industry claims are better dairy management practices, including special diets, confinement, and the elevated use of animal drugs.

Such an increase in milk production over what they would produce naturally just eating grass, is very stressful on the cow, resulting in an increased need for antibiotics and other drugs to keep them producing as much and as long as possible.

Regarding the use of the synthetic growth hormone, bovine somatotropin (BST), the warnings listed on the label concerning its effect on the health of the cow are frightful. According to the manufacturer, use of BST can create difficulties with reproduction, mastitis, increased body temperature unrelated to illness heightening the risk of heat stress, digestive disorders, diarrhea, poor appetite, as well as problems with the cow's knee joints and hooves. Considering that we already have an overproduction of milk, the use of BST crosses the line into cruelty, bad ethics, and greed.

And then there's often the denial of the expression of normal patterns of behavior. Since milk production drops dramatically when they aren't pregnant, dairy cows are usually artificially inseminated to keep them "in the family way." Rather than allowing cows to nurse their calves, in most cases they are separated from their newborns soon after birth so as not to "waste" their milk.

Even worse, some male calves may be sold to veal processors for a pathetic life of confinement. Because they can't grow into milk-producing animals, and because artificial insemination precludes the need of a bull's participation in breeding, the dairy industry regards male calves as useless.

Considering the sacrifices dairy cows make to supply us milk, they deserve better than this.

The Natural Alternative

Although all the concerns about milk purity may make you have second thoughts about using dairy products, the whole industry needn't be implicated. Several dairy farmers take great pride in producing the best milk possible while treating their cows as co-creators of the final product.

While large cooperatives have the potential to be a good source of clean milk free of harmful bacteria and drug residues from humanely treated cows, it may be easier to feel reassured of milk from small local dairies or independent producers. Smaller facilities are certainly no guarantee that the milk they offer is any better, but at least you may have more of an opportunity to talk with the people involved and see the production of milk from start to finish.

An even better choice is to buy milk from certified organic dairy producers. To qualify for organic certification, a dairy farmer must feed her/his cows with 100% organically grown feed produced on land that has not been treated with synthetic fertilizers, pesticides, herbicides, or fungicides for at least 3 successive years prior to harvesting the crop. Since cows are pastured and drink water may be supplied by wells and/or natural bodies of water, the farm must be certified organic as well.

Humane treatment of cows is also a major qualification for organic status. Clean water and comfortable bedding must be provided as well as pasturing and free stalls to allow access to fresh air and exercise. New mothers must be allowed to nurse their calves for at least 3 days after birth. Male calves are not allowed to be sold to veal operations.

Drugs, including growth hormones or other chemicals to alter their growth or milk production patterns, are not allowed to be administered. Should an antibiotic be administered to an otherwise organically raised dairy cow, milk or milk products derived from that particular cow may not be sold or labeled as organically produced for 3 months following the date of application or use.

Milk certified as organic may not be blended or otherwise come into contact with nonorganic milk, a situation which requires that the processing facility has been inspected as thoroughly as the farm itself to assure that organic practices are being followed.

What with humane treatment of the cows and a growth hormone-free environment in addition to the equal or better sanitation standards as required with all milk (including pasteurization), it's hard to come up with a better alternative than certified organic milk.

Exploring Your Options

Our consumption of dairy products goes beyond basic fluid cow's milk. From there it is further processed into dry milk, cultured dairy products, and cheese. Goat milk also has a devoted following.

ACIDOPHILUS MILK

Facts and Features

Acidophilus milk was developed to provide a means to promote beneficial bacteria in the intestines without the sour flavor of yogurt. The sweet flavor of acidophilus milk is obtained by adding acidophilus that has already been cultured on a different medium, directly into the milk with no additional fermentation.

Because acidophilus milk is not cultured, it has the same amount of lactose as regular cow's milk. Therefore, unlike yogurt whose culturing "predigests" some of the lactose, acidophilus milk is not a more easily digested milk for individuals who are lactose-intolerant.

Baking/Cooking Guidelines

Use acidophilus milk as a beverage and in all recipes as you would cow's milk.

GOAT MILK

Facts and Features

Goat milk has a delicious flavor, slightly different from cow's milk. "Goaty-flavored" goat milk is the result of poor dairying or manufacturing practices.

Some people believe they digest goat milk better than cow's milk due to its smaller fat globules. Goat milk also lacks casein, a particular protein in cow's milk that may precipitate allergic reactions. Its lactose content equals that of cow's milk.

Goat milk also has a few drawbacks. It is only sold as whole milk, providing more than 50% of calories from fat. And, although it contains most of the same nutrients as cow's milk, it is deficient in B_{12} and folic acid, two B vitamins essential for the formation of normal red blood cells.

Baking/Cooking Guidelines

Use goat milk as a beverage and in all recipes as you would cow's milk.

COOK MILK LOW AND SLOW

Be sure to heat milk and cream slowly and at low temperatures. The high lactose content in dairy products can caramelize, leaving scorched milk with a burnt taste that leaves an equally irritating mess to clean on the bottom of the pan.

Too high heat also causes the proteins in milk to coagulate on the surface of heated milk, forming a skin that makes the milk lumpy.

NONFAT DRY MILK

Facts and Features

Nonfat dry milk can be reconstituted to make fluid milk or used in its dry form to enrich sauces, cereals, or baked goods. Nonfat, non-instant, spray-dried powdered milk is preferred for several reasons. Full-fat dry milk goes rancid quickly. When reconstituted, instant dry milk has a chalky consistency, so although non-instant dry milk may take more work to reconstitute, it is a better choice for general cooking purposes and for making yogurt.

Because spray-dried milk is dried at lower temperatures than milk processed according to the older roller-drying methods, more of milk's nutrients are retained in the process—including all the lactose.

Baking/Cooking Guidelines

Store powdered milk in an airtight container in the refrigerator. To reconstitute, measure 2/3 cup powdered milk and 1 quart of water. First, add a small amount of water to the dry milk to make a paste. Then, gradually add the remainder of the water and blend. For best flavor, chill at least 2 hours before drinking.

Dry milk is handy at breakfast time when camping or traveling. Just mix a couple of tablespoons with your cereal or granola ahead of time and store in a moisture-proof, air-tight plastic bag or container. When you are ready to eat, add water and stir to create delicious, milk-moistened cereal.

CULTURED DAIRY PRODUCTS

Cultured dairy products provide the same basic nutrients found in milk, protein and calcium, but in a thicker, more tart format. Yogurt that is cultured after the milk is pasteurized has the added benefit of introducing beneficial bacteria into the intestines to inhibit harmful bacteria that may interfere with optimal digestion and elimination. Due to the "predigesting" of lactose that occurs during the culturing process, some cultured products may offer a more easily tolerated form of dairy.

BUTTERMILK

Facts and Features

Buttermilk's distinctive, tangy flavor is the result of the incubation of milk with lactic acid-producing bacteria such as Streptococcus lacti. Unlike the bacteria in yogurt, those used to culture buttermilk do not digest lactose during the fermentation process. Although its thick consistency may make buttermilk appear to be high in fat, its fat content is less than 0.5% by weight, supplying only 2% total calories from fat.

Baking/Cooking Guidelines

Buttermilk can be used as a beverage or to replace sour milk in recipes. When combined in recipes with baking soda, the acidity of buttermilk makes lighter and more tender pancakes and baked goods. If the recipe doesn't already contain baking soda, add 1/2 teaspoon per 1 cup buttermilk to neutralize the milk's acidity. The chemical interaction between the two forms carbon dioxide, which gives baked goods the leavening boost they need.

COTTAGE CHEESE

Facts and Features

Cottage cheese is available in both small and large curds as well as creamy or dry. A few good dairies produce excellent cottage cheese simply made with milk inoculated with lactic acid bacteria, plus cream and salt. The vast majority, however, contain thickeners and stabilizers such as gums and carrageenan, propylene glycol, and the antimicrobial preservatives, potassium sorbate and sodium benzoate.

There's no doubt that the best-quality, best-tasting cottage cheeses contain the least amount of additives. Especially avoid brands with preservatives. Cottage cheese that is sold within a reasonable time has no need for preservatives. Their presence indicates that the manufacturer is trying to stretch its shelf life as long as possible.

Baking/Cooking Guidelines

Dry curd cottage cheese made from low-fat and nonfat milk, is very low in fat and sodium. But, because it lacks the cream and salt found in regular low-fat or farmer-style cottage cheese, it is also dry, crumbly, and bland in flavor. For best results, use dry curd cottage cheese as an ingredient in recipes or season it with herbs or fruit to enhance its flavor.

When processed in a blender or food processor to a smooth consistency, cottage cheese can be used to replace sour cream on potatoes, in spreads, dips, or in salad dress-ings. Or leave it somewhat chunky for an interesting texture.

CRÈME FRAÎCHE

Facts and Features

Crème fraîche is a thick, lightly fermented unpasteurized cream. Its minimum butterfat level of 30% puts it on par with light whipping cream.

Because it is high in fat, crème fraîche should be used judiciously for an occasional treat. While definitely not the same, a lower-fat option is low-fat yogurt produced without thickening gums.

Baking/Cooking Guidelines

The nutty flavor of crème fraîche makes it popular for use in sauces, soups, and as a topping for fresh fruit.

KEFIR

Facts and Features

Kefir, its name originating from the Turkish word meaning "good feeling," tastes like a thick, tangy milk shake. It is made by incubating kefir grains (naturally formed organisms made of milk proteins) overnight in milk. Plain kefir is unsweetened; fruit-flavored kefir is sweetened with fructose or fruit juice concentrate.

Baking/Cooking Guidelines

Kefir is best used as a beverage or as a simple sauce over fruit salads.

SOUR CREAM

Facts and Features

Sour cream is cultured with Streptococcus lacti bacteria, the same type used in buttermilk. It has a minimum of 18% butterfat content. The best brands contain no added thick-

YOGURT CHEESE

1 quart plain yogurt
large wire mesh strainer
cheesecloth

Line the strainer with a double thickness of cheesecloth and place the strainer over a bowl. Spoon in the yogurt and cover the top of the strainer with a plate or plastic. Place the strainer and bowl in the refrigerator and allow the yogurt to drain for at least 8 hours but up to 24 hours. The longer it drains, the more firm the cheese.

Transfer the yogurt cheese to a container and refrigerate, using it within a week. Fresh or dried herbs, garlic, and/or black olives can be mixed in for extra flavor.

Nutrition Facts

Serving Size 2 TB (29 g)
Servings Per Container 12

Amount Per Serving

Calories 30	Calories from Fat 10

	% Daily Value*
Total Fat 1g	**1%**
Saturated Fat 0.5g	**3%**
Cholesterol 5mg	**1%**
Sodium 25mg	**1%**
Total Carbohydrate 3g	**1%**
Sugars 3g	
Protein 3g	

Vitamin A --	•	Calcium 10%

Not a significant source of Dietary Fiber, Vitamin C and Iron.

* Percent Daily Values are based on a 2,000 calorie diet.

Makes 1 1/2 cups.
(Pyramid servings: 1/4 Milk Group, 1 gram Fat)

---

eners such as gums, carrageenan, or modified food starch. Disodium phosphate, a fairly inert, harmless additive, may be added as an emulsifier for a smoother texture.

Baking/Cooking Guidelines

Like buttermilk, baked goods made with sour cream are tangy, moist, and rich-tasting.

It's no secret that a dollop of sour cream is, next to butter, the most popular condiment on potatoes. It's equally delicious as a topping for thick soups like borscht.

For a lower-fat alternative, try the recipe for yogurt cheese mentioned below.

YOGURT

Facts and Features

Yogurts vary according to the type of culture and complexity of ingredients. The bacteria which turn milk into yogurt are Lactobacillus bulgaricus and Streptococcus thermophilus. Another bacterium, Lactobacillus acidophilus, is a more potent, more consistent promoter of beneficial bacteria. Brands that include acidophilus are often suggested to be used to rebalance the digestive system as a preventative for yeast infections, after bouts of diarrhea, and after a course of antibiotics.

Yogurt can be made with goat milk or whole, part skim, or skim cow's milk. Nonfat dry milk is generally added to yogurt made from part skim or skim milk to make up for the creamy texture that is contributed by fat in whole-milk varieties. It also increases the amount of calcium and, to the detriment of those who are lactose intolerant, more lactose to digest. (See "Milk Allergies and Lactose Intolerance" below.) Very occasionally you'll find yogurt made from unhomogenized milk, affording you the pleasure of eating the cream that floats to the top for a moment of real pleasure or stirring it into the rest of the yogurt for a thicker consistency.

Besides nonfat dry milk, several additives may be found in cultured dairy products. To provide a thicker consistency, some yogurts, especially low-fat versions, are stabilized with various vegetable gums, gelatin, and carrageenan.

Sometimes modified food starch is added, a special thickening agent whose starch has been caused by water to expand and by heat, pressure, acid, or enzymes to increase its pectin content. Like corn-starch, modified food starch is pure starch. The structural modification makes it more efficient so less starch is needed when used as a thickener in products.

All of the above may be safe additives, but until you've had yogurt without them, especially those without modified food starch, you haven't tasted the best quality. Sure, it may be a bit more runny, but some yogurts are so thick, it's like eating freshly made plaster of Paris. It also gets to the point that, with all the gums and starches used in some yogurts, milk is almost an afterthought. Do yourself a favor and buy brands that contain the least amount of additives.

Fruit-flavored yogurts are usually highly sweetened, either with honey, maple syrup, corn syrup, sugar, fructose, or artificial sweeteners. For best flavor and optimum nutrition, simply buy fresh or dried fruit and add it to plain yogurt.

Frozen yogurt may contain less fat than ice cream if it is made from low-fat milk, but is usually no better than ice cream in regard to sugar. Viability of the beneficial bacteria supplied by high-quality yogurts with active cultures is very suspect in frozen yogurt.

Baking/Cooking Guidelines

The acidity of yogurt makes it a good addition to marinades to produce extra flavorful, tender meats and poultry.

Besides eating yogurt as a snack plain or with fruit, it is delicious mixed into vegetable salads, dips, and salad spreads as a low-fat substitute for mayonnaise.

Use yogurt instead of milk to moisten cereals and blend it with fruit juice and a frozen banana for a creamy "smoothie."

Yogurt can also be used to make yogurt cheese, a terrific substitute for cream cheese, mayonnaise, and sour cream. It's easily made at home by allowing the yogurt to drain through a cheesecloth-lined strainer, leaving the creamy milk solids behind. A funnel specially made for making yogurt cheese needs no additional liner and is easier to clean.

The liquid whey left behind contains several B vitamins (and a lot of lactose). Use it as a beverage, as a tart liquid in cooking, or to moisten your dog's dry kibble.

Only yogurt free of gums, gelatin, and modified food starch will work for making yogurt cheese since these additives would inhibit the whey from draining. Yogurt which contains pectin is okay to use.

Cheese

ONE OF the most convenient ways to eat dairy is cheese. Nutritionally, cheese is a concentrated form of the protein, calcium, phosphorus, and vitamin A found in milk. The milk's B vitamins, some minerals, and much of the lactose go out with the whey.

NUTRITION

The high sodium content that usually accompanies cheese is a result of its major role in the processing of cheese. Salt helps draw out the whey to reduce moisture content, in effect retarding the growth of microorganisms that promote spoilage and lactic acid bacteria. It also helps control the rate of ripening. The overall effect is a cheese with better flavor, texture, and appearance.

Still, some cheeses are specially made to be lower in sodium. The flavor difference is quite noticeable and refrigerator-life is greatly reduced since salt acts as a natural preservative.

Fat in Cheese

Cheese also contains concentrated amounts of fat and cholesterol. On the average, 65-75% of the calories in cheese are from its fat. What's even more depressing is that much of this fat is highly saturated, the kind that raises blood cholesterol and the risk of heart disease. And yet, it's the fat that gives cheese its creamy texture, rich flavor, and versatility in cooking.

The good news is that manufacturers have managed to remove more than a third of the fat from many cheeses without completely ruining the taste or texture. The newer varieties may not be quite as full-bodied in flavor or as creamy in texture, but many are remarkably delicious, especially when used in cooking.

Even so, most "low-fat" cheeses still derive 45-65% of calories from fat, shaving off only about 2-3 grams of fat per ounce. Typically, only soft, uncured cheeses with a high moisture content such as low-fat cottage cheese, dry cottage cheese, hoop cheese, quark, and nonfat ricotta can meet the recommended U.S. Dietary Goal of 30% calories from fat.

Occasionally, nonfat hard cheeses can be found which rely on skim milk, whey, vegetable gums, and lots of salt to achieve their zero-fat status. Unfortunately, it's not without compromises—flavor and texture often take a back seat to appearances.

A new addition to the low-fat cheese category is cheese made with Simplesse™, the fat substitute made from modified whey proteins. (See Fats and Oils chapter for more information.) Cheese made with Simplesse™ is made the same as regular cheese with the exception that the fat substitute is added to reduced-fat milk after the cream has been separated. Its purpose in the cheese is to transform an insipid, limp cheese into one that has color, flavor, and texture almost like full-fat cheese. Fortunately, the FDA doesn't even consider cheese made with Simplesse™ a real cheese. Since it is made with a whey protein concentrate (the Simplesse™), an ingredient not normally found in cheese, it must be called a "reduced-fat cheese product." Do yourself a favor and eat real cheese or none at all.

Does all this mean that in order to stay healthy, you need to forego Brick, Brie, Gruyere, and all those luscious cheeses that, unfortunately, are high in fat? Absolutely not. Eating low-fat cheese might be the prudent choice for at least some of your meals or snacks, but it's the fat content of the entire day that's most important rather than the fat in a single food or ingredient.

Consider how much fat you've consumed at other snacks and meals during the day. If you've included whole grain breads and cereals, plenty of veggies, and low-fat proteins, you can probably treat yourself to moderate amounts of full-fat cheese and still stay within the suggested 30% calories from fat.

Another trick is to use cheese as a condiment rather than the focal point of the meal. Invest in a cheese plane or cheese slicer to cut super-thin slices of your favorite cheese. Sprinkle on grated cheese instead of melting thick slices of cheese on top of dishes and casseroles. Make low-fat cheese spreads with grated cheese and herbs moistened with yogurt.

HOW CHEESE IS MADE

While admittedly a simplistic, over generalized description of the cheese-making process, cheese is basically made by coagulating the solids in milk with a curdling agent, pressing out the liquid whey, cooking the curds, pressing them into forms, and aging the resulting cheese until ready to eat.

WHAT IS QUARG?

Quarg, whose name is from the German term for curds, is a soft white cheese with a slightly acidic taste and smooth, spreadable texture. A popular cheese in Central Europe, it is easily digested, and low in fat, sodium, and calories.

Use quarg in recipes as a substitute for sour cream, cream cheese, Neufchatel cheese, ricotta, and cottage cheese. It is good in spreads, dips, desserts, and as a topping for baked potatoes.

Quarg's refrigerator life is about 14 days from manufacture. Choose those that are freshly made and free of the mold inhibitor, potassium sorbate.

All cheeses vary according to the kind of milk used (cow, goat, or sheep), the kind of coagulator, the amount of whey removed, and the ripening conditions, including temperature, humidity, and duration.

The color of cheese varies according to the type of milk used, natural molds and bacteria in the cheese, and coloring agents. Most cheeses are pale yellow or white in color. Those that are orange have been colored with safe vegetable coloring from beta-carotene or annatto seed extract.

Rennet/Vegetable Rennet

In the process of making cheese, the protein in milk must coagulate to separate the curds from the whey.

The traditional coagulator is **rennet**, a preparation made from an enzyme extracted from the the lining of calves' stomachs.

About half the cheeses produced are co-agulated with a less-expensive nonanimal-based "vegetable rennet," an enzyme produced from a mold culture. Many cheesemongers claim that cheese made from rennet is superior in flavor; others find little difference. The biggest drawback for these microbial enzymes is that they cannot be used to make cheddar or hard cheeses.

But now there is a nonanimal-based rennet, this time a bio-engineered version. Called chymosin, it was designed to produce a cost-efficient, consistent yield of high-quality cheese. Unlike typical microbial enzymes, chymosin can also be used to make hard cheeses.

Chymosin is produced by a bacterium called Escherichia coli which is altered by the implantation of a gene from a cow carrying the blueprints for rennin. As the bacterium reproduces, it makes copies of the new genetic code which now contains the gene for the cheese-curdling rennin enzyme. The FDA claims that the use of chymosin in cheese is safe; others are not so convinced. (See "Biotechnology" for more details.)

It's going to be tough to differentiate between cheeses made from chymosin and "vegetable rennet" microbial enzymes. The FDA doesn't require that chymosin be listed on the label. Instead, it will be included under the general term "enzymes." One clue that chymosin was used is if cheddar and other hard cheeses list "enzymes" rather than rennet on the label.

TYPES OF CHEESE

Cheese can be categorized in many ways with many variations, but one fairly universal classification method is to divide them according to their consistency and general type. A good cheese shop will include several varieties from all over the world, including those made from goat milk and sheep milk.

Fresh cheeses are unripened and most perishable of the cheeses. Because of this, some brands may contain emulsifiers and other additives. Avoid those with preservatives.

Soft cheeses are ripened for only a short time and have a water content of 45-50%.

Washed rind cheeses ripen from the outside in, curing for months in high humidity and turned regularly in a brine of water, wine, salt, and spices. This helps to keep the cheese moist, soft, and supple and to improve the flavor of the cheese by encouraging certain bacterial cultures and discouraging the growth of certain molds.

Blue cheeses are mold-ripened soft cheeses that ripen from the outside in and have cheese rinds that are edible.

Semi-firm cheeses ripen from the inside out and have a moisture content below 40%.

Firm or hard cheeses are cured a long time, leaving a moisture content well below 40%. The flavor of some firm cheeses corresponds to the length of curing. For example, cheese designated as mild is cured 2-3 months. Mellow cheese is cured 4-7 months. Sharp cheese is cured 8 months or longer.

Pasteurized processed cheeses are made by mixing several aged and unaged natural cheeses with an emulsifier to make a smooth, homogeneous mixture. Pasteurization of the cheese effectively stops the aging process, but because it does not kill all bacteria, preservatives and a great deal of salt are added to improve shelf life.

Pasteurized processed cheese food is made by combining pasteurized processed cheese with whey, cream, milk, non-fat dry milk, or buttermilk. Artificial colors and flavorings may also be included.

STORING CHEESE

Storing cheese properly will save money and frustration. Hard cheeses store longer due to their low moisture content while the softer cheeses have a greater tendency to mold.

Keep cheese in the refrigerator tightly wrapped in foil or plastic wrap to keep it from drying out or from picking up unwanted moisture and odors from other foods. Rewrap in clean foil or plastic each time the cheese is used. If mold appears on your cheese, simply cut it off. If a strange odor accompanies the mold, discard the cheese.

Some cheeses can be frozen but the texture will be crumbly when thawed, making it best for cooking. Cheddar, Gouda, Mozzarella, Muenster, Provolone, and Swiss freeze best. However, a better idea is just to buy what you need and use it fresh while its flavor and texture are at their prime.

BAKING/COOKING GUIDELINES

Cheese is best cooked or baked at low to medium heat since high heat will toughen the cheese. When broiling, keep cheese 4-5 inches away from the heat source and watch it closely to prevent burning.

When cheese is enjoyed on its own, serve at room temperature for the best flavor. Plan on taking the cheese out of the refrigerator about an hour before you intend to use it. Take out only as much as will actually be consumed.

Cheese is easier to grate or shred immediately after it is removed from the refrigerator. Grating warm cheese is an experience you'll not want to repeat.

You can also buy cheese already grated and shredded. Although convenient, its flavor is diminished due to the increased surface area exposure to oxidation. To prevent clumping, microcrystalline cellulose is often

EXPLORING CHEESES

There's more to life than cheddar cheese and mozzarella. Explore the many flavors, consistencies, and the often indescribable, subtle complexities of the following sampling of cheeses.

FRESH
Chèvre
Cream Cheese (natural without gums is the best)
Farmer's Cheese
Fresh Mozzarella (plain and smoked)
Fresh Ricotta (from cow, goat, or sheep milk)
Kefir Cheese
Hoop Cheese
Mascarpone
Montrachet-style Goat Cheese
Roulé

SOFT
Brie
Brillat Savarin
Camembert
Explorateur
Munster
Port Salut
St. André
Teleme

WASHED RIND
Appenzeller
Brick
Chaumes
Limburger
Morbier
Taleggio

EXPLORING CHEESES CONTINUED

SEMI-FIRM
Bel Paese
Canadian Oka
Colby
Daisy Hoop
Edam
Gouda
Havarti
Kasseri
Monterey Jack
Morbier
Mozzarella
Provolone, mild or smoked
Pyrenees
String Cheese
Tilsit
Treccione

FIRM
Aged Gouda
Caerphilly
Cheddar:
   mild, medium, or sharp
   goat cheddar
   farmhouse cheddar
   smoked cheddar
Cotswold
Double Gloucester
Emmenthaler
English Cheshire
Feta (sheep or goat's milk)
Gjetost
Gruyere
Jarlsberg
Leerdammer
Leyden
Raclette
Sage Derby

BLUE
Danish Blue
Gorgonzola
Roquefort
Saga
Stilton
Blue Castello
Maytag Blue
Shropshire Blue

GRATING
Aged Provolone
Argentine Parmesan
Asiago
Dry Jack
Grana Padano (Parmesan)
Parmigiano Reggiano (top quality Parmesan)
Pecorino Romano
Sapsago

REDUCED FAT OR SODIUM
available in:

Cheddar
Fromage Blanc
Gouda
Harvarti light
Jarlsberg light
Lappi
Neufchatel
Quark
Swiss
Yogurt Cheese

added to grated and shredded cheeses. Highly attracted to fat, it coats each shred of cheese, thus preventing the shreds from clinging to one another.

Microcrystalline is a safe, natural additive derived from plant fiber (yes, maybe from wood pulp) that is highly processed to a white crystalline powder. Although it metabolizes like any other fiber that is consumed, its presence in grated cheese is so minute that you won't see any fiber content listed on the label.

Milk Allergies and Lactose Intolerance

NOT EVERYBODY can tolerate dairy products. In fact, milk is one of the most common food allergens, caused by a hypersensitivity to the milk's protein. Symptoms include eczema, ear infections, and upper respiratory problems.

Lactose intolerance is not an allergy to milk. Rather, it is the inability to metabolize some or all of lactose, the primary carbohydrate in milk, into glucose, the usable form of sugar the body requires for energy. Genetic in nature, sometime between weaning and young adulthood, about 70% of the world's population begins to lose their ability to produce lactase, the enzyme produced in the small intestine responsible for digesting the lactose. Symptoms arise from digestive-tract distress, namely cramps, flatulence, and/or diarrhea.

Having a milk allergy or a deficiency in lactase doesn't necessarily preclude a person from being able to drink milk or consume other dairy products. Some sensitivity to milk may be dose-related, with the odds of having problems dependent on frequency and the amount of dairy product consumed at one time. Many people who are lactose-intolerant are able to digest small amounts of dairy, thanks to the friendly bacteria that reside in their large intestines.

The form or type of dairy product can also make a difference in tolerating milk. Ideally, infants should be raised on breast milk. Besides providing nutrients in ideal proportions as required by infants, breast milk also supplies antibodies that promote the growth of the "friendly" bacteria, Lactobacillus bifidus, in the digestive tract to guard against harmful bacteria. Unmodified cow's milk should not be given during the first six months of life since the particular types of proteins found in cow's milk are difficult for an infant's digestive tract to metabolize.

Infant formulas are devised to adjust cow's milk to more resemble the nutrient content in breast milk, but even then using cow's milk as a base may present problems in many infants. Some researchers are suggesting that soy-based formula may be preferable to milk-based versions. Preliminary studies infer that cow's milk during infancy may trigger juvenile diabetes in infants who are genetically prone to diabetes, an immune reaction to a protein in cow's milk. Whether the studies are completely verified or not, breast milk is the best option to create a sound foundation for building strong digestive and immune systems to help protect against the development of allergies to milk or any other foods later on in life.

Past infancy, some people find that goat milk seems to digest better since it lacks casein, the protein in cow's milk that forms a hard curd when exposed to stomach acids. Its small fat globules may also make it more easily digested.

Others have found that they can tolerate certified organic milk better than milk produced according to typical dairying methods. Speculation is that drug residue, even in minute amounts, may be responsible for some of the otherwise unexplained differences between feeling good with organic milk and ill feelings experienced after drinking standard milk.

Still others swear by raw milk or products made from it, claiming that the unaltered state of nutrients provide components that seemingly need to be present for their systems to handle it without problems.

Since cooking milk denatures its protein, some people allergic to the protein in milk may find that they can't drink fresh milk but can handle other processed forms of dairy, such as dairy found in cooked dishes, cheese, and other cultured products, especially yogurt.

Cooking the milk doesn't make much of a difference in breaking down the lactose, but individuals who are lactose-intolerant may find cultured dairy products and cheese a viable option. The bacteria used to culture yogurt, Streptococcus thermophilus and Lactobacillus bulgaricus, can digest some of the milk's lactose both during the culturing process and during its digestion.

Cheese, especially aged cheese with little moisture content, is low in lactose since its lactose-rich whey is separated from the curds during manufacture, with any remaining lactose hydrolyzed during the aging process. Butter, cream cheese, cottage cheese, cream, and sour cream are also lower in lactose than fresh milk.

Frozen yogurt, buttermilk, or sweet acidophilus milk remain high in lactose and, therefore are not good choices for those with lactose intolerance.

The addition of lactase enzymes to milk to "predigest" some of the lactose before it is consumed or the use of supplements before a meal that contains dairy may help those with lactose intolerance. Modified milk already containing the lactase is sold commercially nationwide, under the names Lactaid™ and Dairy Ease™.

Products that contain milk solids, whey, or whey protein concentrate are probably best avoided by both those allergic to milk and those low in lactase.

Non-Dairy Alternatives

MILK AND milk products are not the only way to get the nutrients supplied in dairy. Several vegetables and a few fish and shellfish provide adequate amounts of calcium as well as riboflavin, a B vitamin found in high amounts in milk.

The following chart will illustrate that a wide, varied, nutritious diet may contain more calcium than you think. All values are for the amount you would find in a cooked standard serving size of the food. Consider the vegetables to be cooked from raw, not frozen and then thawed.

As a reference for comparison, the Daily Value for calcium is calculated at 1000 mg. One cup of milk and yogurt or 11/2 oz. of cheese contain approximately 300 mg. of calcium.

NON-DAIRY SOURCES OF CALCIUM

FOOD	AMOUNT	CALCIUM (mg.)
acorn squash, mashed	1/2 cup	33 mg.
almonds	1/4 cup	95 mg.
arame, cooked	1/2 cup	50 mg.
bok choy	1/2 cup	79 mg.
broccoli, chopped	1/2 cup	89 mg.
butternut squash, baked cubes	1/2 cup	42 mg.
carob flour	1/4 cup	98 mg.
collard greens	1/2 cup	57 mg.
corn tortillas	2	80 mg.
figs, dried	2	54 mg.
garbanzo beans	1/2 cup	40 mg.
hijiki, cooked	1/2 cup	20 mg.
kale	1/2 cup	47 mg.
kombu	4" piece	20 mg.
mustard greens	1/2 cup	52 mg.
navy beans	1/2 cup	48 mg.
okra	1/2 cup	75 mg.
orange	1 medium	52 mg.

NON-DAIRY SOURCES OF CALCIUM (CONTINUED)

FOOD	AMOUNT	CALCIUM (mg.)
parsnips	1/2 cup	29 mg.
pinto beans	1/2 cup	43 mg.
quinoa, cooked	1/2 cup	41 mg.
rutabagas	1/2 cup	45 mg.
sardines w/bones (canned)	3 oz.	372 mg.
salmon, pink, canned w/bones	3 oz.	167 mg.
sesame seeds, hulled	1/4 cup	49 mg.
sesame seeds, unhulled	1/4 cup	400 mg.*
shrimp, boiled	3 oz.	274 mg.
soy milk	1 cup	100 mg.
soy milk, fortified	1 cup	200 mg.
spinach, cooked	1/2 cup	122 mg.*
sweet potato	1 medium	32 mg.
sunflower seeds	1/4 cup	42 mg.
tempeh	3.5 oz.	142 mg.
tofu w/calcium sulfate	3 oz.	130 mg.
turnip greens	1/2 cup	99 mg.
wakame, cooked	1/2 cup	54 mg.

*Absorption of calcium may be reduced due to the presence of oxalic acid.

Calcium supplements can also help fill in the gaps, although they don't supply the other nutrients inherent in milk products or vegetables. Certain forms may also be poorly absorbed. Calcium citrate or supplements that supply hydroxyapatite, the major calcium-containing crystal of bone and teeth, may be your best bets.

Exploring Your Options

For drinking, moistening cereal, and as a substitute liquid for cooking and baking several other alternatives for milk are available, including soy milk, rice-based amasake and rice milk, and nut milks. (Note: since these do not contain all the nutrients found in milk, non-dairy milk substitutes should not be the sole source of nutrition for an infant or child.) A nondairy creamed soup base can be made by puréeing rolled oats or couscous that have been cooked in with the soup.

AMASAKE

Facts and Features

Amasake is a sweet, cultured beverage made from rice. Traditional amasake is very thick in texture, although more commercial varieties have consistencies ranging from very thin to milk shake-thick.

Baking/Cooking Guidelines

Use as a beverage, over cereals, or experiment with it in baking. (For more information, see "Amasake" in the Sweets chapter.)

NUT MILKS

Facts and Features

Nut milks can be made at home within minutes from virtually any nut. (For the recipe, refer to the Nuts and Seeds chapter.)

Prepared almond milk packed in shelf-stable aseptic containers is also available in natural foods stores.

Baking/Cooking Guidelines

Use as you would regular dairy milk or soy milk.

SOY MILK

Facts and Features

Soy milk is the most popular nondairy beverage sold in the natural food industry. Because soy milk is vegetable-based, it is lactose-free, cholesterol-free, and low in saturated fats. Accordingly, it provides a viable alternative for those who have difficulty tolerating milk or have been advised to avoid all sources of cholesterol, as well as for those who prefer not to consume dairy for philosophical reasons. Some people choose soy milk simply because they find the flavor enjoyable.

However, nutritionally, it is no match for the calcium, vitamin A, and vitamin D supplied by milk. Some manufacturers are trying to close the gap by fortifying their soy milks with extra calcium, beta-carotene and vitamins D and E.

Commercial production of soy milk goes far beyond the home technique of grinding and cooking soybeans, followed by straining the "milk" from the mixture. Now lipoxidase enzymes and the trypsin inhibitor are modified and deactivated by heat, pressure, and vacuum processing to improve flavor and digestion. The addition of the various ingredients, homogenization, pasteurization, and packaging are all done under sterile conditions. The aseptic packaging used for soy milk allows for a 12-month shelf life that requires no refrigeration until opening.

The many flavors and textures vary from brand to brand according to the techniques and ingredients used by each manufacturer. Choice of sweeteners include honey, rice syrup, malt syrup, malted cereal solids, and maple syrup. Some soy milks are flavored with vanilla, carob, or cocoa. Fat content can also vary, depending on the amount of oil used in manufacture. The addition of sea vegetables such as kombu is used both to enhance flavor and digestion of the protein in soy milk.

Baking/Cooking Guidelines

Use as you would regular dairy milk.

RICE MILK

Facts and Features

Rice milk is produced similarly as amasake. (See "Amasake" in the Sweets chapter for more information.) Naturally sweet, it may also contain an additional sweetener such as rice syrup. Nutritionally, it is very high in carbohydrates but low in calcium, protein, and saturated fat. The addition of oil and carrageenan give rice milk a thicker, more milk-like texture.

TOFU "SOUR" CREAM

16 oz. tofu
2 Tbsp. sesame tahini
2 tbsp. mellow white miso
or 2 tsp. umeboshi paste*

Boil tofu in water for 10 minutes. Drain and process in a blender or food processor with the tahini and umeboshi paste until smooth.

Variations: For extra zip, add 1 Tbsp. lemon juice or rice vinegar. To make tofu ricotta cheese, use the original recipe, mashing the ingredients together instead of blending to a smooth consistency.

Makes 2 cups.
(Pyramid servings: 1/2 Meat/Protein Group, 3 1/2 grams Fat)

*Umeboshi plum paste is the pitted purée of umeboshi plums, the sour green Japanese plums that are pickled with sea salt and shiso, the purple leaves from the beefsteak plant. Umeboshi paste or pitted whole plums impart a sour, salty flavor to foods such as dips, spreads, sauces, grains, and broths.

Nutrition Facts

Serving Size 2 TB. (32 g)
Servings Per Container 16

Amount Per Serving

Calories 60	Calories from Fat 35

	% Daily Value*
Total Fat 3.5g	6%
Saturated Fat 0.5g	3%
Sodium 80mg	3%
Total Carbohydrate 2g	1%
Sugars --g	
Protein 5g	

Calcium 6%	●	Iron 15%

Not a significant source of Cholesterol, Dietary Fiber, Vitamin A and Vitamin C.
* Percent Daily Values are based on a 2,000 calorie diet.

Baking/Cooking Guidelines

Use as you would milk or soymilk as a beverage or in recipes where a sweet flavor would be appropriate.

CHEESE ALTERNATIVES

Imitation cheeses free of lactose and cholesterol are made primarily from soy milk. They can be used just like cheese in any application, but they do not replicate the nutrients or the flavor found in real natural cheese.

Common ingredients also include soy oil, salt, lecithin, citric acid, guar gum, annatto seed (for coloring), and the milk protein, calcium caseinate or casein. If you want your soy cheese to melt, you have to accept the casein, which is not actually a problem unless you are allergic to casein or if you prefer a pure vegan diet. New FDA labeling regulations require that foods like soy cheese which are claimed to be nondairy, must indicate that caseinate is derived from milk.

An almond milk-based cheese is also sold in natural food stores. Its ingredients include milk protein casein, canola oil, salt, sodium and calcium phosphates as safe emulsifiers, citric acid, natural flavoring, carrageenan, and beta-carotene.

Foods that are typically topped with melted cheese can be topped instead with cubed or grated mochi, the "puff-up biscuits" made from sweet brown rice. Just sprinkle the mochi on top of casseroles or vegetables that will undergo steaming or baking, cover, and cook as usual. The mochi will "melt," yielding a texture similar to melted mozzarella.

Tofu can be transformed into substitutes for cream cheese, sour cream, cottage cheese, ricotta cheese, and whipped cream. Digestibility and flavor of the tofu are best when it is boiled for 10 minutes before use, but if the tofu is included in a recipe which will undergo further cooking or baking, the preboiling is unnecessary.

FROZEN TREATS ALTERNATIVES

Urges for ice cream can be fulfilled with those based on soy milk or rice milk. While they are free of lactose and cholesterol, they still contain plenty of fat and sugar. Fruit-sorbet made from unsweetened frozen fruit juice is a better choice for a frozen dessert.

Soy "malteds," thicker and sweeter versions of soy milk, can also be frozen and eaten as a dessert or snack. Thick amasake drinks taste remarkably similar to milk shakes.

Another ice cream alternative is homemade frozen banana custard. Peel and freeze a banana, cut it into chunks, and process in a blender or food processor until the banana becomes creamy. Frozen bananas can also be blended with fruit juice to make "smoothies," nondairy milk shake.

YOGURT ALTERNATIVES

Yogurt alternatives can be made at home with soy milk or nut milk. Several commercial soy-yogurt versions featuring active cultures are available ready-made both plain and with added fruit purée. To make them more palatable, most are highly sweetened with fruit juice concentrate, honey, or brown rice syrup.

FATS, OILS & SWEETS GROUP

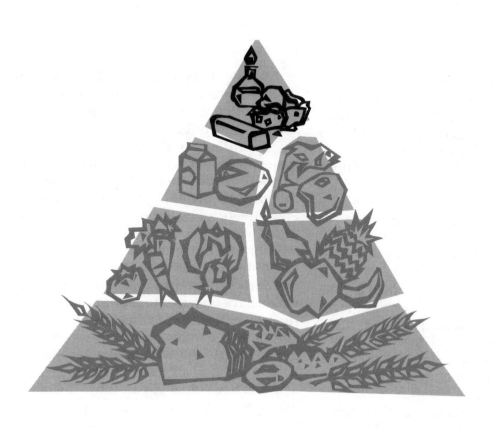

THE LAST group of the Food Guide Pyramid, the Fats, Oils, & Sweets Group, includes two food categories, fats and sugars, both of which are mired in continual controversy concerning their food value and their overconsumption within the average American diet.

The placement of fats and sugars at the tip of the Food Guide Pyramid indicates that foods within these two categories should be used judiciously, as an adjunct to an overall nutritious diet, not as your main source of calories.

Fats and Oils

NUTRITION

In the "old days" few people thought twice about smearing plenty of butter on sandwiches, toast, and vegetables. Nor did they think that cooking chicken, fish, and potatoes in deep-fryers and eating red meat three times a day could be detrimental to one's health.

Now, it's common knowledge that too much fat isn't such a good thing. We're even using words like "hydrogenated," "mono-unsaturated," and "low density lipoproteins" in daily conversation, terminology heretofore expressed primarily by doctors or registered dieticians. The marketplace is overflowing with low-fat and fat-free versions of many of our favorite foods and television talk shows are spreading the word that low fat is the way to go.

And yet, considering that the average American diet still figures out to about 36% of total calories from fat with 13% of fat calories from saturated fats, we have a long way to go before we get our fat intake within healthy guidelines.

According to The National Research Council's landmark study published in 1989, *Diet and Health: Implications for Reducing Chronic Disease Risk* (National Academy Press, 1989), highest priority should be given to reducing fat in our diets to minimize the risks of atherosclerotic cardiovascular diseases, as well as certain forms of cancer, and, of course, obesity. In fact, the researchers would have preferred to suggest a goal much further reduced from their recommended 30% of total calories from fat. However, they reasoned that the 30% level was at least a good interim goal that was within reasonable reach in initial attempts by the American public without dramatically changing their normal diets.

The National Research Council's wish list continues from there. Rather than 10% of calories from saturated fat, they revealed that 7-8% would be even better. Regarding cholesterol, instead of the suggested maximum limit of 300 mg. per day, they believe reductions to 200 mg. or less are optimum.

How Much Fat Do We Really Need?

With all the talk about needing to reduce our fat intake, it's easy to forget how important it is to have some fat in our diets. Besides enhancing the flavor and aroma of foods, fats are carriers of the fat-soluble vitamins A, D, E, and K. These nutrients play a vital role in vision, the health of mucous membranes and skin, bone growth, reproduction, nerves, and clotting of the blood.

Dietary fat is also needed to supply essential fatty acids (EFA). Both linoleic acid (Omega-6 fatty acid) and alpha-linolenic acid (Omega-3 fatty acid) are called "essential" because they cannot be synthesized in your body and must be obtained daily from dietary sources for proper growth, development, and continued maintenance of the body. Essential fatty acids help make cell walls strong and resistant to viruses, bacteria, and allergens. They also keep your hair and skin from getting too dry.

In particular, essential fatty acids serve as precursors to prostaglandins, hormone-like compounds that help regulate vital body functions, including nerve impulses, immunity, mucosal and skin integrity, energy, and clotting of the blood. In order to produce these prostaglandins, linoleic acid converts to gamma-linolenic acid (GLA) which, in turn, generates prostaglandin E_1 (PGE_1). Gamma-linolenic acid can also convert into arachidonic acid, another essential fatty acid. Alpha-linolenic acid converts to eicosapentaenoic acid (EPA) which is then trans-formed into prostaglandin E_3 (PGE_3).

Technically, the average person requires only 4-6% of total calories from fat (the equivalent of about 1 tablespoon of polyunsaturated fats—not saturated or even monounsaturated) to obtain a minimum of essential fatty acids. It's important to remember that you don't have to rely only on oil to supply linoleic or alpha-linolenic acid. Beans, grains, vegetables, nuts, and fruits all contain at least small amounts of polyunsaturated fats. In fact, getting only 4-6% of total calories from fat, even in a seemingly fat-free diet, would be fairly difficult.

Dr. Dean Ornish's famed program for reversing heart disease without using cholesterol-lowering drugs or surgical intervention is based on a holistic program that, along with daily exercise and stress relief, utilizes a nearly total vegetarian diet that provides 10% calories from fat.

Other researchers and dieticians suggest that, for individuals who are healthy and wish to maintain their present weight, a goal of 20% calories from fat is best for optimum health, a figure significantly less than the 30% guideline reluctantly set by the government.

Athletes, too, like to keep their fat intake to no more than 20%. When the cardiovascular system begins to work efficiently, the primary fuel for muscles during aerobic activity switches to fatty acids. Besides the obvious advantage of using up fat stores to maintain an ideal weight, when exercise is fueled by fatty acids, muscle glycogen is spared, thus enabling you to exercise for a longer period of time.

However, even though fat plays an important part in endurance exercise, the goal is to increase your fat utilization through endurance training, not by eating extra fat. Also, since fat takes much longer to digest, too much fat can also impair performance as your working muscles lose out to the energy required by the intestinal tract.

It is very important to note that infants and toddlers under the age of two years old should not be placed on diets restricted in fat and cholesterol. A baby's developing brain and nervous system requires fat to make myelin, a high-cholesterol, fatty substance that protects the nerve fibers. In fact, a diet high in fat and cholesterol is just what Nature intended for the early years of life. About 50% of the total calories supplied in mother's milk come from fat, with about half of the fat calories from saturated fat.

As outlined for adults, children over the age of two should be provided meals and snacks that average out to be less than 30% total calories from fat (less than 10% from saturated fat) and no more than 300 mg. of cholesterol. The progressive buildup of fatty deposits that narrow the arteries and cause heart disease later in life begins in childhood. Diets too high in fat can also lead to obesity. Since eating habits formed in childhood often last a lifetime, a good healthy start can make a significant difference towards achieving a longer, more vigorous and enjoyable life.

LOW FAT/LOW WEIGHT

Fats are a concentrated source of energy, supplying 9 calories per gram of fat, an amount significantly higher than the 4 calories per gram provided by both proteins and carbohydrates. In addition to the weight loss exhibited by Dr. Dean Ornish's heart patients who adopted the 10% calories from fat way of eating, several recent studies have supported the theory that you can eat plenty and still lose weight, as long as the food is high in fiber and low in fat.

In one such clinical trial conducted at Cornell University in 1991, women were allowed to eat all they wanted, provided that fat accounted for about 25% of total calories instead of the 36% fat found in the typi-

cal American diet. The women consistently lost about 1/2 pound per week without hunger pangs, food cravings, or depression as commonly experienced with many other calorie-restricted weight-loss diets. And, they had no decrease in metabolism, the body's response to conserving energy when too few calories are provided to maintain basic autonomic functions within the body. Eating low-fat meals and snacks is definitely the way to get trim and stay that way.

TYPES OF FATTY ACIDS

Fats are classified according to their degree of saturation. Different types of fats have different effects on health, a result of each fat's particular molecular structure. The fat in foods consists of varying proportions of the following kinds of fatty acids. Describing a food as high in a particular type of fatty acid is determined by the predominant fat of which it is composed.

Saturated fats

Fats consist of carbon atoms linked together in a row of varying lengths, depending on the specific type of fat. Except for the carbons situated on either end of the chain, each carbon atom is capable of bonding with two hydrogen atoms.

$$H \quad H \quad H \quad H \quad H \quad H \quad H \quad H \quad H \quad H \quad H \quad H \quad H \quad H \quad H \quad O$$
$$H - C - C - C - C - C - C - C - C - C - C - C - C - C - C - C - C - O - H$$
$$H \quad H \quad H \quad H \quad H \quad H \quad H \quad H \quad H \quad H \quad H \quad H \quad H \quad H \quad H$$

(palmitic acid)

If all the available spaces are filled with hydrogen atoms, the fat is considered **saturated.** Because saturated fat molecules are shaped like a straight line, they can stack together into a compressed mass, making them resistant to oxygen, heat, and light. Accordingly, saturated fats are solid at room temperature and slow to spoil.

They also are the specific type of fat shown to be the major dietary determinant of serum total cholesterol and low-density lipoprotein (LDL) cholesterol levels, thereby associated with elevated risk of coronary heart disease. High intakes of saturated fats, as well as total fats, are also associated with higher incidence and mortality from cancers of the colon, prostate, and breast and also obesity.

Common foods high in saturated fats include full-fat dairy products, meats, poultry-especially if the skin and excess fat is retained, and some vegetable oils, including coconut, palm, and palm kernel oils. Certain varieties of saturated fats, the 16-carbon palmitic acid (as illustrated above), 14-carbon myristic acid, and the 12-carbon lauric acid, raise cholesterol the most.

Monounsaturated fats

Sometimes a carbon atom will not link with a hydrogen atom but will instead form a double bond with the carbon next to it. If a fatty acid contains only one double bond, it is called **mono-unsaturated** ("mono" means "one").

(oleic acid)

In contrast to saturated fat's straight line shape, a monounsaturated fat has a flexible joint occurring at the carbon double bond. This ability to twist and bend at this point makes monounsaturated fats more fluid than saturated fats but still less resistant to oxidation.

Clinical studies have shown that the substitution of monounsaturated fats for saturated fats results in a reduction of serum total cholesterol and LDL cholesterol while preserving the beneficial HDL cholesterol that helps eliminate excess cholesterol. Cultures whose traditional diets depend primarily on monounsaturated fats like olive oil have exhibited lower levels of heart disease than populations who eat a lot of animal proteins and whole milk products.

Monounsaturated fats can easily be distinguished by their liquid state at room temperature that thickens when refrigerated. Oleic acid with its 18-carbon chain is the predominant monounsaturated fatty acid commonly found in food. It is also referred to as an Omega-9 fat which simply describes how far the carbon double bond is from the methyl end of the molecule (the end with the 3 hydrogen atoms).

In addition to olives and olive oil, sources include canola oil, high-oleic safflower and sunflower oils, peanuts and peanut oil, avocadoes and avocado oil, almonds and almond oil, cashews, hazelnuts, macadamia nuts, pistachios, and pecans.

Polyunsaturated fats

A fatty acid with more two carbon double bonds is called **polyunsaturated** ("poly" means "many").

(linoleic acid)

Like monounsaturated fats, each carbon double bond found in the polyunsaturated fatty acid molecule is a flexible joint. Due to the extra double bond, polyunsaturated fats are more fluid, making them liquid at both room temperature and while under refrigeration.

However, the extra double bond also makes it much more chemically unstable and therefore more prone to attack by highly reactive singlet oxygen molecules (also known as "free radicals") drawn randomly from the atmosphere. Encouraged by the effects of heat and light, these free radicals attack the weakened bonds found in polyunsaturated fats to form, not only new compounds, but more free radicals, thus creating the opportunity for a chain reaction. In the process, cell membranes are destroyed, undermining the integrity of various body organs and tissues as a result. It's no surprise that researchers are concerned that individuals whose diets are disproportionately high in polyunsaturated fats may be more prone to cancer.

And, that's not all. Even though substituting some of the saturated fats in your diet with polyunsaturated fats tends to decrease total blood cholesterol and LDL cholesterol, at the same time it also reduces the effect of the beneficial HDL cholesterol.

All that said, it's still very important to include a small amount of polyunsaturated fats in the diet since they also supply linoleic acid, one of the essential fatty acids. Currently, the average intake of polyunsaturated fats in the United States is approximately 7% of calories, an amount that the National Research Council insists should not be increased.

Linoleic acid is also referred to as an omega-6 fatty acid, indicating that its first carbon double bond is 6 carbons from the methyl end of the molecule (the end with the three hydrogens).

Foods high in polyunsaturated fats include regular safflower oil, walnuts and walnut oil, sunflower seeds and regular sunflower oil, corn oil, and soybean oil, brazil nuts, pine nuts, pistachios, pumpkin seeds, sesame seeds, and walnuts. Although both grains and beans are very low in fat, what they contain is primarily polyunsaturated.

Superunsaturated fats

The fourth type of fatty acid has three carbon double-bonds.

Referred to as a **superunsaturated** fatty acid, it is the most fluid of all the fats, remaining liquid even at very cold temperatures. It is also extremely reactive and therefore must be processed in such a way as to shelter the oil from light, heat, and oxygen at all times. Superunsaturated fats must be used only at temperatures below 212° and continously stored in opaque containers.

On food labels, superunsaturated fats are considered a component of polyunsaturated fat. Occasionally you'll see the individual amounts of the two delineated on labels, especially on bottles of oil.

Also known as both alpha-linolenic acid and omega-3 fatty acid (indicating that its first carbon double bond is three carbons from the methyl end of the molecule), it is one of the essential fatty acids that must be obtained from food for cell membrane integrity, energy production, growth, immune response, and reproduction. (The other form of linolenic acid, gamma-linolenic acid, is a derivative of linoleic acid). More commonly supplied in our ancestors' diets, today most people receive an inadequate amount of linolenic acid and an overabundance of linoleic acid (omega-6 fatty acids).

Much excitement was created when the results of studies investigating the diets of the Eskimos in Greenland who have extremely low incidences of heart attacks were revealed. It appeared that their diet, which consisted primarily of fish, supplied them with plenty of omega-3 fatty acids in the forms of eicosapentaenoic acid (EPA) and docosahexaenoic acid (DHA). These fatty acids block the production of thromboxane, a prostaglandin that promotes blood clotting. In contrast, linoleic acid (omega-6 fatty acids) stimulates the synthesis of blood-clotting thromboxane.

Since most heart attacks occur when a blood clot gets stuck in an already-narrowed coronary artery, the importance of omega-3 fatty acids struck a chord with the American public, resulting in increased consumption of fish. Fish particularly high in omega-3 fatty acids include sardines, salmon, mackerel, herring, and trout. Leaner fish supply smaller amounts.

But omega-3 fatty acids in the form of alpha-linolenic acid are also found in plants. Sources include flax seed, chia seed, pumpkin seeds, canola oil, soybeans, and walnuts. When the body has enough alpha-linolenic acid from food, the body's cells can convert it into eicosapentaenoic acid (EPA). So, similar to fish-derived omega-3 fatty acids, in addition to promoting other prostaglandins that help regulate our body's processes, alpha-linolenic acid may stimulate the prostaglandins that block thromboxane.

HYDROGENATION AND TRANS-FATS

New types of fat are synthetically produced through hydrogenation. First developed in 1905 as a less expensive alternative to lard, hydrogenation is a chemical process that transforms liquid vegetable oils into margarine and shortenings that are solid or semi-solid at room temperature. Manufacturers like hydrogenated fats because they are cheap, emulate the consistency and "mouth-feel" of butter and lard, and are more resistant to rancidity so shelf life can be extended much beyond normal expectancy.

During the process of hydrogenation, vegetable oils are combined with hydrogen gas under pressure at high heat. A metal catalyst like nickel, zinc, or copper reacts with the hydrogen gas to break some of the poly-unsaturated fats' carbon double bonds, forcing the carbons to bond with the supplied hydrogen. In effect, this reduces the number of the molecule's double bonds, yielding a saturated fatty acid.

$$-\overset{\text{H}}{\underset{\text{H}}{\text{C}}}=\overset{\text{H}}{\underset{\text{H}}{\text{C}}}- \;+\; \text{H}_2 \;-\; -\overset{\text{H}}{\underset{\text{H}}{\text{C}}}-\overset{\text{H}}{\underset{\text{H}}{\text{C}}}-$$

(complete hydrogenation at a double bond)

However, since complete hydrogenation would produce a very dense and brittle fat, oils are usually partially hydrogenated at various degrees of saturation, depending on the manufacturer's desired finished product.

Here's where the term "trans-fatty acid" enters the picture. During partial hydrogenation, hydrogen is not added at all of the carbon double bonds. Instead, at the remaining double bonds, a major transformation occurs in the placement of the hydrogen atoms that were originally present at the double bond.

Chemists refer to the normal flexible carbon double bond in which both hydrogens are on the same side as a "cis-configuration." During partial hydrogenation, the double bonds that do not add hydrogens are broken and reformed into a new shape in which one of the existing hydrogens at the double bond is flipped and rotated. Therefore, the hydrogens at the double bond are now on opposite sides of the carbon chain. As a result, the joint of the carbon double bond changes from a flexible joint to a straight, more rigid molecule, thus making the oil behave like a saturated fat.

```
   H    H              H H   H
 -C-C=C-C-           -C-C=C-C-
   H H H H            H    H H
```

"cis-configuration"   "trans-configuration"

While hydrogenation may be a fascinating process, it should never go beyond the laboratory. Trans-fats are not metabolized in our bodies like the naturally occurring "cis-form." As the body tries to incorporate these foreign trans-fatty acids into its cell membranes (in effect, taking the place of essential fatty acids and blocking them from performing their biological functions), deformed cellular structures may result, increasing cancer risks, accelerating aging and degenerative changes in tissues, and, as research now shows, increasing potential for heart disease.

The study that initially raised major concern throughout the nation was one conducted in 1990 by Dutch scientists. Results published in The New England Journal of Medicine reported that these hydrogenated fats not only raise "bad" low-density lipoprotein (LDL) cholesterol but also reduce the otherwise protective "good" high-density lipoprotein (HDL) cholesterol—something even saturated fat doesn't do.

At the request of the Institute of Shortening and Edible Oils trade association who complained that the Dutch study fed participants three to six times more trans-fats than the average American eats per day, the USDA conducted a study in 1992 using more realistic amounts of trans-fats. Much to the chagrin of the shortening trade association, the USDA research corroborated the Dutch study. Furthermore, they found that diets averaging only 10-20 grams of trans-fats per day, the average amount in a typical American diet, raises serum cholesterol as much as a diet high in saturated fat.

The final clincher was the Harvard Nurses Study whose results hit the headlines in 1993. An ongoing analysis of the diets of 90,000 nurses, found that women who frequently use products containing hydrogenated fats, such as margarine, have more than a 50% higher risk of heart disease than those who rarely use them. The more they used, the higher their risk.

Given their widespread consumption throughout the United States, the implications of the problems associated with trans-fatty acids are mind-boggling. Today, we use nearly four times as much margarine as butter on our bread, pancakes, and vegetables. And the marketplace is saturated with foods made with hydrogenated oils. Ironically, in response to previous nutritional concerns about highly saturated lard and tropical oils such as coconut oil and palm kernel oil, not too long ago most manufacturers made the switch to partially hydrogenated fats for baked goods, salty snacks, puddings, frozen fish sticks, imitation cheeses, chicken nuggets, and ready-made frostings.

While other countries require labels to list the amount of trans-fats contained within a product, no direct provision was mandated in the FDA's newly revised labeling system. The FDA did, however, write in regulations that acknowledge that trans-fats are significantly different than other unsaturated fats.

Although, technically, trans-fats are considered unsaturated, voluntary listings of monounsaturated and polyunsaturated fats may not include trans-fats in their totals. So, provided that the label lists the voluntarily reported amounts of monounsaturated and polyunsaturated fats in addition to the mandated saturated fats, you can actually figure out how much trans-fats a product may contain. Simply add up the listed amounts of saturated, monounsaturated, and polyunsaturated fats and then subtract them from

THE ORIGINS OF MARGARINE

Margarine was first developed in 1869 by a French pharmacist in response to Napoleon III's promise of a substantial prize to the first person to produce a synthetic, edible fat. At the time, a European cattle plague had made butter both scarce and expensive. The Frenchman's first prototype, a mixture of beef fat, milk, chopped sheep's stomachs and cow's udders, was named after a newly discovered fatty acid, margaric acid (a name derived from the Greek word for "pearl"), believed to have been found in the animal fat he used. Calling the synthetic fat "margarine" was doubly appropriate since not only did the isolated substance from animal fat form pearly drops, the original margarine was hard, white, and glossy.

After the hydrogenation process was developed in 1905, vegetable oils were used to make margarine. Chemical additives to improve spreadability, appearance, and flavor were added in the 1920s.

In the United States, both the American government and the dairy industry did everything they could to undermine margarine's popularity. It was heavily taxed and grocery stores had to obtain a license just to sell it. The armed forces were not allowed to use it. And, some states required that margarine be sold uncolored in its natural white state to further differentiate it from real butter. Instead, the yellow dye was provided in a separate packet for the consumer to mix in at home. Not until 1950 were federal taxes on margarine abolished. It wasn't until 1967 that Wisconsin allowed the sale of predyed yellow margarine.

Originally just a cheap alternative to butter, margarine won increased respect as doctors and dieticians become convinced of the dangers of saturated fats and cholesterol. Unfortunately for margarine, the bad news about trans-fatty acids raising serum cholesterol as much as saturated fats is making its fame short-lived.

---

the total amount of fat listed. The remaining number will indicate whether a product contains trans-fats and the exact amount.

Another regulation stipulates that a product that bears a "saturated fat-free" claim must contain less than half a gram of trans-fat. Since trans-fats have been found to raise cholesterol as much as saturated fats, it makes sense that trans-fats content should be negligible.

Given all we know about the serious health concerns surrounding trans-fatty acids, it's highly doubtful that hydrogenation would be approved if the process had been just recently discovered. Still, we're left with the fact that it's now in many of our processed foods and that for years many people have been led to believe that using a hydrogenated fat such as margarine was the healthy way to go.

So, what do you do now? Start reading labels to eliminate foods that contain partially hydrogenated oil or vegetable shortening, the primary source in the typical American diet for trans-fatty acids. Switch to higher-quality foods either fat-free or made with small amounts of natural oils.

Instead of margarine, look at other op-

FAT AND CHOLESTEROL: WHAT DOES IT MEAN?

Cholesterol: A waxy substance made primarily in the liver and in cells lining the small intestine, is an essential constituent of cell membranes and nerve fibers, and a building block of certain hormones. It is found in all body tissues, but the cholesterol that circulates in the blood creates the most concern.

Fats (triglycerides) and cholesterol are transported through the bloodstream in protein-wrapped clusters called lipoproteins which are assembled in the liver and intestinal tract. These lipoproteins are labeled according to their "density," based on their proportion of triglycerides, phospholipids, cholesterol, and protein.

It is believed that 20-30% of the population are genetically hypersensitive to dietary cholesterol and, therefore, have blood cholesterol levels which increase with the intake of high cholesterol-containing foods. Since there is no simple test for cholesterol hypersensitivity, it is suggested that, to be on the safe side, everyone should keep their daily intake of dietary cholesterol below 300 mg.

Cholesterol is found only in foods of animal origin: meat, eggs, fish, and dairy products, including butter. Fruits, vegetables, grains, and legumes contain no cholesterol.

Low Density Lipoproteins (LDL): contain 45% cholesterol, 25% protein, 10% triglycerides, and 22% phospholipids. These are the lipoproteins that have become known as "bad" cholesterol because after they deliver the cholesterol actually needed by the cells, they deposit any excess in arterial walls and other tissues.

High Density Lipoproteins (HDL): contain the highest amount of protein (45-50%) along with 5% triglycerides, 20% cholesterol, and 30% phospholipids. Also known as "good" cholesterol, HDL lipoproteins pick up the cholesterol deposits and bring them to the liver for recycling or disposal. A higher proportion of HDL lipoproteins to LDL lipoproteins represents more active cholesterol, a lower risk of developing atherosclerosis, and a lower risk of heart attack and stroke.

tions. Better restaurants offer cruets of herb-infused olive oil for use on bread. Flax seed oil can be drizzled on baked potatoes for a tasty and much more nutritious alternative.

It's also a good time to learn to cut down on all fats in general. Whole bread is delicious without margarine or butter. Lemon juice and seasonings can more than adequately enhance the flavor of vegetables. Cookies and cakes can also be made with liquid vegetable oils.

If you insist on using margarine, minimize your intake of trans-fatty acids by choosing soft tub-like or liquid "squeeze" margarines instead of the more hydrogenated stick versions. The first ingredient listed on the label should be a liquid vegetable oil rather than partially hydrogenated fat.

Better yet, margarine aficionados should try Spectrum Spread™, a non-hydrogenated soft margarine substitute made by Spectrum Naturals, Inc. Available at many natural food stores throughout the country, Spectrum Spread™ is based on expeller-pressed canola oil and water, thickened and emulsified with soy protein isolate, xanthan gum, and guar gum, flavored with sea salt and natural butter flavor, colored with natural annatto bean and turmeric, and stabilized with natural citric acid and a synthetically derived sorbic acid.

While it is generally best to avoid synthetic preservatives whenever possible, it appears that without the addition of sorbic acid, mold could form on the surface of Spectrum Spread™ due to the fact that water is a necessary part of the patented non-hydrogenation production process. Since it is metabolized by the body as if it were a natural fat, sorbic acid's effect on the body is, at least, fairly innocuous as preservatives go. If you want to eat margarine, you may find that the product's benefits far outweigh its use of a synthetic preservative, especially considering that most other margarines also contain sorbic acid but can't lay claim to Spectrum Spread™'s laudable zero trans-fatty acids content.

Where does butter fit in with the controversy about margarine and its trans-fatty acid content? Overall, it still contains a higher percentage of cholesterol-raising fats as well as 25-30 milligrams of cholesterol per tablespoon. However, unlike any of the manufactured fats, it has a centuries-old track record and is completely natural. Still, since it's best to cut down on all fats in general and minimize foods high in saturated fat, butter, if used at all, should be used judiciously and only in small amounts.

HOW OILS ARE PRODUCED

The natural oils in seeds, nuts, beans, and even some fruits (avocado and olives) have been extracted since ancient times. The Chinese made sesame oil by first grinding roasted sesame with a mortar and pestle and then waiting until the liberated oil rose to the surface.

Fortunately, oil processing has become easier and more efficient throughout the years. Depending on the particular oil being extracted, as well as its intended use, certain methods of processing are superior to others.

Stone-pressing is the traditional method of extracting oil from some seeds and, especially, olives. The method is still used at least partially for some brands of olive oil. Stone pressing generates little heat and protects the olives' natural antioxidants that preserve the integrity of the oil.

Hydraulic pressing is used for soft-fleshed fruits (avocados), olives, and walnuts in which the oil is squeezed out from the ground-up material by means of a weight applied from above with the aid of a crank or lever. Hydraulic pressing remains the typical method of producing extra virgin olive oil.

After World War II, the oil industry shifted from extensive hydraulic pressing to the more economical methods of mechanical pressing and solvent extraction.

Mechanical pressing, also known as expeller pressing, removes oil through the use of continuously driven screws that crush the seed or other oil-bearing material into a pulp from which the oil is expressed. Friction created in the process can generate heat between 120-190° F. Therefore, the use of the term "cold-pressed," sometimes used in reference to mechanical pressing, is a misnomer.

Except for the specialized modified atmosphere packing extraction system (see below), the mechanically pressed method is the best, most health-promoting extraction system we currently have available to us. Unless an oil is labeled as "100% mechanically pressed" or "100% expeller pressed," assume it is solvent-extracted. Their increased cost can be attributed to the fact that it takes more raw material to produce an equivalent amount of mechanically pressed oil compared to solvent. Look for it in natural food stores and some gourmet stores.

Solvent extraction was invented in Germany in 1870 as a way to maximize the efficient removal of oil from the raw material, especially since the pulp left over from mechanical pressing has about 5-13% residual oil remaining. During solvent extraction, flaked and cooked kernels are exposed to hexane, a highly flammable, colorless, volatile solvent that dissolves out the oil, leaving only 1-3% oil remaining in the residual meal. Hexane compounds are considered carcinogenic by the Environmental Protection Agency (EPA) and are classified as a hazardous substance. Oil manufacturers repeatedly claim that the hexane is flashed off when the oil/solvent blend is heated to 212° F. and distilled to remove all traces of hexane. Still, microscopic parts of up to 25 parts per million may remain in the meal. Full refining of an oil will generally remove most traces of hexane.

While undoubtedly the most efficient extraction will yield a less expensive oil, there are several nutritional and environmental concerns about the use of hexane.

First, the use of a known carcinogen in the processing of a food is unnerving, no matter if it could ever be guaranteed that all traces have been removed.

Second, the residual meal is sold as animal feed. Since the meal doesn't go through further refining as may be administered to an oil, some hexane residues likely remain. In fact, excessive amounts of solvent in residual meal are known to cause anemia in livestock. Accordingly, there are strict regulations to keep hexane contamination from exceeding toxic levels. Oil meal produced

without the use of hexane would be even better for the animals.

Third, hexane is a hydrocarbon polluter, contributing to ozone and air pollution when it is vented into the atmosphere in the flash-off cycle. Fortunately most manufacturers are now recycling the hexane.

Since a nonchemical extraction alternative is readily available, it makes sense to choose an oil processed without hexane. Assume all oils are solvent-extracted unless labeled as "100% mechanically pressed" or "100% expeller pressed."

Combination mechanical/solvent extraction, subjecting the oil-bearing material to mechanical pressing followed by solvent extraction, is the most efficient method of all. Oils resulting from this combination process are called **"integrated oils."** Assume all oils are at least partially solvent-extracted unless labeled as "100% mechanically pressed" or "100% expeller pressed."

Modified Atmosphere Packing (MAP) is a specialized mechanical extraction system in which the oil is extracted in a non-oxygen, light-free atmosphere at temperatures as low as 70° F. using processing equipment, tanks, lines and valves made only from non-reactive metals such as stainless steel. This type of processing is necessary to keep nutrients and freshness intact for oils containing the highly reactive superunsaturated fatty acids, such as fresh flax seed oil. The elimination of light during production prevents the color bodies in the oil from starting the free radical cycle.

Cold temperatures are used to preserve the natural vitamin E and to minimize free radical initiation from whatever source.

Canola, borage, safflower, sunflower, sesame, and hazelnut oils referred to as "fresh" may also be processed in this method. The oils are packed in opaque inert black plastic bottles or encapsulated to protect them from the destructive influences of light in shipping, on display, and after purchase. Continuous refrigeration from extraction to the store ensures oil freshness. The best "fresh" oils processed under the modified atmosphere packing system are from organically grown oil-bearing materials. Look for these oils in the refrigerated sections of natural food stores or health food stores.

UNREFINED VS. REFINED OILS

Choosing the Right Oil for the Right Job

Once extracted, oils will either be lightly filtered to remove any obvious extraneous particles before bottling or subjected to further processing or refinement. Both unrefined and refined oils are appropriate but for different reasons and, consequently, for different applications.

Unrefined oils are highly valued for their nutrient content. (Note: Since minute amounts of solvent can still be found in solvent-extracted oils before the refining process, it is critical that you only buy 100% mechanically pressed unrefined oil.) The heat generated during expeller pressing stays below 200° F., therefore unrefined oil retains most of the nutrients originally found in the natural oil, including vitamin E, carotenes (vitamin A precursors), chlorophyll, phytosterols, and phospholipids, most notably lecithin. These and other biochemical compounds in the oil also provide unrefined oil's characteristic full-bodied flavor, enticing aroma, and deep, rich color.

On the other hand, it's these same compounds, as well as the oil's free fatty acids which remain intact, that limit the uses of the oil and shorten its stability and shelf life.

As soon as a bottle of oil is opened, the fatty acids in the oil combine with oxygen, creating the conditions for gradual chemical breakdown of the oil, a process hastened even more by exposure of the oil to both light and heat.

Photons, the electromagnetic rays that carry the energy of light, can pass through clear glass or plastic to destroy some of the oil's molecules, resulting in the formation of free radicals. These highly reactive oxygen molecules begin a chain reaction in which they seek to bond with other molecules, destroying them in the process and creating more free radicals. After enough time goes by, the oil will begin to smell and taste rancid, not to mention subjecting more of your body's cells, and, on a larger scale, your organs and tissues to the gradual deteriorative effects of the free radicals.

This process of light deterioration is even quicker in unrefined oils, owing to the increased number of free fatty acids found in unrefined oils. The color bodies act as catalysts between light rays and the oil's fatty acid molecules to start the process of free radical chain reactions. As the oil begins to deteriorate, the nutritive components found in the oil decline, as well.

Using unrefined oils at temperatures above 320° F. also accelerates oxidation of the oil to transform fatty acids and destroy nutrients. Therefore, unrefined oils should only be used under low and moderate heat applications such as steaming, light sautéing, sauce or salad dressing-making, or for drizzling over cooked vegetables or grains. Because the internal temperatures of cookies, cakes, and breads remains below 320° F. when baked in an oven heated to 350° F., unrefined oils can be used at low to medium baking temperatures. (Refined oils should always be used, however, to oil baking pans since their temperature will exceed the maximum temperature allowed for refined oils.)

For maximum flavor and nutrition, you should only buy unrefined oils whose bottles have been flushed with nitrogen or, preferably, argon gas. Both harmless, they are used to flush the bottle before the oil is added to get rid of any oxygen already present in the bottle and then to top off the filled bottles of oil before they are tightly sealed. Thus, the oxidation process is put on hold while the bottle sits on the shelf waiting to be opened. Argon is the better of the two because it is inert and completely arrests oxidation. Nitrogen reacts slightly with the oil and, therefore, serves only to slow down oxidation rather than completely preventing it. (Nitrogen is still the best gas to use when packing grains. Unlike its slight reaction with oils, nitrogen remains inert with grains.)

Always store unrefined oils in the refrigerator to retard oxidation and extend the life of the oils. Ideally, unrefined oils should be packaged in opaque, nonreactive, inert containers to protect them from light decay. However, once they are in the refrigerator, light decay isn't a problem until you bring them out for use. For optimum refrigerator shelf life, be sure to return unrefined oils to refrigeration as quickly as possible.

Once open, refrigerated shelf life varies according to the type of oil. Unrefined oils high in monounsaturated fats can be kept up to 8 months. Unrefined oils high in the more reactive polyunsaturated fats may last only half as long, up to 4 months. Superunsaturated oils like flax seed oil last only 6-8 weeks refrigerated; however, these oils can be successfully stored in the freezer to delay oxidation significantly longer. (They won't freeze; rather they become like a thick paste that is spreadable.) To remind you of the day you broke the oil bottle's inner seal, it's a good idea to write the date directly on the bottle with a pen or indelible marker.

The comparison between unrefined and refined oils is very similar to that between whole wheat flour and white flour. Both white flour and refined oil provide calories and, beyond that, minimal nutrition. While it's true that refined oil contains essential fatty acids, it remains devoid of the other supporting nutrients that facilitate the transformation of both linoleic acid and alpha-linolenic acid into prostaglandins. The more processing an oil undergoes, the more nutritionally compromised it becomes.

Despite all the precautions and special conditions required for the safe and savory use of unrefined oils, nutritionally speaking, they remain the oils of choice for cooking below 320°F and when baking at temperatures no higher than 350°F. Except for extra virgin or virgin olive oils, which are available at most good-quality grocery stores, you'll most likely find other unrefined oils in a natural food store or gourmet shop.

Refined oils are the way to go when you are cooking at higher heats. An oil is refined to remove all the bioactive components found in unrefined oil that make it more prone to oxidation, including the color, odor, and flavor bodies, free fatty acids, as well as components that make the oil cloudy and less manageable. While extensive processing significantly reduces their nutritive content (the oil's essential fatty acids remain) and makes them bland in flavor, aroma, and color, they are much more chemically stable, making them suitable for high-heat cooking.

The full refining process involves many steps. First, oils high in phosphatides are **"degummed,"** using water and citric acid or phosphoric acid to remove the lecithin and phosphatides that can make the oil thick and cause the oil to darken at high temperatures. The degumming process occurs under temperatures ranging from 90-120° F. The lecithin removed from soy oil is sold as a food supplement and as an emulsifier in food processing.

The **"refining"** stage (not to be confused

with the general term for the entire process) combines an alkali such as caustic soda with the oil to reduce free fatty acids and peroxides that can accelerate the oxidation of the oil. The interaction of the alkali and the free fatty acids creates soap, which is separated from the oil by means of a high-speed centrifuge. The soap stock is sold to the personal care industry for further processing. Refining processing temperatures do not exceed 150° F.

During **"bleaching,"** the oil is mixed with diatomaceous earth or clay to remove colors and some odors. Temperature during bleaching is usually 230° F.

Further clarification is accomplished through **"deodorizing."** In this process, steam is blown through the oil under a high vacuum at temperatures up to 470° F. to remove flavors and remaining odors.

Oils that contain high amounts of waxes or stearines are **"winterized"** to reduce cloudiness. When subjected to temperatures around 45° F., the waxes or stearines solidify and are separated from the liquid oil through a filtering process.

Some brands of oil may also add preservatives such as BHA, BHT, or TBHQ to enable consumers to store the oil unrefrigerated and to slow down oil degradation in general. Methyl silicone is sometimes added as a defoamer to prevent the oil from bubbling over during deep frying. Common sense dictates that these additives are unnecessary. It is rare that anyone who would be cooking with an oil would not have access to a refrigerator. Furthermore, oils should not be subjected to such high temperatures that they would be prone to foam up in the first place. Oils that contain preservatives and defoamers should be avoided.

Like unrefined oils, for maximum flavor and nutrition, only buy refined oils that have been flushed with either nitrogen or argon gas before they are tightly sealed to make sure that oxidation hasn't already started before you ever open the bottle.

All refined oils may be used for medium-high to high temperature applications (325-400° F.) such as stir-frying, quick sautéing, and high temperature baking. A few refined oils, namely avocado oil and refined high-oleic safflower and sunflower oils, can withstand higher temperatures, up to 450° F.

To maximize shelf life, store refined oils in the refrigerator. Refined oils high in monounsaturated fats have a refrigerator shelf life of up to 1 year. Refined oils high in polyunsaturated fats last only half as long, up to 6 months.

Smoking Point: What Does It Mean?

In their hurry to cook foods quickly, many people consistently cook at too high a temperature. Especially with unrefined oils, but even with refined, high heat can cause volatile degradation products that not only can ruin the flavor of the dish but also harm your health, causing gastric distress, irritated lungs and mucous membranes, and the release of toxic substances into the food and atmosphere. The reuse of frying oils compounds the problem. Therefore, an attempt to save money by filtering the oil and storing it to use again can, in terms of your health, be more costly in the long run.

An oil's smoking point is the temperature to which an oil can be heated before it smokes and discolors, a visual indication of the oil's decomposition. The smoking point varies from oil to oil. Always keep the temperature low enough so that the oil never begins to smoke.

COOKING LOW FAT

We use fat in our cooking for more reasons than as a way to get our required essential fatty acids. We use it to create smooth, rich textures that not only serve to bind ingredients but also to carry and enhance flavors in our food. There's an old restaurant adage that says, "Cook anything with enough fat and salt and it's sure to be a hit."

Fortunately, as more people finally get the message that for optimum health and performance we need to keep our diets low in fat, high-fat cooking is gradually going by the wayside. But it requires a whole different set of cooking habits than we've been accustomed to, as well as a whole new outlook on low-fat cooking. Rather than a diet of deprivation, it's one that enhances the wonderful flavors inherently found in food. The transition from high fat to low fat is easier than you may imagine.

Baking: Fat is used in cakes, muffins, and cookies to make them light and tender. To reduce fat, you need to use ingredients that can stabilize the air bubbles that the leavening provides. In most cake and muffin recipes, up to half of the oil or butter in the recipe can often be substituted with applesauce, mashed ripe bananas, tofu, or prune purée without significantly altering the original taste and flavor. Just remember to keep the same proportion of liquid to dry ingredients.

To make 1 cup prune purée, combine 11/3 cups (8 oz.) of pitted prunes in a food processor with 6 tablespoons of water. Pulse on and off, puréeing until the prunes are finely chopped.

Cookies made with less fat will turn out less crisp but remain satisfying. Commercially prepared low-fat cookies are soft due to the extra amount of water added to partially substitute for the oil found in higher-fat cookies. Also, many commercially prepared low-fat or fat-free baked goods are very high in sugar, including fruit juice sweeteners, to compensate for the otherwise reduced flavor and to help coat the gluten strands in the flour to trap the air bubbles for a lighter texture. There is a point, however, when in trying to remedy one problem, you create another. If you feel it is absolutely necessary, perhaps add a bit, but not a lot more sweetener. Try adding more natural flavorings instead.

Sautéing: Vegetables can be sautéed with only 1 teaspoon of oil and still taste great. If the vegetables are going to be added to a recipe that already contains oil, instead of sautéing them in oil, steam or liquid-sauté them. Substitute 3 tablespoons of vegetable broth, water, tomato juice, dry sherry, or wine for each tablespoon of butter or oil omitted. Bring the liquid to a boil first and then add the vegetables or other ingredients you wish to "sauté."

Sauce-making: Use low-fat milk, buttermilk, or yogurt in cream sauces, adding 1 teaspoon of cornstarch or arrowroot per cup of dairy product to prevent curdling.

Or change your conception of a cream sauce or soup. Cook potatoes or other starchy vegetables in water or broth either with or separate from the other components of the sauce or soup. Purée the cooked vegetables in a blender or food processor and return to your original recipe.

Salsa or other fresh vegetable sauces can also serve as an accompaniment to entrées instead of cream, or butter-based sauces.

Cooking Oil Sprays

Just how safe and effective are cooking oil sprays? Typical ingredients include some kind of oil (count on it being solvent-extracted), lecithin, alcohol, a propellant, and sometimes a butter flavor. Lecithin is a slippery phosphatide that helps replace some of the oil. The spray's propellant contains carbon and hydrogen, substitutes for the formerly popular chlorofluorocarbons that were banned because they contributed to the destruction of the atmosphere's ozone layer.

Your best bet is to skip the propellant altogether. Even though there is minimal propellant in each can of cooking spray, it's still creating more air-polluting hydrocarbons to add to the amount we already create with car exhaust. Instead, look for an oil in a spray pump dispenser that dispenses without propellants. Or invest in an cooking oil brush to spread a thin coating on pots and pans.

FAT SUBSTITUTES

Where there is a perceived need, there is always someone or some company to fulfill it. And, it's no different when it comes to providing fat substitutes. Some fat substitutes, like guar gum, xanthum gum, and starch-based fat replacers like malto-dextrin and tapioca have been used for years, previously as a cheaper alternative to real fats but now marketed as a new fat-reducing revelation, to simulate the body and creamy-smooth texture of fat.

The newest kid on the block in starch-based fat substitutes is hydrolyzed oat flour, developed by the U.S. Department of Agriculture in 1993 and now licensed to a couple of large food manufacturers. It is a carbohydrate fiber made with natural enzymes that can be used as a fat substitute in such foods as cheeses, ground beef, cookies, and muffins. In comparison to the nine calories normally supplied per gram of fat, hydrolyzed oat flour contains only one calorie per gram. Since it naturally contains the fibers amylodextrin and beta-glucan, it has the added benefit of helping reduce cholesterol.

Other fake fats get a bit more complex and contrived. Simplesse™ is made by cooking and blending egg whites and whey protein into microparticulated proteins, tiny round particles similar to the shape and size of fat globules but so small that the tongue perceives them as fluid rather than individual particles. Applicable to dips, puddings, yogurt, soups, cheesecake, sour cream, cakes, pies, and salad dressings, once in the mouth these proteins function like little ball bearings that simulate the creaminess of fat but without the calories.

Another kind of fat substitute approved for use in candies and confectionary coatings for nuts, fruits, and cookies is caprenin. It is a totally restructured fat in which three different fatty acids (capric, caprylic, and behenic acids) that contribute less than 9 calories per gram are attached to the glycerol backbone. The result is a cocoa butter-like fat that contributes 5 calories per gram instead of the usual 9.

Yet another fat substitute, Olestra™, is a sucrose polyester in which sugar is used to replace the usual fat's glycerol backbone to which as many as 8 fatty acids are joined. Because of the extra fatty acids, it cannot be digested by lipase, the fat enzyme that normally breaks down fat. Otherwise, it looks, tastes, and behaves like standard fat. As this is such a new concept that raises several questions, the FDA has delayed its approval. Previous tests with lab animals suggested concerns about increased rates of cancer, liver damage, and other serious problems.

Have we gone too far? Can't we learn some new eating habits rather than depend on altered fat molecules to reduce our fat intake? The fact is, no studies have proven that using fat substitutes helps cut down on fat; instead people generally make up for the fat deficit by eating more of something else.

When it comes right down to it, the most effective way to cut down on high-fat, high-calorie foods is to rediscover the flavors and textures of whole grains and breads, legumes, fruits, veggies, low-fat dairy products, lean fish, and poultry eaten without the skin. If it's weight loss you're also after, eating good, health-promoting, nutritious food is the best way to lose body fat, too.

You can also invest in gadgets that help remove excess fat from food such as gravy pitchers that cause the fat to rise to the top for you to discard and ladles that skim fat from the top of the liquid. Collapsible steamers allow you to steam vegetables and cook fish and poultry fat-free. A yogurt funnel creates a low-fat-cream cheese-like soft cheese from yogurt that can be used as a spread on bagels or as an ingredient in spreads, dips, and salad dressings.

Exploring Your Options

ALMOND OIL

Facts and Features
Almond oil is derived from bitter almonds and almond kernels. Pale, light in color, its flavor is mildly sweet and nutty. Almond oil is available mechanically extracted and only refined. As evidenced by its fatty acid profile of 9% saturated, 26% polyunsaturated, and 65% monounsaturated, almond oil is considered a monounsaturated fat.

Baking/Cooking Guidelines
Refined almond oil has a smoking point of 495° F., indicating that it can withstand high-heat cooking. Almond oil is best for general cooking, sautéing, and for making sauces and salad dressings.

AVOCADO OIL

Facts and Features
Avocado oil is pale in color and has a nutty, sharp flavor. With its fatty acid profile of 20% saturated, 10% polyunsaturated, and 70% monounsaturated, avocado oil is undoubtedly considered a monounsaturated fat. Avocado oil is available mechanically extracted and only refined.

Baking/Cooking Guidelines
Avocado oil has a smoking point of 520°, making it the oil that can withstand the most heat. Use it in general cooking, sautéing, sauces, and, especially, for making salad dressings.

CANOLA OIL

Facts and Features
Canola oil is derived from a specially bred variety of rapeseed, a plant in the mustard family. Although rapeseed oil has been a traditional cooking oil in China, Japan, and India for many years, a study conducted in 1970 raised concerns whether erucic acid, a predominant type of fatty acid found in conventional rapeseed plants, could lead to heart damage as was demonstrated in rats who were fed large amounts of the high erucic-acid variety of rapeseed.

In their quest for an oil with an ideal fatty acid profile, plant geneticists from Canada developed a new variety of rapeseed that is 6% saturated, 60% monounsaturated, 24% polyunsaturated, and 10% superunsaturated omega-3 fatty acids. They also bred out the erucic acid content from its original 45% down to less than 0.5%, an amount so low that its effects, if any, would be virtually nil. (Subsequent studies have failed to show any detrimental effect on humans.) The name for the oil expressed from the new low-erucic acid rapeseed, canola oil, is derived from the words "Canadian oil" in honor of the Canadian scientists who developed it.

Canola oil has a mild flavor and aroma. It is available mechanically pressed and, as a cooking oil, is always sold refined. As shown above, its fatty acid profile makes canola oil a monounsaturated fat with the extra bonus of omega-3 fatty acids. A "fresh" unrefined canola oil extracted under the modified atmosphere expeller extraction method is also available and used as a therapeutic dietary supplement oil.

Baking/Cooking Guidelines

Canola oil has a smoking point of 400° F., making it stable at medium-high heat cooking temperatures. If you have only one oil in your refrigerator, this is the one to have. Canola oil is an excellent all-purpose oil suitable for all types of cooking, baking, frying, sautéing, and salad-making, bland enough to allow the flavors of the entrées and baked goods to come through.

COCONUT OIL

Facts and Features

Coconut oil is derived from dried coconut meat. It is only available solvent-extracted and refined. The fatty-acid profile of coconut oil shows why it is a favorite of many food manufacturers: 92% saturated, 6.5% monounsaturated, 1.5% polyunsaturated. Because it is so saturated, it is used in coatings for ice cream bars, nondairy creamers, as lubricants in caramels, nougats, and in other applications needing an increased shelf life. Coconut oil is also used for frying potato chips, nuts, and other snacks, particularly movie theater popcorn, due to its flavor appeal and the crisp texture it imparts.

However, because it is so saturated, foods made with it should be avoided.

Baking/Cooking Guidelines

Coconut oil is not recommended for baking or cooking. It is best used in body-care applications such as skin creams.

CORN OIL

Facts and Features

An old American standby, corn oil has a buttered popcorn flavor that is either quite pronounced or subtle, depending if the oil is unrefined or refined. Corn oil extracted only from the germ of the corn is light yellow while that extracted from the entire kernel is dark orange.

Corn oil's fatty-acid profile is 13% saturated, 27% monounsaturated, and 60% polyunsaturated, making it primarily a polyunsaturated fat. It is available mechanically pressed and, although it is available both unrefined and refined, research shows you're likely better off using only unrefined corn oil. Studies of diets high in refined polyunsaturated fats suggested rapid tumor formation and suppression of the immune system. Perhaps some of the naturally occurring constituents allowed to remain in refined oil provide a synergistic effect where the whole is more healthy than the sum of its parts. For peace of mind and better health, stick to unrefined corn oil.

Baking/Cooking Guidelines

Corn oil has a smoking point of 320° F. if unrefined and 450° if refined. Because of its tendency to foam and smoke at high heat, corn oil should not be used for deep-frying.

The favorite use of corn oil is with baking and sautéing. When using unrefined corn oil, be sure to use a light saute' and an oven temperature no higher than 350° F.

COTTONSEED OIL

Facts and Features

Cottonseed oil is derived from the seeds of the cotton plant that remain after the downy cotton has been removed for use in manufacturing fabric. It was first used as a food oil during the 1860s. The original Crisco™ shortening was introduced in 1911, made entirely from hydrogenated cottonseed oil. In fact, cottonseed oil was the most important food oil in the United States until the 1940s when production of soybean and other oils began to increase. Even though cottonseed oil is not sold at retail on its own merits, it continues to be used as an ingredient or processing aid in commercial food production for its flavor, high smoke point, and its ability to resist oxidation. It is used as a common frying medium for potato chips and other snack foods. Combined with other hydrogenated vegetable oils, cottonseed oil helps improve the flavor, odor, consistency and shelf life of shortenings. It is also used as a base in many salad dressings and as an ingredient in cookies.

Cottonseed oil's fatty acid profile lists 26% saturated, 18% monounsaturated, 52% polyunsaturated with 4% other minor fatty acids. While high in polyunsaturated fats, it also contains a significant amount of saturated fats, mostly palmitic acid which is the type of saturated fat most known to elevate cholesterol.

Traditionally, natural food advocates have not held cottonseed oil in high regard for several reasons. First, compared to other oil-bearing plants, cotton is more heavily sprayed with pesticides and herbicides. Legitimate rebuttals from the cottonseed industry counter that since cotton is considered both a food crop and a fiber, pesticides used on cotton are restricted as on any other oilseed or food crop. And, technically, most pesticide residues that may linger are supposedly removed during the refining process. However, given that other oils are available that have much fewer pesticides used during the growth of the oilseed, individuals who avoid products with cottonseed oil are essentially emphasizing the growing belief that the use of pesticides adversely affects the environment and that they need to be curtailed significantly in our food crops. If you have the choice, it makes sense to buy organically grown oils or those derived from sources known to be grown with fewer pesticides.

Secondly, very little cottonseed oil is left unhydrogenated, presenting the fact that products that use cottonseed oil as an ingredient or processing aid also contain cholesterol-raising trans-fatty acids beyond their own naturally occurring levels of saturated fats. For this fact alone, many people avoid cottonseed oil in favor of oils left in their natural, unhydrogenated state. (Obviously, using this criterion, products made with another commonly used ingredient, partially hydrogenated soybean oil, should also be avoided.)

Baking/Cooking Guidelines

Cottonseed oil is used only as an ingredient or processing aid in foods and is not available on its own for retail sale.

FLAXSEED OIL

Facts and Features

Flaxseed oil has a golden color and nutty, buttery flavor. It is prized as containing 57% alpha-linolenic acid, the highest plant-based source of omega-3 fatty acids. Alpha-linolenic acid is one of the essential fatty acids that are needed for proper growth, development and maintenance of the body. It also serves as a precursor to prostaglandins, hormone-like compounds that help regulate vital body functions. Through its conversion into eicosapentaenoic acid (EPA), the synthesis of a prostaglandin called thromboxane can be blocked, thus allowing the blood to run "thin" as a way that may help reduce the incidence of heart attack. Flaxseed oil's fatty acid profile also contains 9% saturated, 16% monounsaturated, and 18% polyunsaturated fats.

To ensure that it retains its nutrients, including vitamin E and naturally occurring compounds that assist in the digestion of fats, and remains as stable as possible, flaxseed oil must be extracted under the light-free, oxygen-free, reactive metal-free, low-heat, modified atmosphere packing, mechanical pressing method.

Baking/Cooking Guidelines

Flaxseed should only be used in no-heat recipes or added to foods that register less than 212° F. It makes a delicious and healthy replacement for butter or margarine on baked potatoes, steamed vegetables, or drizzled on bread or cooked grains. Use flaxseed oil to make salad dressings, sandwich spreads and dips. For extra flavor and nutrition, add a teaspoon or so to shakes and smoothies.

GRAPESEED OIL

Facts and Features

Grapeseed oil is made from the seeds of grapes after wine is pressed. Because grapeseed oil has a very high smoke point, 485°F., it works well in French cooking that characteristically involves searing and pan-frying over very high heat. Organoleptically speaking, grapeseed oil has a very nutty flavor and a faint bouquet.

Nutritionally, grapeseed oil is primarily polyunsaturated (76%), rounded out with 9% saturated fat and 15% monounsaturated fat. Some publications are elevating grapeseed oil as the next miracle food to decrease the potential for heart disease. They claim it

is one of the only foods known not only to decrease low density lipoproteins, the "bad" cholesterol, but also to raise high density lipoproteins, the "good" cholesterol. However, many question whether grapeseed oil is that much better than any other oil, citing that it's difficult to depend on just a few studies as evidence of proof and that much of the information appears generated by companies interested in marketing the product.

While traditional chemical-free processing of grapeseed oil may be found on a local basis in some wine-producing areas of France and Italy, unfortunately, most grapeseed oil currently available on a commercial scale is solvent-extracted. For high heat cooking, an excellent alternative is expeller-pressed avaocado oil which has a smoke point of 520°F.

Baking/Cooking Guidelines

Refined grapeseed oil has a smoking point of 485° F. Unrefined grapeseed oil, if ever available, would have a smoking point of 320° F. Grapeseed oil can be used in general cooking, baking, and sautéing, and for salad dressings and marinades.

OLIVE OIL

Facts and Features

Olive oil varies in flavor, color, and aroma depending on the variety of olive used, the soil and climate in which it was grown, when it was picked, and how it was pressed.

Generally, the greener the olive oil, the more fruity and pungent the flavor. Yellowish olive oil, so colored because it is pressed from more ripe olives, has a sweeter, more subtle, nutty flavor. It takes 1300-2000 olives to make one quart of olive oil.

According to internationally recognized guidelines, virgin olive oil must be obtained from olives exclusively by mechanical or other physical means (stone-pressing, or more commonly, hydraulic-pressing) under conditions, particularly in regards to heat, that do not lead to deterioration of the oil. It may not be subjected to any treatment other than washing, decantation, centrifugation, and filtration. Solvents may not be used to extract the oil nor may the virgin olive oil be blended with any other kinds of oils.

Grades within virgin olive oils are classified according to its acidity, in other words, the percentage of free fatty acids present in the oil. **"Extra virgin olive oil"** is the ultimate in flavor and aroma, exhibiting no more than 1% acidity. **"Virgin olive oil"** has good flavor but with an acidity level of more than 1% but less than 2%. Both are considered unrefined oils.

Quality can vary within the ranks of extra virgin and fine virgin olive oils. Some of it is purely subjective; depending on personal preferences regarding specific characteristics exhibited in the oils. It's best to try several and discover which you prefer.

The question of decanted or undecanted oil is a case in point. Decanted olive oil has been stored in urns for 6 months to allow olive skin and pulp particles to settle. The oil that rises to the top is then bottled. While some people like the lighter flavor and texture of a decanted oil, others prefer the more cloudy, stronger flavor of undecanted olive oil.

Estate-bottled olive oil is obtained from olives grown solely at the particular estate listed on the bottle. Generally speaking, estate-bottled olive oil is considered excellent quality. It's also the most expensive way to go with olive oil, although price or name is not always indicative of a good-quality oil.

Sometimes the vintage year is printed on the label. Unlike fine wines that are stored to mature, olive oil should be opened within two years of production. Once opened, it should be used within a year.

Virgin olive oil that has an off-taste or an acidity level higher than 3% must be refined and then blended with a small percentage of better quality virgin olive oil in order to be palatable. Previously labeled as "pure olive oil", since January 1991, the International Olive Oil Council now classifies such oil as **"olive oil."** Since the refining process removes not only excess oleic acids but also the distinctive color, aroma, and flavor components from the oil, the organoleptic qualities of the final product will vary from brand to brand according to the amount of virgin olive oil blended in by the manufacturer. The percentage of virgin olive oil added is more a matter of taste rather than price since there is little difference between the price a manufacturer pays for virgin olive oil and for refined olive oil.

Infused and flavored olive oils will generally be based on "olive oil" since the natural fruity flavors of extra virgin or virgin oils tend to mask any added flavors. Quality varies widely. Look for brands that depend on fresh ingredients such as garlic, real lemon, herbs, peppers, or mushrooms rather than artificial flavors. Or make your own.

"Olive pomace oil" is derived from the portion of the olive that remains after pressing or centrifuging. Unlike virgin oils or olive oil, solvents may be used to extract even more oil from the pomace. Olive pomace oil is then refined and, for palatability, blended with small amounts of virgin olive oil. Since the pomace starting material is inexpensive compared to whole olives as used in virgin oils, the final product will also be much cheaper. However, when considering overall health and gastronomical enjoyment, olive pomace oil is no bargain.

Unfortunately, conscious mislabeling of olive oil does occur within the olive oil industry. Since the classification of extra virgin olive oil is largely based on its acidity level, some unscrupulous manufacturers are blending refined and virgin oils to achieve an acidity level of less than 1% and then passing it off as extra virgin rather than "olive oil." Others are cheating on labeling of the oil's origin. Although olive oil from Spain can be of excellent quality, some of it is sent to other countries, including Italy, for packaging and then labeled as a product of that country. Depend on knowledgeable retailers to advise you on brands recognized for their high quality and integrity.

Like all unrefined oils, extra virgin and virgin olive oils should be kept out of light and kept cool. For optimum shelf-life, especially in hot climates, keep refrigerated. Although it will cloud under refrigeration, it will liquify quickly at room temperature.

Besides being a superior culinary oil, on the average, about 77% of olive oil's fatty acids are heart-healthy monounsaturated fats that reduce LDL cholesterol but maintain levels of HDL cholesterol. Rounding out olive oil's fatty acid profile are 14% saturated and 9% polyunsaturated fats. Mediterranean cultures who use large amounts of olive oil in their cooking and few foods high in saturated fats tend to exhibit lower rates of heart disease.

Baking/Cooking Guidelines

Olive oil has a smoking point of 350° F. Use it in low- to medium-heat cooking applications such as light sautéing, savory breads, and sauces. Olive oil is especially good in marinades, salad dressings, drizzled on bread, pasta, pizza, and vegetables.

PALM/ PALM KERNEL OIL

Facts and Features

Palm oil and palm kernel oil come from the fruit of the oil palm tree that grows in Southeast Asia, Africa, and Central and South America. Palm oil is isolated from the pulp. Palm kernel oil is derived from the kernel.

The oils have different fatty acid profiles. Palm oil is 51% saturated, 39% monounsaturated, and 10% polyunsaturated. Palm kernel oil is 84% saturated, 14% monounsaturated and 2% polyunsaturated.

Because both are so high in saturated fats, they are used in similar food manufacturing applications as coconut oil, especially candies and coatings, including carob-based confections. Despite the fact that, as vegetable-based fats, palm oils contain no cholesterol, they are rich in palmitic acid and lauric acid, particular types of saturated fats that significantly raise cholesterol levels in the blood. Therefore, products made with palm or palm kernel oil should be avoided.

Fractionated palm kernel oil is often found in carob candies to imitate the consistency and texture of chocolate. When palm kernel oil is fractionated the liquid oil is separated from the solid fat to produce a hard butter suitable for transforming carob into a solid candy or coating.

First, the oil is melted and then slowly cooled. As the oil cools, a solid layer of fat rises to the surface, much like the home process of removing fat from gravy. The big difference is that instead of discarding the fat as you would at home, the manufacturers collect the various layers that rise throughout the process and combine certain ones to yield a manipulated fat with a higher melting point.

Although fractionated palm kernel oil is reportedly used instead of a hydrogenated fat, it's certainly nothing to brag about. The bottom line is that it remains a highly saturated fat that should be avoided or at least rarely eaten and then only in very small amounts. If truth be told, the fat in real chocolate candies is less saturated and likely easier to digest.

Palm oil and palm kernel oil are always sold to manufacturers refined.

Baking/Cooking Guidelines

Palm oil is sold in some ethnic markets for traditional recipes prepared in the countries in which the oil palm tree grows.

Considering its saturated fat, you're better off using other more heart-healthy oils in your cooking.

PEANUT OIL

Facts and Features

Peanut oil has long been used for stir-frying and, considering its fatty acid content, it's little wonder: 19% saturated, 51% monounsaturated, and 30% polyunsaturated. The saturated fat, fairly high for a nontropical oil, increases the stability of peanut oil. Its monounsaturated fat content adds to the stability and gives peanut oil its distinction as a monounsaturated oil.

Peanut oil is available mechanically pressed, both unrefined and refined.

Baking/Cooking Guidelines

The smoke point for unrefined peanut oil is 320°. Stir-frying (and the occasional deep-frying) should only be done with refined peanut oil whose smoke point registers at 450° F. Peanut oil is also good for sautéing and baking.

SAFFLOWER OIL

Facts and Features

Safflower oil is expressed from the seeds of a thistle-like plant sometimes referred to as "false" saffron. Unrefined safflower oil has a unique nutty flavor and golden color. Its refined version has very little flavor and is very light in color.

Safflower oil was particularly popular in the 1970s when current nutritional theory at that time praised the virtues of polyunsaturated fats. A look at its fatty acid profile shows that safflower oil contains the highest percentage of polyunsaturated fats of all commercially sold oils: 8% saturated, 13% monounsaturated, and 78% polyunsaturated fats. Now it is believed that polyunsaturated fats should be used in moderation since oils high in polyunsaturated fats, particularly safflower, are very vulnerable to oxidation.

Safflower oil is available mechanically pressed, both unrefined and refined.

Baking/Cooking Guidelines

The smoking point of unrefined safflower oil is 320° F. Refined oil has a smoking point of 450° F. but it should not be used for deep-frying since its already high rate of oxidation escalates with increased temperatures.

Use safflower oil in general cooking, baking, and sautéing. Many people also use safflower oil in salad dressings, but due to its greasy texture you may want to combine it with other oils.

HIGH OLEIC SAFFLOWER OIL

Facts and Features

High oleic safflower oil has been dubbed "the new safflower oil." Thanks to a new strain of seed developed to provide a more heart-healthy and stable spectrum of fatty acids, high oleic safflower oil contains 8% saturated, 76% monounsaturated, and 16% polyunsaturated fats. The name "high oleic" refers to its high percentage of monounsaturated fats (oleic acid).

Accordingly, high oleic safflower oil is much less susceptible to oxidation than regular safflower oil, an important fact you should consider when buying your next bottle of safflower oil.

High oleic safflower oil is available mechanically pressed, both unrefined and refined.

Baking/Cooking Guidelines

The smoking point of high oleic safflower oil is the same ar regular safflower oil for both unrefined and refined, respectively

320° F. and 450 F. The difference is that you can use high oleic safflower up to these temperatures and not worry as much as with regular safflower oil about oxidation. In fact, if you deep-fry foods, high oleic safflower oil can take the heat.

SESAME OIL

Facts and Features

Sesame oil has a rich, nutty flavor and golden color that are more pronounced if purchased unrefined. Its fatty acid profile is 13% saturated, 46% monounsaturated, and 41% polyunsaturated. The monounsaturated aspect of sesame oil makes it more resistant to oxidation than a polyunsaturated oil. Its polyunsaturated content makes it a source of linoleic acid.

Toasted sesame oil is from sesame seeds that are toasted before the oil is extracted. With its richer taste and aroma, it is used most often as a condiment rather than a cooking agent.

Sesame oil and toasted sesame oil are available mechanically pressed, both unrefined and refined.

Baking/Cooking Guidelines

The smoking point for unrefined sesame oil is 320° F. and as high as 410°F. for refined. Sesame oil is terrific in general cooking, baking, sautéing, and for making sauces and salads. If stir-frying, stick with refined sesame oil.

SOY OIL

Facts and Features

Soy oil was considered inedible until the early 1940s, probably due to its development of flavors which can only be described as grassy, painty, or fishy-tasting when used in its unhydrogenated state. Hydrogenation remedied the problem then but now a new

TIPS FOR REDUCING FAT BUT NOT THE FLAVOR

• Heat cooking oil before adding food. The food will cook quicker and have less time to absorb the fat.

• Use a pastry brush to coat pans and skillets with oil. Even half a teaspoon of oil can go a long way.

• Rely on herbs and spices to flavor foods instead of butter, gravies, and dressings.

• Use a small amount of the "real thing" rather than a lot of a low-fat or no-fat substitute. It's often more satisfying. For example, a quick grating of a high-quality Parmesan cheese will do the trick much more than several ounces of a blander-tasting, low-fat alternative.

• Substitute fruit juices or wines for part of the oil in dressings and marinades.

• Splash salads with a high-quality, flavorful vinegar as an alternative to dressings.

• Use more grains to bulk up the meal and balance fat and protein calories.

• Buy produce in season. Fruits and veggies at the peak of the season are so flavorful they need little enhancement.

• Explore the different varieties of mustards to add moisture and flavor to sandwiches rather than fat-laden spreads.

• A teaspoon of a full-bodied unrefined oil on a salad or drizzled over an entrée can be just as or even more satisfying than a high-fat dressing or sauce.

technology for extracting soy oil can remove the enzymes responsible for the off-flavors.

Some of the off-flavor problem can also be attributed to soy oil's high (50%) polyunsaturated fat content. Its fatty acid profile also contains 14% saturated, 28% monounsaturated, and an impressive 8% omega-3 fatty acids. Soy oil is also prone to oxidation. Since hydrogenation helps to stabilize oil, much soy oil is partially hydrogenated for use in shortenings, margarines, and salad dressings.

Soy oil is solvent-extracted and always refined.

Baking/Cooking Guidelines

Soy oil has a smoke point of 450° F. It can be used in general cooking and baking but, since it is solvent-extracted and so many other excellent oils are available, why bother?

SUNFLOWER OIL

Facts and Features

Sunflower oil tastes just like eating a handful of raw sunflower seeds—as long as it is extremely fresh. However, since it is second only to safflower oil in terms of its high amount of polyunsaturated fats, it is an unstable oil whose flavor can taste very rancid quickly after processing. That's why you'll only see sunflower oil refined. Removing the bioactive components from the oil retards oxidation (and makes it taste bland). As evidenced by its fatty acid profile, 12% saturated, 19% monounsaturated, and 69% polyunsaturated, it's about as unstable as regular safflower oil. Sunflower oil is available mechanically pressed, only refined.

Baking/Cooking Guidelines

The smoking point for sunflower oil is 450° F. Similar to regular safflower oil, it can be used for general cooking, baking, and sautéing but not for deep-frying. Sunflower oil is particularly good in salad dressings and when cooking vegetables.

HIGH OLEIC SUNFLOWER OIL

Characteristics

Like high oleic safflower oil, a new seed was specially bred to produce a sunflower oil with a fatty acid content that was more resistant to oxidation. High oleic sunflower oil contains 8% saturated, 81% monounsaturated, and 11% polyunsaturated fats. When considering stability of the oil, high oleic safflower oil is a better choice than regular sunflower oil.

High oleic safflower oil is available mechanically pressed, both unrefined and refined.

Baking/Cooking Guidelines

The smoking point for unrefined high oleic sunflower oil is 320° F. that increases to 450°F. for refined. Use for cooking, baking, sautéing, salad dressings, and for the occasional deep-frying.

WALNUT OIL

Facts and Features

Walnut oil has a subtle, nutty flavor that is a favorite for salad dressings. Its fatty acid profile is 16% saturated, 28% monounsaturated, 51% polyunsaturated, and 5% omega-3 fatty acids, making it a polyunsaturated fat.

Walnut oil is available mechanically pressed, only as refined.

Baking/Cooking Guidelines

Walnut oil's smoking point is 400° F. It is excellent in salad dressings, sauces, sautéing, and baking.

Sweets

WE ALL know that too much sugar isn't good for us, yet there's no denying that sometimes nothing hits the spot more than something really sweet.

Blame it on our genes. Since poisonous plants generally contain bitter alkaloids, scientists speculate this penchant for sweets may have evolved as a protective mechanism to ensure that our primitive ancestors ate enough high-calorie but nontoxic foods to survive through times of scarcity. These days, however, this innate calorie-seeking radar can get us into trouble, especially when surrounded by a plethora of pastries, pies, and puddings.

According to the USDA, the average American ate more than 133 lbs of sugar in 1991. While some of these sugars are naturally occurring in fruits, vegetables, milk (lactose), and to a small degree in legumes and grains, the major percentage of our intake is from sugar added to foods prepared in the home or consumed indirectly as additives in cereals, frozen dinners, canned fruits and vegetables, breads, french fries, ketchup, and almost every processed packaged food that is available today.

Interestingly enough, our actual consumption of white sugar, about 60 lbs. per year, hasn't changed all that much since the turn of the century. It's the huge increase in other types of sweeteners, including high fructose corn sweeteners, fruit juice sweet-eners, and artificial sweeteners, that accounts for the ever-increasing average intake of simple sugars in proportion to complex carbohydrates.

NUTRITION

Because added sugars supply calories and virtually nothing else, the 1990 U.S. Dietary Goals for the United States urges us to return to more balanced proportions in our total carbohydrate consumption by increasing our daily intake of nutrient-dense complex carbohydrates and moderating our use of added sugars to lower than the present 11% of total calories.

New food labels list the grams of sugar found in each food, an amount that includes both the simple sugar content that occurs naturally in foods and added simple sugars found in sweets and processed foods. While the inclusion of both naturally occurring and added sugars under this one listing may seem to imply that there is no difference between a banana and a candy bar, the fact of the matter is that nutritional analysis can't actually differentiate between the sources of the sugars. Common sense will dictate that a naturally occurring sugar in a food which comes with a package deal including other nutrients is a better choice.

As there appears to be no proof of a specific appropriate or inappropriate percentage of sugars in the diet, especially given that both naturally occurring and added sugars are listed together, the Nutrition Facts label lists no Daily Value for sugars.

However, in "The Food Guide Pyramid" booklet prepared by the Human Nutrition Information Service branch of the USDA, it is suggested that added sugars (not naturally occurring) be limited to an average equivalent of 6 teaspoons per day for a 1,600 low-calorie diet, 12 teaspoons for a 2,200 moderate-calorie diet, and 18 teaspoons for a 2,800 higher-calorie diet. The suggested simple sugar guidelines are intended to be averages over a period of time. Depending on the circumstances, some days you may have more, some days less.

Since there are 4 grams of sugar in each teaspoon, to figure out how many teaspoons of sugar there are in a particular product you enjoy, divide the number of sugar grams listed on the label by 4.

The USDA's suggested simple sugar guidelines represent an approximate 6-10% of total calories from simple sugars. However, many experts recommend 5-6% as the preferable goal. While the 6 teaspoons recommended in the 1600-calorie diet match this level, the number of simple sugar teaspoon equivalents for a 2200-calorie diet would need to be reduced to about 8 teaspoons or 32 grams of sugar. At 6% of total calories, a 2800-calorie diet would allow for about 11 teaspoons or 44 grams of sugar.

Which sugar is best?

So what is the best type of simple sugar to use? Most nutritionists would say that it doesn't matter whether you eat treats sweetened with white sugar, brown sugar, honey, maple syrup, or fruit juice sweetener. During digestion, all eventually break down into the same simple component: glucose, commonly known as "blood sugar," the basic fuel for the body essential to the functioning of all cells.

Furthermore, despite the fact that some "natural" sweeteners contain some nutrients, the amount they offer is merely a trace, not enough to be considered truly nutritious.

Factoring in an individual's reactions to sugars

And yet, while neither of these facts can be refuted, equally valid is the way each of us feels after ingesting particular forms of sugar. Some people may feel irritable, excitable, unfocused, or even sleepy after eating a cookie sweetened with white sugar but experience a more balanced response with one sweetened with brown rice syrup. Others may be fine with treats sweetened with maple syrup but feel out of control when ingesting those made with fruit juice concentrate.

These varied responses to sugar among people can be explained by the fact that hormones that help to control blood sugar levels are affected by diet, lifestyle factors, and also by each person's individual biochemistry and state of health.

The release of sugar into the blood depends upon four different processes, each of which can be affected by diet: 1) the rate at which the stomach empties, 2) the rate of digestion of starch and sugar in the intestines, 3) the rate of absorption of the sugars, and 4) the speed at which the liver releases sugars into the bloodstream.

Simple Sugars

The sweet flavor in any food is basically a functional property of the proportions of any of the six different simple sugars commonly found in foods. These include the single sugar monosaccharides: glucose, fructose, and galactose, and the disaccharides: sucrose, maltose, and lactose, sugars that are pairs of monosaccharides linked together.

Absorption rates of sugars and the foods that contain them can be estimated by the particular sweetener's sugar profile which indicates the percentage of each simple sugar of which it is comprised.

Glucose is absorbed into the bloodstream most quickly, requiring insulin to keep blood sugar levels in balance.

In contrast, fructose must first be transported in the bloodstream to the liver to be converted into glucose before it can be used as an energy source for the cells. Not only is the metabolism of fructose into the cells a slower process than occurs with glucose, its other claim to fame is that it has no need of insulin in the process, thus causing little fluctuation in blood glucose levels.

Sucrose or table sugar is hydrolyzed by enzymes in your digestive tract into its equal components of glucose and fructose. Due to its glucose content, it absorbs quite rapidly, requiring the balancing work of insulin. Honey and maple syrup react in the body in much the same manner.

Maltose, composed of two glucose units linked together, is a more complex sugar than glucose or fructose. Since it takes time for your digestive enzymes to hydrolyze the maltose into 2 glucose units before they are absorbed into the blood, foods sweetened with barley malt and brown rice syrup, both of which contain significant amounts of maltose, will be digested with little noticeable effect in blood sugar levels.

When too much simple sugar enters the bloodstream faster than can be assimilated, the body responds by releasing a large burst of insulin from the pancreas. This overreaction results in a glucose level even lower than it was to start with, causing the "let-down," fatigue, and irritability people often experience after eating or drinking something too sweet. Consequently, the next urge is to eat something sweet in order to raise the blood sugar level, thus starting the cycle over again.

Rates of digestion

A diet high in minimally processed, complex carbohydrates helps slow the release of sugar from the meal into the blood. Eating a cookie or a piece of pie soon after a meal featuring a cooked whole grain such as millet, quinoa, or brown rice, accompanied by vegetables and a source of protein (legumes, fish, meat, poultry, or dairy products) will minimize the sweet's potentially erratic effect.

In contrast, having dessert or a snack after eating highly refined, low-fiber carbohydrates with minimal protein such as a breakfast consisting of a sugary cereal, a doughnut, and fruit drink or a lunch of a white bread sandwich, french fries, and a soft drink will exaggerate any consequences an individual may experience with a particular sweetener.

Studies have shown that unbalanced carbohydrate meals can be linked to the attention problems sometimes observed in children after they have consumed something sweet. In one such test, both children with normal behavior and those diagnosed as hyperactive were given three breakfast options: a refined carbohydrate meal of buttered toast, a protein meal of scrambled eggs, or no meal at all. Following the breakfast, each child was given sugar or an artificial sweetener. Results indicated that children who were given sugar following a refined carbohydrate breakfast did poorly on tasks that measured attention and reaction time. Those who had the protein breakfast or nothing at all were less affected by the sugar.

Even if one eats a well-balanced diet, biochemical individuality remains a major factor when responding to a particular type of sweetener. Each person has unique ways of releasing the hormones that control blood sugar levels after eating, resulting in sensitivity to certain sweeteners, even to particular fruits. Therefore, the assumption that everyone should react the same to any sweetener, that "sugar is sugar is sugar," has no validity. While an individual's preference for a particular type of sweetener could be based on a personal philosophical belief, personal physiological factors are very real considerations.

General State of Being

One's state of health is also involved in response to sweeteners in general. A reasonably happy, relatively healthy individual experiencing only the minor stressers that come with everyday living has better odds of reacting to any type of sugar on a more even keel. If your adrenal glands are pushed to the limits from overwork, overindulgences, and emotional upheaval, there's a chance you will eventually lose the normal resilience required to respond to periodic bursts of sweetness.

ARTIFICIAL SWEETENERS

Artificial sweeteners are not the answer to dealing with our desires for sugar. The primary reason people choose to use artificial sweeteners is to lose weight. As high-intensity sweeteners ranging from 30 to 600 times the sweetness of table sugar, significantly less is needed, thus significantly reducing the number of calories that would have been provided by the sugar. Some artificial sweeteners are also calorie-free.

But weight gain from eating too many sweets can largely be attributed to the high amounts of fat that usually accompany foods that contain a lot of sugar. In fact, numerous studies show that individuals who substitute artificial sweeteners actually end up gaining weight rather than losing it as they had hoped. Instead of replacing other sugary, high-fat, high-calorie foods, artificially sweetened foods are often simply added to an already fat-laden diet.

There are more serious concerns, however, than weight gain. Seizures, headaches, mood swings, blurred vision, and other problems have been linked with artificial sweeteners. Long-term use of ever-increasing amounts of several kinds of artificial sweeteners used in processed foods has many scientists concerned.

Despite the problems that are currently being experienced by an increasing number of people who use artificial sweeteners, many have been approved for use by the FDA. More details on artificial sweeteners can be found under the specific artificial sweeteners throughout the rest of the chapter.

Exploring Your Options

ACESULFAME-K

Facts and Features

Acesulfame-K, also known as acesulfame potassium, is 200 times as sweet as sucrose. Since it is not metabolized in the body, it is calorie-free.

Even though laboratory tests showed that it caused cancer in rats, it was approved by the FDA in 1988. The FDA claims the cancer occurred spontaneously due to the specific type of rat used in the study. Some scientists still believe acesulfame-K is inadequately tested for its safety in humans.

Acesulfame-K is now allowed in hard and soft candies, dry beverage mixes, dry dessert mixes, dry dairy products, chewing gums, and as a tabletop sweetener. Food manufacturers like it because it blends very well with other sweeteners and mixtures and, unlike aspartame, is heat-stable and shelf-stable.

Baking/Cooking Guidelines

Because some doubt remains about the safety of acesulfame-K, it is not recommended for home use or in commercially prepared products.

AMASAKE

Facts and Features

Amasake (pronounced ah-mah-ZAH-key) is a creamy rich beverage that, if left undiluted, doubles as a sweetener.

A cultured food hailing from Japan, amasake is traditionally made by inoculating cooked sweet rice with koji, rice that has been inoculated with spores of the mold called Aspergillus oryzae. After an incubation period of 6-10 hours, the koji reacts with the grain's starch, transforming it primarily into maltose and glucose, making it sweet and easy to digest.

Some small producers in the United States continue to manufacture amasake by the original method but, more often than not, the amasake you buy will be made from a less labor-intensive, more predictable process substituting part or all of the koji with enzymes made from sprouted grain, specially grown and isolated to create a specific sugar profile, flavor, and texture.

Both traditional and modern enzyme processing methods of amasake are acceptable, but there is a distinct difference in flavor and texture. Although the quality and wholesomeness of traditional amasake is unsurpassed, enzyme-cultured amasake is much milder in flavor and smoother in texture, characteristics that tend to make it more versatile as a "milk" to pour over breakfast cereals or as a thick, malt-like beverage. The different brands of amasake also vary in consistency, ranging from liquids resembling a thin gruel to those resembling skim milk.

Because of its high glucose and maltose content, athletes find amasake a light, nourishing, easily digested, low-fat, high-carbohydrate drink that is invaluable before or after workouts. Although each brand may vary in its dilution factor, 8 oz. of plain amasake typically contains about 200 calories, 3 grams of protein, .5 gram of fat, and 45 grams of carbohydrates.

Baking/Cooking Guidelines

Thicker versions of amasake make excellent, subtle sweeteners for breads, pancakes, muffins, cookies, and cakes. Even diluted amasakes can be substituted for the liquid required in any sweet recipe. You'll find that amasake has the added benefit of making baked goods more moist.

It also makes a good base for creamy puddings, pies, salad dressings, and other recipes where a liquid similar to sweet condensed milk would be appropriate.

Drink as is for a beverage similar to a malt or a shake, or use it to make your own smoothies. Several brands are available in different flavors including almond, apricot, and mocha. For a soothing drink on a cold day or night, try amasake the traditional Japanese way served warm, topped with a pinch of freshly grated ginger.

ASPARTAME

Facts and Features

Aspartame is an artificial sweetener made by combining two amino acids, aspartic acid and the methyl ester of phenylalanine. Ounce for ounce it has as many calories as sugar, but since aspartame is 180-200 times sweeter, much less needs to be used, giving products that contain it the distinction of being labeled as low-calorie or sugar-free.

Unlike some other artificial sweeteners, aspartame has no aftertaste and does not cause diarrhea. It also does not promote tooth decay.

Initially approved by the FDA for use as a tabletop sweetener in 1981, it is now used in over 4500 products including soft drinks, flavored gelatins, candy, yogurt, and desserts.

Despite its apparent positive aspects, aspartame has the dubious honor of being the food ingredient that has been the subject of more complaints about adverse reactions than the FDA has ever received regarding any other single ingredient. While studies have shown that it breaks down into its original constituents plus methanol in the digestive tract and is metabolized through regular pathways in the body, many people have reported problems of blurred vision, headaches, dizziness, mood swings, difficulty breathing, high blood pressure, and seizures.

A warning is listed on the labels of aspartame-sweetened products as unsuitable for individuals with phenylketonuria (PKU), a metabolic defect that affects about 20,000 babies born in the United States each year. Lacking an enzyme for breaking down phenylalanine, one of the components in aspartame, an accumulation of the amino acid within a young child's body can lead to brain damage and mental retardation.

Many scientists are concerned that large amounts of phenylalanine can have irreversible and toxic effects on the fetal brain even if the infant would not test positive for PKU, possibly contributing to mental retardation or other problems. Accordingly, to be on the safe side, pregnant women, nursing mothers, and infants under six months of age should especially avoid products sweetened with aspartame.

Since the amino acids used to make aspartame react with the neurotransmitters in the brain that control moods, thinking, and behavior, many scientists believe that the use of aspartame could affect these aspects in people of all ages.

Problems with aspartame may even be dose-related, creating problems in individuals who may not be aware of any obvious symptoms after occasionally drinking or eating products that contain aspartame. Considering that the amount of aspartame used in a product is not listed on its label and that an increasing number of products contain it, it may be easier to get to the FDA's safety limit of 50 mg. aspartame per every kilogram (2.2 lbs) of body weight without even knowing it. Children are particularly at risk to exceed the FDA limits.

Baking/Cooking Guidelines

Because some doubt remains about the safety of aspartame, it is not recommended for home use or in commercially prepared products.

BARLEY MALT

Facts and Features

Barley malt is a thick, sticky, dark-colored sweetener with a distinctively malty, molasses-like flavor. It is made from sprouted barley which is dried, mixed with water, and cooked slowly until a syrup is produced.

Barley malt is considered one of the best, whole food-based sweeteners around. The sprouting of barley transforms the grain's starch into a sweetener consisting primarily of complex, slowly digesting sugars, yielding a sugar profile of 72% maltose, 25% glucose, 2% sucrose, and 1% fructose.

Some barley malt consists of a blend of 60% barley malt and 40% corn malt syrup, thus increasing the glucose content of the syrup and, accordingly, its sweetness and absorption into the body.

Baking/Cooking Guidelines

Barley malt is best used in foods that take well to strong, molasses-like flavors, such as baked beans, cookies, muffins, and some cakes. It is particularly good combined with ginger, carob, or chocolate.

Substitute barley malt 1 to 1 for white sugar, reducing the recipe's liquid content by 1/4 cup for every cup of barley malt used.

BROWN RICE SYRUP

Characteristics

Brown rice syrup, like barley malt, is one of the most balanced, unrefined sweeteners available. Based on whole or partially polished brown rice, not starch as is the case when making corn syrup, the process is also devoid of any chemicals. Its high maltose and complex carbohydrate content makes it extremely easy on your blood sugar levels, providing a steady, slowly absorbed sweet.

Traditionally, it is made by adding a small amount of sprouted barley (or rarely sprouted rice) to cooked brown rice. The diastatic enzymes from the sprouted barley break down the starches of the rice into about 45% maltose, 3% glucose, and 50% complex carbohydrates. It is then strained and cooked to yield a mildly sweet, caramel-flavored, golden syrup. Traditionally made rice syrup can be identified by the terms "sprouted barley," "malted barley," "sprouted rice," or "malted rice" printed in the list of ingredients.

Sweet Cloud™, a popular domestically-made brown rice syrup, is manufactured in the traditional manner with the exception of the use of partially polished brown rice instead of whole rice for a more honey-like consistency and lighter flavor.

Many varieties of brown rice syrup now on the market are made by using enzymes isolated from sprouted barley rather than adding the sprouted barley directly to the cooked rice. With the ability to control the amount and particular type of enzyme, different types of rice syrups can be created according to the specifications of the various companies who use rice syrup in the manufacturing of candies and baked goods. In general, enzyme-manufactured rice syrup is sweeter than malted rice syrup with an average sugar profile of 20-40% maltose, 20-35% glucose, and 30-40% complex carbohydrates. Even though malted rice syrup involves more of a whole-food process, the lower price of enzyme-treated rice syrups makes them more affordable. This type of rice syrup can be identified by the term "cereal enzymes" on the ingredient label or simply "brown rice, barley, water" or "brown rice, water."

Baking/Cooking Guidelines

The most significant difference between traditional malted rice syrup and enzyme-treated rice syrup is apparent in baking. Rice syrup is very humectant, much more so than honey. As a result, cakes and muffins made with baking powder and/or baking soda as rising agents and a moderate amount of liquid have a higher tendency to remain fairly flat and goopy on the inside. Fortunately, this is only a problem with the enzyme-treated rice syrups, possibly due to enhanced invert sugar characteristics from the enzymes' digestion of the starch which retards the crystallization of the sugars present in the rice syrup during baking. Therefore, when making cakes and muffins, always use malted rice syrups. Because cookies contain a low moisture content and aren't expected to rise to a large extent, they can be sweetened with either malted rice syrups or enzyme-treated rice syrups.

Likewise, sweet and sour sauces or puddings thickened with arrowroot or kuzu are

COCONUT WALNUT CHIP COOKIES

3/4 cup walnuts
1/4 tsp. baking soda
1/4 tsp. salt
1 1/2-1 3/4 cups whole wheat
    pastry flour
1/4 cup canola oil
1/3 cup rice syrup or
    honey
1 egg, slightly beaten
1/2 tsp. vanilla extract
1/2 tsp. coconut extract

Preheat oven to 350° F. Chop walnuts and add to soda, salt, and 1 1/2 cups flour. In a separate bowl, beat oil and syrup together. Then add egg, vanilla, and coconut extract and beat well. Combine oil mixture to flour mixture. The dough should be very stiff; add extra flour, if necessary. Drop dough by rounded teaspoonfuls onto lightly oiled cookie sheets. Press cookies with a fork to about 1/2 inch thickness. Bake for 12-15 minutes or until the undersides of cookies are golden. Remove and cool cookies on a wire rack.

Nutrition Facts

Serving Size 1 cookie (17 g)
Servings Per Container 24

Amount Per Serving

Calories 80	Calories from Fat 45

	% Daily Value*
Total Fat 5g	8%
Cholesterol 10mg	3%
Sodium 40mg	2%
Total Carbohydrate 8g	3%
Dietary Fiber 1g	3%
Protein 2g	

Iron 2%

Not a significant source of Saturated Fat, Sugars, Vitamin A, Vitamin C and Calcium.
* Percent Daily Values are based on a 2,000 calorie diet.

Makes 24 cookies.
(Pyramid servings: 1/2 Bread/Grain Group, 5 grams Fat, 3 grams Sweets)

---

best sweetened with malted rice syrups. Marinades, salad dressings, toppings, and spreads can be made with either malted rice syrups or enzyme-treated rice syrups.

To substitute for sugar, use equal amounts and reduce the recipe's liquid content by 1/4 cup per 1 cup rice syrup used. Even though rice syrup is much less sweet than honey, maple syrup, or corn syrup, start by using equal proportions of rice syrup when substituting for any of the more intense sweeteners. You may find less sweet treats are just as satisfying.

Rice syrup can be stored without refrigeration, but keeping it cool will reduce the tendency for rice syrup to grow surface molds if condensation takes place in the jar.

CORN SYRUP

Facts and Features

Corn syrup, called glucose syrup in Europe, is produced from refined corn starch using strong acids and enzymes such as Aspergillus oryzae (the one used to make koji, the catalyst used to make traditional amasake) to hydrolyze long-chain starch molecules into shorter chain lengths. In the process, the starch is converted to glucose and maltose in varying proportions, depending on the length of time and conditions under which the starch is broken down. The longer it is processed, the more glucose is produced, ranging on the low end with a glucose content of 20% or less (referred to as malto-dextrins) up to 95% for special applications. Retail versions of corn syrup are absorbed similarly to white sugar.

Corn syrup is used in food processing as an inexpensive sweetener to help retain moisture within bakery products, increase browning of foods, prevent simple sugars from crystallizing in candy, and to impart a thick, chewy texture to foods.

Another type of process using amylolytic enzymes, such as the alpha and beta amylases, produces a corn syrup with a higher proportion of maltose.

Baking/Cooking Guidelines

Equal amounts of corn syrup can be used to replace white sugar, requiring a recipe reduction of 1/4 cup liquid for every 1 cup corn syrup substituted. However, considering that you have access to sweeteners that are much less refined and made without the use of strong acids, such as barley malt and rice syrup, minimal or no use of corn syrup is advised.

CYCLAMATES

Facts and Features

Cyclamates, an artificial sweetener discovered in 1937, is 30 times sweeter than sucrose. It is metabolized in the body with its by-products excreted by the kidneys.

In response to a study that raised concerns whether cyclamate was a possible cancer-causing agent, it was banned by the FDA in 1970. Several other countries allow cyclamates for use in low-calorie foods. Canada restricts its use to tabletop sweeteners and for use in pharmaceuticals. There is speculation that at some point it may be reapproved by the FDA.

Baking/Cooking Guidelines

Cyclamates are unavailable in the United States. Since artificial sweeteners have not been proven to be beneficial in weight loss, their primary reason for being, as well as having no long-term human use to actually confirm its safety, any artificial sweetener should be avoided.

DATE SUGAR

Facts and Features

Date sugar is made from dates (usually ones that are cosmetically imperfect) dehydrated down to 3-5% moisture level and ground into powder. While it contains virtually all the minerals and flavor supplied by dried dates, it also is quite high in sucrose, making its effect on blood sugar levels almost as dramatic as refined and unrefined sugars. Therefore, like all sweeteners, it should be used in moderation.

Baking/Cooking Guidelines

To counter the insolubility of date sugar, before using it in baked goods, date sugar should be combined with enough hot water to make a syrup. It can then be used similarly to honey, maple syrup, or rice syrup.

Like brown sugar, date sugar is very good sprinkled on hot cereals and yogurt. When used as a sweet ingredient in streusel and crumb toppings, it should be added after baking to prevent burning.

Substitute date sugar 2/3 to 1 for white sugar, reducing the liquid by 1/4 cup for every cup of date syrup used. You many need to increase the recipe's dry ingredients by 1/3 cup for every 2/3 cup of date sugar used.

FRUCTOSE

Facts and Features

Although its name may imply fruit as its source, commercially prepared fructose is a highly processed sweetener either produced from corn syrup treated with an enzyme called glucose isomerase, isolated from refined sugar, or sometimes, as noted on some sport energy bars, from a combination of pears, grapes, and/or corn.

Its sweetness and effect on the body depends on the proportions of fructose and glucose that result from the specific formulations produced.

Crystalline fructose is 99.5% pure, making it perform in the body as you would typically expect from fructose. It absorbs slower than glucose or sucrose with no need for insulin in the process, thus creating little fluctuation in blood sugar levels. Individuals with blood sugar disorders, including diabetics and people with reactive hypoglycemia, may find foods sweetened with fructose particularly appealing.

On the other hand, other sweeteners often referred to as fructose but rightly named **high fructose corn syrup,** metabolize just as fast as, if not a little faster than, sucrose. And it's no wonder. The sugar profile of high fructose corn syrup, 55% fructose and 44% glucose, is very similar to sucrose. Unlike crystalline fructose, high fructose corn syrup requires insulin for its metabolism, an important distinction that diabetics and others sensitive to sugar should note. Manufacturers like using high fructose corn syrup in soft drinks, candy, and bakery products due to its cheap cost, carbohydrate functionality, and stability of supply. Nutritionally, it offers only calories, nothing more.

Fructose has a tendency to be converted into fat rather than glycogen, the storage form of glucose in the liver and muscle cells. Therefore, too much fructose in the diet may lead to elevated triglyceride levels in the blood, increasing the risk of arteriosclerosis.

Baking/Cooking Guidelines

Crystalline fructose is about 60% sweeter than sugar, requiring only half to two-thirds as much to achieve the same sweetening power as sucrose. Since application of heat reduces fructose's level of sweetness, you'll likely need to use more, in this case about equal amounts as sucrose. However, best results occur with recipes specifically formulated with fructose in mind rather than trying to substitute it in a favorite family recipe.

FRUIT JUICE CONCENTRATES

Facts and Features

Fruit juice concentrates are increasingly being used as sweeteners in cookies, jellies, syrups, beverages, muffins, cereals, and granolas. Owing to the high regard we have for the nutritional attributes of fruit, at first glance the use of fruit juice concentrates as a sweetener may appear to be an optimum choice. And yet, a closer inspection will reveal that, like other concentrated sweeteners, its nutritional attributes are fairly negligible and its sugar profile looks suspiciously similar to refined sugars from other sources. Depending on the specific fruit or blend of fruits used, fruit juice concentrates contain primarily sucrose with some fructose. Sweeteners based on white grape juice are high in glucose and therefore are absorbed into the bloodsteam very quickly.

Some fruit juice sweeteners are better than others. Manufacturers who are as concerned about quality as they are about making a profit insist on concentrates made from juice evaporated in a vacuum, much like the process for making unrefined sugar from sugar cane juice. To keep the aroma and flavor of the fruit, the fruit's essence is captured from the water vapor and returned to the concentrate. Only a small amount of nutrients are lost in the process. To make the concentrate more neutral in flavor, vacuum-evaporated fruit juice concentrates may also

APPLE CINNAMON COUSCOUS CAKE

2 cups apple juice
1 cup water
pinch of salt
1 1/4 cups couscous
1 tsp. ground cinnamon
1/2 cup chopped roasted
    walnuts
1/2 tsp. vanilla extract

Combine juice, water, and salt in a saucepan and bring to a boil. Add couscous and cinnamon, stir, and adjust heat to low. Simmer for 10 minutes. Remove pan from heat, add walnuts and vanilla, and allow flavors to mingle for another 10 minutes. Rinse an 8" X 8" baking dish with water. Do not dry. Add couscous mixture and pack down. Allow "cake" to cool before serving.

Serves 8.
(Pyramid servings: 1 Bread/Grain Group, 1/2 Fruit Group, 5 grams Fat)

Nutrition Facts

Serving Size 1 piece (129 g)
Servings Per Container 8

Amount Per Serving

Calories 190   Calories from Fat 45

                        % Daily Value*

Total Fat 5g	8%
Sodium 40mg	2%
Total Carbohydrate 31g	10%
Dietary Fiber 2g	8%
Sugars 8g	
Protein 5g	

Vitamin C 2%   •   Calcium 2%

Iron 4%

Not a significant source of Saturated Fat, Cholesterol and Vitamin A.

* Percent Daily Values are based on a 2,000 calorie diet.

---

be altered through a charcoal filtration process. More nutrients are lost during filtration.

But using vacuum-evaporated fruit juice concentrates can be tricky since the flavors aren't neutral or predictable like sugar or corn syrup. That's why some manufacturers resort to "stripped" juice concentrates. These are ultra-clarified to remove all natural color, flavor and nutrients from the juice by passing them through two ion-exchange columns. In one column, the juice's positively charged minerals are replaced with hydrogen atoms. In the other column, the negatively charged acids as well as flavor and color components are replaced with a hydroxyl group, molecules of oxygen and hydrogen bound together. What's left are the simple sugars originally found in the juice.

Knowing which kind of fruit juice sweetener is being used will be easier with the new labeling laws. Fruit juice labels must now indicate the percentage of real fruit juice found in the product. "Stripped" juices cannot be included as part of the juice content. Other foods sweetened with "stripped" juices must be labeled as containing a "modified" juice sweetener to differentiate it from real juice concentrates.

No matter what quality of fruit juice concentrate used, the bottom line is that they are at least 2/3 as sweet as sucrose and can affect blood sugar levels accordingly. Products sweetened with them should be used in moderation.

Baking/Cooking Guidelines

At home you can experiment by substituting thawed, undiluted frozen juice concentrates in place of sugar. Use equal amounts of fruit concentrate to sugar, reducing the recipe's liquid content by 1/3.

Sugar content can also be reduced by substituting unsweetened fruit juices for part or all of the liquids called for in a recipe.

To counter the acidity of fruit concentrates or juices, when baking add 1/4-1/2 tsp. baking soda per cup of juice.

FRUITSOURCE™

Facts and Features

FruitSource™ is the name for a brand of sweetener made from a blend of grape juice concentrate and brown rice syrup. Light amber in color with a pleasant, sweet taste, it is available in both granular and liquid forms.

At 80% of the sweetening power of refined sugar, most of the sweetness comes from the grape juice concentrate. The rice syrup adds mostly complex carbohydrates, a great addition to the products's sugar profile. FruitSource's granular form has 22-27% glucose, 20-25% fructose, 5-11% maltose, 0-6% sucrose, and 35-45% complex carbohydrates, providing an initial surge in energy that is more sustained than sucrose.

There are two versions of liquid FruitSource™. Original FruitSource™ Liquid has an almost identical sugar profile as the granular form: 22-27% glucose, 20-24% fructose, 8-10% maltose, 0-5% sucrose, and 35-45% complex carbohydrates.

FruitSource™ Liquid Plus sweetener is designed for uses where a sweetness similar to sucrose is desired. Therefore, not surprisingly, FruitSource™Liquid Plus is higher in glucose and maltose: 40-45% glucose, 23-27% fructose, 20-24% maltose, 0-6% sucrose, and appreciably lower in complex carbohydrates: 7-10%. The longer-digesting higher-maltose component helps to compensate for the increased glucose percentage and reduction in complex carbohydrates.

Baking/Cooking Guidelines

FruitSource™ works very well in any recipe that calls for refined sugar or liquid sweetener, including cakes, cookies, puddings, toppings, and pies. Commercial food production use includes many candies and confections, baked goods, and sports endurance bars.

Use the liquid form of FruitSource™ as you would honey, rice syrup, or corn syrup in a 1 to1 ratio as required in a recipe. To make your own liquid FruitSource™ from the granular form, mix 2 cups of the granular with 1/2 cup water in a very heavy 3-4 quart saucepan. Let it stand 5 minutes, stirring occasionally. Then cook it over medium heat to 225°F. as measured with a candy thermometer, stirring constantly. Remove from the heat, pour into a sterilized glass jar, cover, and store in the refrigerator until use.

Use the granular form of FruitSource™ in a 1 to 1 ratio to the amount of refined sugar required in a recipe. For best results, first mix FruitSource™ with the wet ingredients in the recipe until well-blended. Let stand for about 5 minutes while preparing the dry ingredients. Then beat the wet ingredients again for 15 seconds before gradually adding the dry ingredients.

Recipes with FruitSource™ bake best at 325-350° F. to avoid overcooking since products made with the sweetener will bake quickly.

The humectant qualities of Fruit-Source™ not only help increase shelf life of baked goods, you will also be able to reduce fat content in the recipe by 25%, with only minor changes in formulation (a bit more flour or less liquid as necessary).

HONEY

Characteristics

Honey is extracted from flower nectar and converted by bees into a sweetener that is about 25-50% sweeter than refined sugar. Its range in colors and flavors depends on the particular plant visited by the bees and the environmental conditions in which it is grown. Dark honeys such as buckwheat or heather are much stronger in flavor than light-colored orange blossom and clover honeys.

Good-quality honey is natural and unrefined, heated only enough to extract it from the comb and strained only to remove beeswax and the occasional bee. Some producers use more heat and filtering to facilitate packing, retard crystallization, and to produce a more crystal-clear product. In fact, the voluntary U.S. grading of honey merely indicates the degree of filtration the honey has been subjected to, not its overall quality. The higher the grade, the more filtered the honey. Overprocessed honey is less flavorful due to the deterioration of enzymes and proteins present in the honey. It also removes the valuable bee pollen and propolis, the bee's version of antibiotics, from the honey.

Creamed honey has been allowed to crystallize and is then blended to a spreadable consistency. All honey will eventually crystallize. When this happens and you prefer it in its liquid state, simply place the jar in a pan of lukewarm water.

Contrary to popular belief, honey is metabolized in the body similarly to refined sugar, causing major fluctuations in blood sugar levels when used in excess. Honey's sugar profile includes 31% glucose, 38.5% fructose, 7.2% maltose, 1.5% sucrose, and 4.2% other sugars. Minute amounts of nutrients are present but not enough to be significant. The real significance in honey lies in the fact that, compared with refined sugars, fructose, corn syrup, sorbitol, and artificial sweeteners, it is one of the least refined sweeteners we have available. Even so, honey should be used in moderation.

It is very important to note that raw honey should never be given to a child under the age of one on pacifiers, in beverages, or in food. Spores of clostridium botulinum can be found in raw honey which can germinate and grow in infants whose internal defense systems are still underdeveloped. When the toxins are absorbed into the bloodstream, initial symptoms include constipation, difficulty feeding, and lethargy. If left unchecked, it can progress to a point where hospitalization is required, with possibly fatal results.

Baking/Cooking Guidelines

Honey is a favorite simply spread on bread or used to sweeten cakes, cookies, puddings, and muffins. Baked goods made with honey keep moist longer; cookies are more soft than crisp. It also makes great barbeque sauces and marinades, helping to produce tender, succulent results and when the honeyed foods are grilled or roasted, rich, caramel-like colors.

Substitute 1/2-2/3 cup honey per 1 cup sugar. Cut liquid by 1/4 cup for each 1 cup honey used. For improved volume in baked goods, add 1/4 tsp. baking soda per 1 cup honey to neutralize its acidity. If the recipe already calls for sour milk, yogurt, or sour cream, no extra baking soda is needed.

Since honey caramelizes at lower temperatures, when baking with honey reduce oven temperature by 25° F.

Store honey tightly sealed at room temperature.

JAMS AND JELLIES

Facts and Features

All jams and jellies have one common element—the presence of at least some fruit or fruit juice. However, the quality of fruit, the sweetener used, and flavor separate the mediocre from the really delicious, more healthy varieties.

Jams and jellies require fruit, acid, pectin, and a sweetener to jell. Pectin is a carbohydrate that is present in most fruits, especially tart blackberries, boysenberries, concord grapes, crab apples, cranberries, green gooseberries, loganberries, plums, fresh prunes, quince, red currants, sour guavas, and tart apples. Fruits low in pectin include apricots, blueberries, cherries, figs, peaches, pears, pineapples, raspberries, and strawberries. Good jams and jellies can be made from low-pectin fruits if they are combined with high pectin fruits or commercial pectin.

In order to jell effectively, jams made with commercial pectin require substantial amounts of some type of sugar in addition to the sugar that is already included in the powdered or liquid pectin formulas. The result is a product that masks the full flavor of the fruit and transforms the jam or jelly merely into a thick sugar product with some fruit flavor. Honey is used to sweeten some jams and jellies, however, its use results in a loosely textured product with a distinctly strong honey flavor. High quality jams and jellies rely upon the fruit itself to carry the flavor.

Two factors determine the amount of natural pectin available from a fruit—the stage of ripening and the processing temperature. Fruit that is almost at its peak of ripeness contains more pectin than underripe or overly ripe fruit. Too much heat destroys the natural pectin.

Perfectly ripe fruit also has the higher acid content that is needed to make a good jam or jelly. Lemon juice or other acids are added if the acid content is too low.

Applesauce and apple butter are the most familiar naturally sweetened spreads. The FDA regulates the proportions of fruit, juice, and sugars used in manufacturing jams, jellies, and preserves. Most reduced-sugar varieties and those made with fruit juice sweeteners don't fit within these standards and therefore cannot be labeled as a jam or a jelly. The words "spread," "conserve," or "butter" will alert you to products made with alternative sweeteners or those low in sugar. Most of these products seem as sweet as the sugar/corn syrup varieties.

Despite the fact that jams and jellies contain fruit, most of their calories come from concentrated simple sugars and therefore should not be counted as a fruit serving.

Baking/Cooking Guidelines

Most jams and jellies are enjoyed as bread spreads, but they can also be baked as a surprise into muffins. Try mixing them with nut butters as a frosting or filling for layer cakes.

MAPLE SYRUP

Facts and Features

Maple syrup is concentrated from the special sap of the maple tree that flows only during the late winter and early spring. It takes about 51/2 days for a tree to produce enough sap, approximately 40 gallons, for 1 gallon of maple syrup.

Quality is determined by color, flavor, and sugar content—all dependent on the the health of the tree, the weather during sugaring time, the skill of the producer, the cleanliness of the sugarhouse, and how the syrup is stored. In general, the darker and more concentrated in flavor, the longer the sap has been boiled.

There are three grading systems used today, U.S. standards, Vermont's own quality standards, and Canadian standards.

U.S. standards classify all maple syrups in only two categories, Grade A and Grade B. Maple syrups that have a light amber color and more delicate flavor are considered Grade A. Darker, thicker, stronger-tasting syrup is sold as Grade B.

In contrast, Vermont and Canadian standards are much more precise, using five classifications instead of two. Vermont Fancy/Canadian AA maple syrup is pale gold in color with a very sweet, delicate maple flavor. Vermont Grade A Medium Amber/Canadian Grade A has a medium gold color and true full-bodied maple flavor that is terrific for pancakes. Vermont Grade A Dark Amber/Canadian Grade B has a dark golden color whose maple flavor has undertones of caramel, a good choice for strong-flavored dishes. Vermont Grade B/Canadian Grade C is darker still, with a strong caramel flavor and some maple taste. Darkest of all is Vermont Commercial/Canadian Grade D whose flavor is even more caramel-like with only hints of maple.

Starting with sap that consists of 2-3% sucrose content, the final product consists of 62% sucrose, 35% water, 1% glucose, and 1% malic acid. Consequently, maple syrup is 2/3 as sweet as white sugar and metabolized similarly in the body.

Unlike the production of many other sweeteners, maple syrup is one of the least refined, basically requiring only boiling down of the sap. The concern that some producers may use formaldehyde pellets to prevent the tree from healing over at the tap is currently misfounded. Vermont, the top producing state for maple syrup, outlawed it in the early 1970s. Furthermore, the very few that used the pellets found that it hurt the trees. Defoamers used to keep the syrup from boiling over during the concentration of sap to syrup only include such aids as oil, butter, or cream, using only about 4 oz. of them per 160,000 gallons of sap at that. While occasionally a maple tree may be fertilized, more often than not it needs nothing more than what Nature provides. Pesticides aren't even an option.

Don't buy maple syrup in bulk. Its high water content can cause slow fermentation if left unsealed and unrefrigerated, leaving a syrup with compromised flavor. Even though maple syrup in tins may have a quaint old-fashioned feel, it can also give the syrup a metallic flavor. Your best bet is maple syrup in glass jars. Refrigerate it after opening and use within one year. Any crystallization that appears can be dissolved by gently warming the syrup.

Maple sugar is maple syrup that has been boiled down and evaporated to 93% solids.

Products labeled simply as "pancake syrup" contain no more than 2-3% real maple syrup with corn syrup and artificial flavoring and coloring making up the balance.

Baking/Cooking Guidelines

Besides topping pancakes and hot cereals, maple syrup can be used to sweeten cookies, cakes, muffins, and granola.

Substitute 1/2-2/3 cup maple syrup and decrease the liquid in the recipe by 1/4 cup per one cup sugar called for in a recipe.

Maple sugar can be used in a 1 to 1 ratio with granulated sugar.

MOLASSES

Facts and Features

Molasses is thick, strong-tasting cane sugar syrup manufactured either as a by-product from making sugar or directly for the molasses itself.

Blackstrap molasses is the final syrup left from crystallizing the sucrose from the sugar cane. Its dark color is the result of the caramelization of the sugars from the high temperatures repeatedly reached through boiling. Very strong, slightly bitter in flavor, it also contains a significant amount of minerals, particularly calcium, iron, magnesium, and potassium. However, blackstrap's sticky texture makes taking it by the tablespoon a risky venture for your teeth.

Unfortunately, blackstrap molasses has several other downsides. As the final extraction of sugar refining, it contains residues from the chemicals used during the growing and processing of the sugar, including sulfur dioxide. A preservative used as an anti-browning agent for the sugar, its residues can cause allergic reactions in sensitive individuals.

Blackstrap molasses is about half as sweet as white sugar.

Barbados molasses is made by slowly boiling the filtered sugar cane juice down into a syrup, not as a by-product of sugar refining. Its mellow, light flavor has significantly fewer nutrients than blackstrap molasses, but on the positive side, less chemical residue. Barbados molasses contains no sulfur dioxide and therefore is sometimes referred to as "unsulfured molasses".

Barbados molasses is about 2/3 as sweet as white sugar.

Sorghum molasses is the concentrated juice of the sweet sorghum plant, a grain that looks similar to millet. Popular in years past, it became more scarce as a sweetener with the increased production of sugar beets in the northern United States.

Sorghum tastes similar to molasses but is light and more tart and fruity. Its mineral content and sweetening power (65% of sucrose) is similar to barbados molasses.

Baking/Cooking Guidelines

All types of molasses, especially blackstrap, should be used to bake or cook foods that can handle a strong flavor, such as rye breads, cookies, corn muffins, and gingerbread.

Substitute for sugar in a recipe with a 1 to 1 ratio, reducing liquid by 1/4 cup for each cup of molasses used.

SACCHARIN

Facts and Features

Saccharin is an intensely sweet, calorie-free artificial sweetener produced by the Sherwin-Williams Co., made from the oxidation of toluene. Discovered in 1878, it was initially used as an antiseptic and food preservative. During World Wars I and II, it was used as a sugar substitute to counter sugar shortages and rationing.

Criticized in the early 1900s because it had no food value, it remained approved for use in the United States primarily because then-president Teddy Roosevelt liked it as a sugar substitute in his tea and coffee.

Until cyclamates came into use during the 1950s, saccharin was the country's major artificial sweetener. When cyclamates were banned in 1970 out of concern for their possible carcinogenicity, saccharin once again came into the limelight. But, soon after, studies unequivocally showed that saccharin causes bladder cancer in test animals during long-term feeding studies.

The FDA tried to ban saccharin in 1977 but, under pressure from consumers and the food industry, Congress stepped in and exempted saccharin from the country's food safety laws which prohibited the use of carcinogenic food substances.

As a compromise, the following warning continues to be placed on all food products sweetened with saccharine: "Warning: Use of this product may be hazardous to your health. This product contains saccharin which has been determined to cause cancer in laboratory animals."

In December 1991, after years of extended moratoriums on the removal of saccharin, the FDA officially withdrew its proposed federal ban on the artificial sweetener.

There still is no denying that saccharin has been shown to be carcinogenic. Why would you want to use a sweetener with a confirmed safety profile like that?

Baking/Cooking Guidelines

Due to its confirmed carcinogenicity, saccharin or products containing saccharin should not used. Since artificial sweeteners have not been proven to be beneficial in weight loss, their primary reason for being, as well as having no long-term human use to actually confirm their safety, any artificial sweetener should be avoided.

SORBITOL

Facts and Features

Sorbitol is a sugar alcohol, a class of carbohydrates that are metabolized into glucose more slowly than other sugars. Likewise, sugar alcohols are not metabolized as quickly by bacteria in the mouth, so they don't promote tooth decay. All sugar alcohols (sorbitol, mannitol, and xylitol) are more naturally metabolized than artificial sweetners.

Although sorbitol was first isolated from the berries of the mountain ash tree, it is made commercially from the hydrogenation of corn glucose. Sorbitol is most commonly found as a sweetening agent in diabetic foods, due to the fact that its delayed metabolism means that it requires little, if any, insulin.

Since it is not fully absorbed in the intestines, amounts over 1 oz. may cause diarrhea.

Baking/Cooking Guidelines

Sorbitol is only used in commercial food production and is not available as a tabletop sweetener for use in home recipes.

STEVIA

Facts and Features

Stevia is an intensely sweet natural substitute for sugar obtained from the South American herb known as yerba dulce or "sweet leaf." A plant from the genus Stevia, the only known species in the genus that is commercially used for its sweet flavor is Stevia rebaudiana.

Stevia has a flavor reminiscent of dark molasses. Considering that it is 100-200 times sweeter than sugar, very little is needed in a recipe. It also is calorie-free since its sweetness is from a glucoside that our bodies cannot completely metabolize.

Used for centuries in South America and as a popular sweetening agent in Japan for the past 20 years, unfortunately the FDA has restricted its use in the United States. In May 1991, the FDA issued an import alert on Stevia in an attempt to try to stop it from being imported to the United States.

Despite long-term historical use and several short-term and long-term safety studies conducted on Stevia in Japan, the FDA still considers it an unsafe food additive and seems resistant to examine studies that have been provided to vouch for its safety. After 20 years of use in Japan, there have been no reports of adverse effects from the use of Stevia products by humans.

Ironically, artificial sweeteners such as aspartame which have been the cause of innumerable health complaints, and saccharin, which is known to cause cancer in lab animals, have won approval by the FDA.

Baking/Cooking Guidelines

Currently, Stevia is not available for use in the United States. However, to get an idea about its relative sweetness, 1 cup of liquid sweetener can be made from mixing 1 rounded teaspoon of Stevia in 1 cup of water.

SUGARS: REFINED/UNREFINED

Characteristics

Refined sugar commonly refers to granulated sweeteners made from sugar cane or sugar beets highly refined to remove not only impurities in the sugar (soil, bacteria, lint, molds, pesticide residues, and insect parts) but also flavoring and color components contributed from its naturally occurring molasses. Most nutrients originally found in the sugar cane are removed, as well. Brown sugar and white sugar are considered fully refined sugars. In the process, the amount of sucrose found in the sugar cane juice, comprising approximately 15%, is concentrated down to yield about 96% sucrose in brown sugar and 99.9% in white sugar. Brown sugar is white sugar that is sprayed with molasses or caramel coloring.

Unrefined sugar refers to granulated sweeteners in which the juice extracted from sugar cane or sugar beets is evaporated under vacuum until the sucrose crystallizes. It is then ground to the desired size of sugar crystal. The various types of unrefined sugars are classified according to their moisture content, granular quality, color, and flavor.

In contrast to refined crystalline sugar, unrefined sugars have more depth of color and flavor owing to the preservation of the molasses which is naturally present in the cane juice. Sucrose content ranges from about 85-95%, with the remaining sugar profile including 1-4% fructose, and 1-3% glucose, making it little different than refined sugars in its absorption rates and effects on blood sugar levels.

Small amounts of minerals may also be present, retained from the minimal processing of the cane juice to its crystalline form. Because trace elements such as potassium, magnesium, and calcium form alkaline salts that help neutralize mouth acids, in theory, but not necessarily in reality, individuals who use unrefined sugar instead of comparable amounts of refined sugar may find reduced incidence of cavities. Some people also believe the naturally occurring amounts of chromium present in unrefined sweetener aid in the metabolism of the sugar. However, it's unlike a few more minerals is going to make a significant difference. When it gets down to it, don't try to convince yourself that unrefined crystalline sugars are nutritious. They remain a concentrated sugar that should be used in moderation.

Because unrefined sugars are not fully refined to remove almost all flavor, color, nutrient components, as well as agricultural chemicals, any pesticide residues that may linger on the sugar cane or beets will be concentrated once the juice is crystallized. Therefore, unrefined sugars that are organically grown are a better buy not only for the environment but also for your health.

Included within the unrefined sugar category are: demarara sugar, sugars sometimes referred to as evaporated cane juice, light and brown muscovado sugars, and turbinado sugar.

Demarara sugar is cane juice that has been evaporated and coarsely ground into large golden crystals that are slightly sticky. Its texture makes demarara sugar good for cookies, sprinkled on cereals, and for crunchy toppings on coffee cakes and other baked goods.

Evaporated cane juice, a term that is interchangeable with **unrefined sugar**, simply refers to the fact that it has not been subjected to the extreme refinement, as occurs in the process to make white and brown sugar, that removes most nutrients and flavor and color components originally found in the sugar cane. Unlike demarara and muscovado sugars, evaporated cane juice and brands that advertise themselves as unrefined sugar typically feature finely ground, light brown crystals that have a mild molasses flavor. Look for brands that are organically grown .

Muscovado sugars are the product of the third crystallization process in which the second concentration of molasses is boiled down and crystallized. Since the crystals are so small, rather than being centrifuged they are placed in a tall sugar filtering bin with a fine mesh bottom. Molasses then slowly filters through the mesh, leaving the unrefined sugar in the bottom. Light muscovado sugar is taken from the top of the bin. Dark muscovado sugar is removed near the bottom where the molasses is much more concentrated.

Unlike brown sugar which is sprayed with molasses, muscovado sugar incorporates the molasses within its crystals. It is also more coarse and sticky. Use muscovado sugars in recipes where a strong caramelized-molasses flavor is acceptable, such as cookies and some barbeque sauces.

Turbinado sugar is made from the first crystallization of the cane juice, retaining some of the molasses, which accounts for its golden-brown color. Its crystals are more finely ground than demarara sugar and more appropriate for general baking needs.

Baking/Cooking Guidelines

All refined and unrefined sugars have the same relative sweetness and, allowing for varying concentrations of molasses, can be used interchangeably in recipes.

XYLITOL

Characteristics

Xylitol is a sugar substitute extracted from birchwood chips and other hemicellulose sources. Like other sugar alcohols (see Sorbitol), it is more naturally metabolized by the body than artificial sweeteners.

Its most significant characteristic is its ability to help clean and protect teeth from decay. Xylitol's cool aftertaste stimulate salivation which, in turn, neutralizes acids in the mouth that demineralize tooth enamel.

Xylitol has the same relative sweetness as sucrose, but because of its cooling effect, it is used primarily in chewing gums.

Baking/Cooking Guidelines

Xylitol is used only in food manufacturing. It is not available for home use.

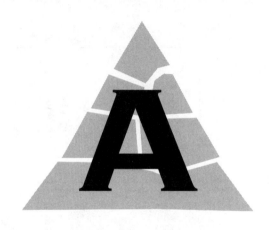

Good Food
NUTRITION FACTS

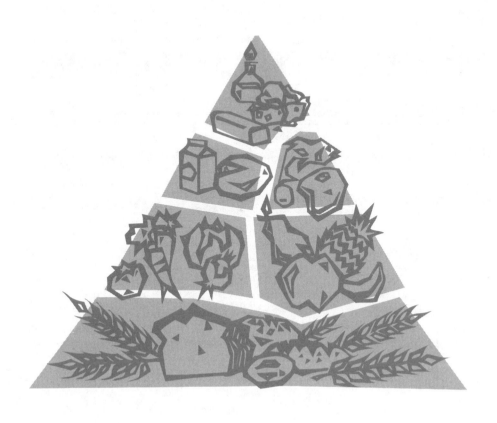

Food	Weight Per Serving	Calories	Calories from Fat	Fat	% Daily Values	Saturated Fat	% Daily Values	Cholesterol	% Daily Values	Sodium	% Daily Values
GRAINS (1/2 cup cooked)											
amaranth	127 g.	129	14	1.5 g.	2.5%	0.5 g.	2.5%	0 mg.	0%	0 mg.	0%
barley, pearled	100 g.	100	0	0 g.	0%	0 g.	0%	0 mg.	0%	0 mg.	0%
barley, rolled flakes	100 g.	55	5	0.5 g.	1%	0 g.	0%	0 mg.	0%	0 mg.	0%
barley, whole	100 g.	140	10	1 g.	2%	0 g.	0%	0 mg.	0%	0 mg.	0%
buckwheat (kasha)	90 g.	104	7	1 g.	1%	0 g.	0%	0 mg.	0%	0 mg.	0%
bulgur wheat	68 g.	123	0	1 g.	1%	0 g.	0%	0 mg.	0%	0 mg.	0%
couscous	89 g.	100	0	0 g.	0%	0 g.	0%	0 mg.	0%	0 mg.	0%
granola (1/2 cup dry)	52 g.	230	80	9.5 g.	15%	1.5 g.	8%	0 mg.	0%	0 mg.	0%
kamut, rolled flakes	85 g.	65	2.5	0.5 g.	1%	0 g.	0%	0 mg.	0%	0 mg.	0%
kamut, whole	90 g.	110	9	1 g.	1.5%	0 g.	0%	0 mg.	0%	0 mg.	0%
millet	95 g.	54	5	0.5 g.	1%	0 g.	0%	0 mg.	0%	0 mg.	0%
oat groats	100 g.	121	20	2 g.	3.5%	0 g.	0%	0 mg.	0%	0 mg.	0%
oats, rolled flakes	117 g.	70	10	1 g.	2%	0 g.	0%	0 mg.	0%	0 mg.	0%
oats, steel-cut	114 g.	102	18	2 g.	2.5%	0 g.	0%	0 mg.	0%	0 mg.	0%
quinoa	129 g.	130	20	2.5 g.	4%	0 g.	0%	0 mg.	0%	10 mg.	0%
rice, brown basmati	97 g.	116	7	1 g.	1%	0 g.	0%	0 mg.	0%	0 mg.	0%
rice, brown long	97 g.	116	7	1 g.	1%	0 g.	0%	0 mg.	0%	0 mg.	0%
rice, white basmati	102 g.	116	0	0 g.	0%	0 g.	0%	0 mg.	0%	0 mg.	0%
rice, white long enriched	102 g.	111	0	0 g.	0%	0 g.	0%	0 mg.	0%	0 mg.	0%
rice, wild	100 g.	92	0	0 g.	0%	0 g.	0%	0 mg.	0%	0 mg.	0%
rye, whole	90 g.	98	0	0 g.	0%	0 g.	0%	0 mg.	0%	0 mg.	0%
spelt, whole	90 g.	100	0	1 g.	1%	0 g.	0%	0 mg.	0%	0 mg.	0%
spelt rolled flakes	71 g.	77	0	0.5 g.	1%	0 g.	0%	0 mg.	0%	0 mg.	0%
teff	115 g.	102	5	0.5 g.	1%	0 g.	0%	0 mg.	0%	0 mg.	0%
wheat, rolled flakes	120 g.	70	0	0 g.	0%	0 g.	0%	0 mg.	0%	0 mg.	0%
wheat, whole hard red winter	90 g.	98	0	0 g.	0%	0 g.	0%	0 mg.	0%	0 mg.	0%

Carbohydrates	% Daily Values	Fiber	% Daily Values	Sugars- Natural and Added	Protein	Vitamin A	% Daily Values	Vitamin C	% Daily Values	Calcium	% Daily Values	Iron	% Daily Values
22 g.	7%	2 g.	9%	0 g.	5 g.	0 i.u.	0%	0 mg.	0%	60 mg.	6%	2.7 mg.	15%
22 g.	7%	2.5 g.	10%	1 g.	2 g.	0 i.u.	0%	0 mg.	0%	N/S**	0%	.54 mg.	3%
14 g.	4.5%	2.5 g.	10%	1 g.	2 g.	0 i.u.	0%	0 mg.	0%	N/S	0%	.54 mg.	3%
30 g.	10%	6 g.	25%	1 g.	4 g.	0 i.u.	0%	0 mg.	0%	20 mg.	2%	1.08 mg.	6%
12 g.	4%	2.5 g.	10%	1 g.	3.5 g.	0 i.u.	0%	0 mg.	0%	N/S	0%	1.08 mg.	6%
22 g.	7%	3.5 g.	14%	0 g.	5 g.	0 i.u.	0%	0 mg.	0%	N/S	0%	1.44 mg.	8%
21 g.	7%	1 g.	5%	1 g.	3 g.	0 i.u.	0%	0 mg.	0%	N/S	0%	.36 mg.	2%
32 g.	11%	4 g.	16%	6 g.	6 g.	N/S	0%	N/S	0%	20 mg.	2%	1.8 mg.	10%
15 g.	5%	2.5 g.	10%	0 g.	2.5 g.	0 i.u.	0%	0 mg.	0%	N/S	0%	.54 mg.	3%
26 g.	8.5%	2.3 g.	9%	0 g.	4 g.	0 i.u.	0%	0 mg.	0%	N/S	0%	2.7 mg.	15%
11 g.	3.5%	1 g.	4%	0 g.	1.5 g.	0 i.u.	0%	0 mg.	0%	N/S	0%	1.08 mg.	6%
22 g.	7%	3 g.	12%	0 g.	4.5 g.	0 i.u.	0%	0 mg.	0%	N/S	0%	1.36 mg.	7%
13 g.	4%	2 g.	8%	N/S	3 g.	N/S	0%	0 mg.	0%	N/S	0%	.72 mg.	4%
17.5 g.	6%	3 g.	12%	0 g.	3.5 g.	0 i.u.	0%	0 mg.	0%	N/S	0%	1.08 mg.	6%
29 g.	10%	3 g.	10%	N/S	6 g.	N/S	0%	N/S	0%	20 mg.	2%	3.6 mg.	20%
25 g.	8%	N/S	0%	0 g.	3 g.	0 i.u.	0%	0 mg.	0%	N/S	0%	.72 mg.	4%
25 g.	8%	2 g.	8%	0 g.	3 g.	0 i.u.	0%	0 mg.	0%	N/S	0%	.72 mg.	4%
25 g.	8%	0.5 g.	2%	0 g.	3 g.	0 i.u.	0%	0 mg.	0%	N/S	0%	.72 mg.	4%
25 g.	8%	0.5 g.	2%	0 g.	3 g.	0 i.u.	0%	0 mg.	0%	20 mg.	2%	1.08 mg.	6%
19 g.	6%	2.5 g.	10%	1 g.	3.5 g.	0 i.u.	0%	0 mg.	0%	N/S	0%	1.08 mg.	6%
24 g.	8%	2 g.	8%	1 g.	4 g.	0 i.u.	0%	0 mg.	0%	N/S	0%	.72 mg.	4%
26 g.	8.5%	3.5 g.	14%	0 g.	4 g.	0 i.u.	0%	0 mg.	0%	N/S	0%	1.08 mg.	6%
15 g.	5%	2.5 g.	10%	0 g.	3 g.	0 i.u.	0%	0 mg.	0%	N/S	0%	.72 mg.	4%
20 g.	7%	4 g.	15%	0 g.	3 g.	0 i.u.	0%	0 mg.	0%	50 mg.	5%	2.3 mg.	13%
16 g.	5%	2 g.	8%	0 g.	2 g.	0 i.u.	0%	0 mg.	0%	N/S	0%	.72 mg.	4%
24 g.	8%	2 g.	8%	0 g.	4 g.	0 i.u.	0%	0 mg.	0%	N/S	0%	.36 mg.	2%

Food	Weight Per Serving	Calories	Calories from Fat	Fat	% Daily Values	Saturated Fat	% Daily Values	Cholesterol	% Daily Values	Sodium	% Daily Values
FLOUR (1/4 cup)											
amaranth flour	30 g.	110	15	1.5 g.	2%	0 g.	0%	0 mg.	0%	0 mg.	0%
arrowroot flour	32 g.	110	0	0 g.	0%	0 g.	0%	0 mg.	0%	0 mg.	0%
barley flour	25 g.	75	5	0.5 g.	0%	0 g.	0%	0 mg.	0%	0 mg.	0%
buckwheat flour	30 g.	100	10	1 g.	1%	0 g.	0%	0 mg.	0%	0 mg.	0%
carob flour	26 g.	100	0	0 g.	0%	0 g.	0%	0 mg.	0%	10 mg.	0%
chickpea flour	35 g.	130	20	2.5 g.	4%	0 g.	0%	0 mg.	0%	0 mg.	0%
cornmeal	35 g.	120	10	1 g.	2%	0 g.	0%	0 mg.	0%	0 mg.	0%
cornmeal, blue	35 g.	130	15	1.5 g.	2%	0 g.	0%	0 mg.	0%	0 mg.	0%
cornstarch	32 g.	120	0	0 g.	0%	0 g.	0%	0 mg.	0%	0 mg.	0%
garbanzo flour	30 g.	110	15	2 g.	3%	0 g.	0%	0 mg.	0%	5 mg.	0%
gluten flour	30 g.	110	5	0.5 g.	1%	0 g.	0%	0 mg.	0%	0 mg.	0%
kamut flour	35 g.	110	5	0.5 g.	1%	0 g.	0%	0 mg.	0%	0 mg.	0%
millet flour	35 g.	110	10	1 g.	2%	0 g.	0%	0 mg.	0%	0 mg.	0%
oat flour	23 g.	83	11	1.5 g.	2%	0 g.	0%	0 mg.	0%	0 mg.	0%
rice (brown) flour	39 g.	140	10	1 g.	2%	0 g.	0%	0 mg.	0%	0 mg.	0%
rice (white) flour	35 g.	130	5	0.5 g.	1%	0 g.	0%	0 mg.	0%	0 mg.	0%
rye flour	30 g.	100	0	1 g.	1%	0 g.	0%	0 mg.	0%	0 mg.	0%
semolina flour	35 g.	120	5	0.5 g.	0%	0 g.	0%	0 mg.	0%	0 mg.	0%
soy flour	21 g.	90	40	4.5 g.	7%	0.5 g.	3%	0 mg.	0%	0 mg.	0%
spelt flour	35 g.	100	5	0.5 g.	1%	0 g.	0%	0 mg.	0%	0 mg.	0%
teff flour	35 g.	120	5	0.5 g.	1%	0 g.	0%	0 mg.	0%	5 mg.	0%
triticale flour	35 g.	120	5	0.5 g.	0%	0 g.	0%	0 mg.	0%	0 mg.	0%
wheat bran	15 g.	30	5	0.5 g.	1%	0 g.	0%	0 mg.	0%	0 mg.	0%
wheat germ	25 g.	90	20	2.5 g.	4%	0 g.	0%	0 mg.	0%	0 mg.	0%
white flour, unbleached	34 g.	121	4	0 g.	0%	0 g.	0%	0 mg.	0%	0 mg.	0%
whole wheat flour	35 g.	130	5	0.5 g.	1%	0 g.	0%	0 mg.	0%	0 mg.	0%

Carbohydrates	% Daily Values	Fiber	% Daily Values	Sugars- Natural and Added	Protein	Vitamin A	% Daily Values	Vitamin C	% Daily Values	Calcium	% Daily Values	Iron	% Daily Values
19 g.	6%	2 g.	8%	N/S	4 g.	0 i.u.	0%	0 mg.	0%	40 mg.	4%	7.2 mg.	40%
28 g.	9%	1 g.	4%	0 g.	0 g.	0 i.u.	0%	0 mg.	0%	20 mg.	2%	N/S	0%
19 g.	6%	3 g.	14%	0 g.	3 g.	N/S	0%	N/S	0%	N/S	0%	.72 mg.	4%
21 g.	7%	3 g.	12%	1 g.	4 g.	0 i.u.	0%	0 mg.	0%	N/S	0%	.72 mg.	4%
23 g.	8%	10 g.	41%	??	1 g.	N/S	0%	N/S	0%	80 mg.	8%	.72 mg.	4%
21 g.	7%	1 g.	5%	4 g.	7 g.	N/S	0%	0 mg.	0%	40 mg.	4%	2.7 mg.	15%
27 g.	9%	3 g.	13%	0 g.	3 g.	200 i.u.	4%	0 mg.	0%	N/S	0%	1.08 mg.	6%
25 g.	8%	3 g.	13%	0 g.	3 g.	0 i.u.	0%	0 mg.	0%	N/S	0%	.72 mg.	4%
29 g.	10%	N/S	0%	0 g.	0 g.	N/S	0%	0 mg.	0%	N/S	0%	N/S	0%
18 g.	6%	1 g.	5%	1 g.	6 g.	N/S	0%	1.2 mg.	2%	40 mg.	4%	1.8 mg.	10%
14 g.	5%	0 g.	0%	0 g.	12 g.	N/S	0%	0 mg.	0%	20 mg.	2%	N/S	0%
25 g.	8%	4 g.	16%	0 g.	4 g.	0 i.u.	0%	0 mg.	0%	N/S	0%	.72 mg.	4%
26 g.	9%	2 g.	9%	0 g.	4 g.	0 i.u.	0%	0 mg.	0%	N/S	0%	2.7 mg.	15%
15 g.	5%	3 g.	14%	0 g.	4 g.	0 i.u.	0%	0 mg.	0%	20 mg.	2%	1.08 mg.	6%
30 g.	10%	2 g.	7%	??	3 g.	0 i.u.	0%	0 mg.	0%	N/S	0%	.72 mg.	4%
28 g.	9%	1 g.	3%	0 g.	2 g.	0 i.u.	0%	0 mg.	0%	N/S	0%	N/S	0%
20 g.	7%	4 g.	16%	0 g.	5 g.	0 i.u.	0%	0 mg.	0%	20 mg.	2%	1.44 mg.	8%
25 g.	9%	2 g.	8 %	5 g.	4 g.	N/S	0%	N/S	0%	N/S	0%	.54 mg.	3%
7 g.	2%	N/S	0%	2 g.	8 g.	N/S	0%	0 mg.	0%	40 mg.	4%	1.44 mg.	8%
24 g.	8%	5 g.	19%	0 g.	4 g.	0 i.u.	0%	0 mg.	0%	N/S	0%	1.08 mg.	6%
25 g.	8%	5 g.	20%	0 g.	4 g.	N/S	0%	N/S	0%	0 mg.	0%	2.7 mg.	15%
25 g.	8%	5 g.	18%	1 g.	4 g.	0 i.u.	0%	0 mg.	0%	20 mg.	2%	1.08 mg.	6%
10 g.	3%	6 g.	26%	1 g.	2 g.	0 i.u	0%	0 mg.	0%	20 mg.	2%	1.44 mg.	8%
13 g.	4%	3 g.	13%	3 g.	6 g.	0 i.u.	0%	0 mg.	0%	N/S	0%	1.44 mg.	8%
25 g.	8%	0 g.	0%	0 g.	4 g.	0 i.u.	0%	0 mg.	0%	N/S	0%	1.44 mg.	8%
25 g.	8%	4 g.	17%	0 g.	5 g.	0 i.u.	0%	0 mg.	0%	20 mg.	2%	1.08 mg.	6%

Food	Weight Per Serving	Calories	Calories from Fat	Fat	% Daily Values	Saturated Fat	% Daily Values	Cholesterol	% Daily Values	Sodium	% Daily Values
whole wheat pastry	23 g.	76	0	0 g.	0%	0 g.	0%	0 mg.	0%	0 mg.	0%
BREADS (1 slice/each or as noted)											
bagel, Alvarado St. Bakery™ sprouted spelt**	94 g.	262	27	3 g.	5%	.5 g.	4%	0 mg.	0%	400 mg.	17%
bagel, Alvarado St. Bakery™ sprouted wheat**	94 g.	260	10	1 g.	2%	0 g.	0%	0 mg.	0%	400 mg.	17%
bagel, white*	68 g.	200	10	1 g.	2%	0 g.	0%	0 mg.	0%	380 mg.	16%
bagel, whole wheat*	55 g.	140	5	1 g.	1%	0 g.	0%	0 mg.	0%	270 mg.	11%
crackers, rye crispbread (1)	8 g.	30	0	0 g.	0%	0 g.	0%	0 mg.	0%	75 mg.	3%
crackers, rye thin crisp(4)	8 g.	30	0	0 g.	0%	0 g.	0%	0 mg.	0%	70 mg.	3%
crackers, stoned wheat (2)	8 g.	30	0	1 g.	2%	0 g.	0%	0 mg.	0%	45 mg.	2%
french bread	35 g.	100	10	1 g.	2%	0 g.	0%	0 mg.	0%	210 mg.	9%
mochi, Grainaissance™ plain* (1 piece)	45 g.	110	0	1 g.	2%	0 g.	0%	0 mg.	0%	0 mg.	0%
mochi, Grainaissance™sesame garlic* (1 piece)	45 g.	110	0	1.5 g.	2%	0 g.	0%	0 mg.	0%	20 mg.	1%
mochi, Grainaissance™ raisin-cinnamon* (1 piece)	45 g.	120	0	1 g.	2%	0 g.	0%	0 mg.	0%	35 mg.	1.5%
naan, Garden of Eatin™ **	71 g.	200	35	4 g.	6%	1 g.	5%	0 mg.	0%	330 mg.	14%
pita, whole wheat *	45 g.	120	10	1 g.	2%	0 g.	0%	0 mg.	0%	240 mg.	10%
pita, white unenriched*	60 g.	160	5	0.5 g.	1%	0 g.	0%	0 mg.	0%	320 mg.	13%
rice cake, Lundberg™ no salt	17g.	60	0	0 g.	0%	0 g.	0%	0 mg.	0%	0 mg.	0%
rice cake, Lundberg™ w/salt	17 g.	60	0	0 g.	0%	0 g.	0%	0 mg.	0%	120 mg.	5%
rye bread, typical	25 g.	60	5	1 g.	1%	0 g.	0%	0 mg.	0%	160 mg.	7%
rye sourdough bread*, French Meadow Bakery™	44 g.	103	6	1 g.	1%	0 g.	0%	0 mg.	0%	138 mg.	6%
tortilla, blue corn (2)*	47 g.	110	15	1.5 g.	2%	0 g.	0%	0 mg.	0%	0 mg.	0%
tortilla, corn (2) *	47 g.	120	15	1.5 g.	2%	0 g.	0%	0 mg.	0%	0 mg.	0%
tortilla, flour	35 g.	105	24	2.5 g.	4%	.5 g.	2.5%	0 mg.	0%	135 mg.	5.5%
tortilla, spelt*	56 g.	160	20	3 g.	4%	0 g.	0%	0 mg.	0%	280 mg.	16%
tortilla, Alvarado St. Bakery™ sprouted wheat*	47 g.	130	9	1 g.	1.5%	0 g.	0%	0 mg.	0%	250 mg.	10%
tortilla, whole wheat	35 g.	70	0	0 g.	0%	0 g.	0%	0 mg.	0%	170 mg.	7%
white bread	25 g.	70	10	1 g.	1%	0 g.	0%	0 mg.	0%	135 mg.	6%

* 1 whole counts as 2 servings grain   ** 1 whole counts as 3 servings grain

Carbohydrates	% Daily Values	Fiber	% Daily Values	Sugars- Natural and Added	Protein	Vitamin A	% Daily Values	Vitamin C	% Daily Values	Calcium	% Daily Values	Iron	% Daily Values
17 g.	6%	2 g.	10%	0 g.	3 g.	0 i.u.	0%	0 mg.	0%	20 mg.	2%	1.08 mg.	6%
49 g.	16%	1 g.	8%	4.5 g.	9.5 g.	300 i.u.	6%	1.2 mg.	2%	20 mg.	2%	3.6 mg.	20%
54 g.	18%	2 g.	9%	24 g.	9 g.	N/S	0%	N/S	0%	20 mg.	2%	2.7 mg.	15%
38 g.	13%	1 g.	6%	1 g.	7 g.	N/S	0%	N/S	0%	20 mg.	2%	1.08 mg.	6%
30 g.	10%	5 g.	22%	1 g.	6 g.	N/S	0%	N/S	0%	20 mg.	2%	1.8 mg.	10%
6 g.	2%	1 g.	5%	N/S	1 g.	N/S	0%	N/S	0%	N/S	0%	.36 mg.	2%
6 g.	2%	1 g.	5%	N/S	1 g.	N/S	0%	N/S	0%	N/S	0%	.36 mg.	0%
5 g.	2%	1 g.	3%	N/S	1 g.	N/S	0%	N/S	0%	N/S	0%	.36 mg.	2%
18 g.	6%	1 g.	4%	N/S	3 g.	N/S	0%	N/S	0%	20 mg.	2%	.72 mg.	4%
24 g.	8%	2 g.	8%	0 g.	2 g.	N/S	0%	0 mg.	0%	N/S	0%	.72 mg.	4%
23 g.	8%	2 g.	8%	0 g.	2 g.	N/S	0%	0 mg.	0%	N/S	0%	.72 mg.	4%
25 g.	8%	3 g.	12%	3.5 g.	2 g.	N/S	0%	0 mg.	0%	N/S	0%	.72 mg.	4%
35 g.	12%	4 g.	16%	2 g.	7 g.	N/S	0%	N/S	0%	20 mg.	2%	1.8 mg.	10%
25 g.	8%	3 g.	14%	1 g.	4 g.	N/S	0%	N/S	0%	N/S	0%	1.44 mg.	8%
33 g.	11%	1 g.	4%	1 g.	5 g.	N/S	0%	N/S	0%	60 mg.	6%	.72 mg.	4%
14 g.	5%	2 g.	7%	0 g.	1 g.	N/S	0%	N/S	0%	N/S	0%	N/S	0%
14 g.	5%	2 g.	5%	0 g.	1 g.	N/S	0%	N/S	0%	N/S	0%	N/S	0%
12 g.	4%	2 g.	6%	2 g.	2 g.	N/S	0%	N/S	0%	20 mg.	2%	.72 mg.	4%
22 g.	8%	3 g.	11%	0 g.	2 g.	N/S	0%	N/S	0%	20 mg.	2%	.54 mg.	3%
22 g.	7%	2 g.	7%	0 g.	3 g.	0 i.u.	0%	N/S	0%	60 mg.	6%	1.44 mg.	8%
29 g.	10%	5 g.	20%	0 g.	3 g.	0 i.u.	0%	0 mg.	0%	80 mg.	8%	.36 mg	2%
19 g.	6%	1 g.	4%	N/S	2.5 g.	0 i.u.	0%	0 mg.	0%	20 mg.	2%	.55 mg.	3%
30 g.	10%	1 g.	2%	4 g.	6 g.	0 i.u.	0%	0 mg.	0%	0 mg.	0%	1.44 mg.	8%
26 g.	9%	1 g.	4%	12 g.	4 g.	N/S	0%	N/S	0%	N/S	0%	1.26 mg.	7%
20 g.	7%	2 g.	8%	N/S	3 g.	0 mg.	0%	0 mg.	0%	20 mg.	2%	.72 mg.	4%
12 g.	4%	1 g.	2%	1 g.	2 g.	N/S	0%	N/S	0%	20 mg.	2%	.72 mg.	4%

Food	Weight Per Serving	Calories	Calories from Fat	Fat	% Daily Values	Saturated Fat	% Daily Values	Cholesterol	% Daily Values	Sodium	% Daily Values
whole wheat bread	35 g.	90	15	1.5 g.	2%	0 g.	0%	0 mg.	0%	180 mg.	8%
PASTA (1/2 cup cooked)											
cellophane noodles	95 g.	80	0	0 g.	0%	0 g.	0%	0 mg.	0%	0 mg.	0%
corn pasta	70 g.	100	5	0 g.	0%	0 g.	0%	0 mg.	0%	0 mg.	0%
egg noodles, enriched	80 g.	110	10	1 g.	2%	0 g.	0%	25 mg.	9%	5 mg.	0%
fresh pasta	70 g.	120	10	1 g.	2%	0 g.	0%	30 mg.	10%	10 mg.	0%
sifted wheat ribbons (Eden™)	70 g.	110	5	0.5 g.	1%	0 g.	0%	0 mg.	0%	0 mg.	0%
kamut pasta	70 g.	105	8	1 g.	1%	0 g.	0%	0 mg.	0%	0 mg.	0%
macaroni, enriched	70 g.	100	0	0 g.	0%	0 g.	0%	0 mg.	0%	0 mg.	0%
macaroni, whole wheat	70 g.	90	0	0 g.	0%	0 g.	0%	0 mg.	0%	0 mg.	0%
brown rice pasta (Mrs. Leeper's™)	70 g.	101	7	1 g.	1%	0 g.	0%	0 mg.	0%	8 mg.	0%
soba (40% buckwheat)	70 g.	95	0	0 g.	0%	0 g.	0%	0 mg.	0%	245 mg.	10%
somen	88 g.	120	0	0 g.	0%	0 g.	0%	0 mg.	0%	140 mg.	6%
spaghetti, spinach enriched	70 g.	90	0	0 g.	0%	0 g.	0%	0 mg.	0%	10 mg.	0%
spaghetti, whole wheat	70 g.	90	0	0 g.	0%	0 g.	0%	0 mg.	0%	0 mg.	0%
spelt pasta (Vita-Spelt™)	70 g.	100	5	1 g.	1%	0 g.	0%	0 mg.	0%	0 mg.	0%
udon noodles	70 g.	95	7	1 g.	1%	0 g.	0%	0 mg.	0%	330 mg.	14%
vegetable pasta enriched	70 g.	100	0	0 g.	0%	0 g.	0%	0 mg.	0%	10 mg.	0%
VEGETABLES (1/2 cup raw or cooked, 1 1/2 cup chopped lettuce, or as noted)											
alfalfa sprouts	17 g.	5	0	0 g.	0%	0 g.	0%	0 mg.	0%	0 mg.	0%
artichoke, steamed (1)	120 g.	60	0	0 g.	0%	0 g.	0%	0 mg.	0%	115 mg.	5%
arugula, chopped	10 g.	0	0	0 g.	0%	0 g.	0%	0 mg.	0%	0 mg.	0%
asparagus, cooked	90 g.	22	0	0 g.	0%	0 g.	0%	0 mg.	0%	0 mg.	0%
beets, cooked, diced	85 g.	35	0	0 g.	0%	0 g.	0%	0 mg.	0%	65 mg.	3%
bell pepper, green- 1 med.	74 g.	20	0	0 g.	0%	0 g.	0%	0 mg.	0%	0 mg.	0%
bell pepper, red-1 med.	74 g.	20	0	0 g.	0%	0 g.	0%	0 mg.	0%	0 mg.	0%
bok choy, steamed	85 g.	10	0	0 g.	0%	0 g.	0%	0 mg.	0%	30 mg.	1%

Carbohydrates	% Daily Values	Fiber	% Daily Values	Sugars- Natural and Added	Protein	Vitamin A	% Daily Values	Vitamin C	% Daily Values	Calcium	% Daily Values	Iron	% Daily Values
16 g.	5%	2 g.	10%	1 g.	3 g.	N/S	0%	N/S	0%	20 mg.	2%	1.08 mg.	6%
20 g.	7%	N/S	0%	N/S	0 g.	N/S	0%	N/S	0%	N/S	0%	.36 mg.	2%
17 g.	6%	3 g.	11%	N/S	2 g.	N/S	0%	N/S	0%	N/S	0%	N/S	0%
20 g.	7%	1 g.	4%	1 g.	4 g.	N/S	0%	N/S	0%	N/S	0%	1.44 mg.	8%
23 g.	8%	2 g.	7%	1 g.	5 g.	N/S	0%	N/S	0%	N/S	0%	1.44 mg.	8%
22 g.	7%	1.5 g.	6%	N/S	4 g.	N/S	0%	N/S	0%	20 mg.	2%	.72 mg.	4%
19 g.	6%	3 g.	11%	1 g.	5 g.	N/S	0%	N/S	0%	N/S	0%	2.7 mg.	15%
20 g	7%	1 g.	4%	1 g.	3 g.	N/S	0%	N/S	0%	N/S	0%	.72 mg.	4%
19 g.	6%	3 g.	12%	1 g.	4 g.	N/S	0%	N/S	0%	20 mg.	2%	.72 mg.	4%
21 g.	7%	1 g.	4%	N/S	2 g.	N/S	0%	N/S	0%	N/S	0%	.63 mg.	3.5%
18.5 g.	6%	1.5 g.	6%	1 g.	4 g.	N/S	0%	N/S	0%	20 mg.	2%	.9 mg.	5%
24 g.	8%	1 g.	4%	1 g.	4 g.	N/S	0%	N/S	0%	N/S	0%	.36 mg.	2%
18 g.	6%	2 g.	6%	1 g.	3 g.	100 i.u.	2%	N/S	0%	20 mg.	2%	.72 mg.	4%
19 g.	6%	3 g.	13%	1 g.	4 g.	N/S	0%	N/S	0%	20 mg.	2%	.72 mg.	4%
20 g.	7%	2 g.	10%	2 g.	4 g.	N/S	0%	N/S	0%	N/S	0%	.72 mg.	4%
19 g.	6%	1.5 g.	6%	2.5 g.	4 g.	N/S	0%	N/S	0%	N/S	0%	.72 mg.	4%
21 g.	7%	3 g.	14%	1 g.	4 g.	N/S	0%	N/S	0%	N/S	0%	1.08 mg.	6%
1 g.	0%	N/S	0%	N/S	1 g.	N/S	0%	1.2 mg.	2%	N/S	0%	N/S	0%
13 g.	4%	6 g.	26%	1 g.	4 g.	200 i.u.	4%	12 mg.	20%	60 mg.	6%	1.44 mg.	8%
N/S	0%	N/S	0%	N/S	0 g.	200 i.u.	4%	1.2 mg.	2%	20 mg.	2%	N/S	0%
4 g.	1%	2 g.	8%	2 g.	2 g.	500 i.u.	10%	25 mg.	41%	20 mg.	2%	.60 mg.	3%
8 g.	3%	1 g.	6%	6 g.	1 g.	N/S	0%	3.6 mg.	6%	20 mg.	2%	.72 mg.	4%
10 g.	2%	1 g.	5%	2 g.	1 g.	500 i.u.	10%	66 mg.	110%	N/S	0%	.36 mg.	2%
5 g.	2%	2 g.	7%	2 g.	1 g.	4000 i.u.	80%	138 mg.	230%	N/S	0%	.36 mg.	2%
2 g.	1%	1 g.	5%	0 g.	1 g.	2250 i.u.	45%	21 mg.	35%	80 mg.	8%	.72 mg.	4%

Food	Weight Per Serving	Calories	Calories from Fat	Fat	% Daily Values	Saturated Fat	% Daily Values	Cholesterol	% Daily Values	Sodium	% Daily Values
broccoli (1 stalk, raw)	148 g.	40	5	0.5 g.	1%	0 g.	0%	0 mg.	0%	40 mg.	2%
broccoli, (1 stalk, cooked)	180 g.	50	5	0.5 g.	1%	0 g.	0%	0 mg.	0%	45 mg.	0%
brussels sprouts, steamed	78 g.	30	0	0 g.	0%	0 g.	0%	0 mg.	0%	15 mg.	1%
cabbage, cooked, shredded	75 g.	15	0	0 g.	0%	0 g.	0%	0 mg.	0%	5 mg.	0%
cabbage, green, raw, shredded	35 g.	8	0	0 g.	0%	0 g.	0%	0 mg.	0%	8 mg.	0%
cabbage, red, raw, shredded	35 g.	10	0	0 g.	0%	0 g.	0%	0 mg.	0%	0 mg.	0%
carrot (1 med.)	78 g.	35	0	0 g.	0%	0 g.	0%	0 mg.	0%	25 mg.	1%
cauliflower, cooked	62 g.	15	0	0 g.	0%	0 g.	0%	0 mg.	0%	10 mg.	0%
cauliflower, raw flowerets	50 g.	12	0	0 g.	0%	0 g.	0%	0 mg.	0%	7 mg.	0%
celery (2 med. stalks)	110 g.	20	0	0 g.	0%	0 g.	0%	0 mg.	0%	95 mg.	4%
celery root, cooked	78 g.	20	0	0 g.	0%	0 g.	0%	0 mg.	0%	45 mg.	2%
chard, cooked	88 g.	20	0	0 g.	0%	0 g.	0%	0 mg.	0%	160 mg.	7%
cilantro (1/4 cup)	4 g.	2.5	0	0 g.	0%	0 g.	0%	0 mg.	0%	0 mg.	0%
collard greens, cooked	64 g.	15	0	0 g.	0%	0 g.	0%	0 mg.	0%	10 mg.	0%
corn (1 med. ear cooked)	90 g.	100	10	1 g.	2%	0 g.	0%	0 mg.	0%	15 mg.	1%
cucumber + peel (1/3 med.)	99 g.	15	0	0 g.	0%	0 g.	0%	0 mg.	0%	0 mg.	0%
daikon radish, raw slices	22 g.	5	0	0 g.	0%	0 g.	0%	0 mg.	0%	0 mg.	0%
eggplant, cubed, steamed	48 g.	15	0	0 g.	0%	0 g.	0%	0 mg.	0%	0 mg.	0%
escarole, chopped (11/2 cup)	75 g.	15	0	0 g.	0%	0 g.	0%	0 mg.	0%	15 mg.	1%
green beans, cooked	62 g.	20	0	0 g.	0%	0 g.	0%	0 mg.	0%	0 mg.	0%
green beans, raw	55 g.	15	0	0 g.	0%	0 g.	0%	0 mg.	0%	0 mg.	0%
green onions, raw (1/4 cup)	25 g.	10	0	0 g.	0%	0 g.	0%	0 mg.	0%	0 mg.	0%
jerusalem artichoke, raw	75 g.	60	0	0 g.	0%	0 g.	0%	0 mg.	0%	0 mg.	0%
jicama, raw	60 g.	25	0	0 g.	0%	0 g.	0%	0 mg.	0%	0 mg.	0%
kale, cooked	65 g.	20	0	0 g.	0%	0 g.	0%	0 mg.	0%	15 mg.	1%
kohlrabi, cooked	83 g.	25	0	0 g.	0%	0 g.	0%	0 mg.	0%	15 mg.	1%
leeks, cooked	52 g.	15	0	0 g.	0%	0 g.	0%	0 mg.	0%	5 mg.	1%

Carbohydrates	% Daily Values	Fiber	% Daily Values	Sugars- Natural and Added	Protein	Vitamin A	% Daily Values	Vitamin C	% Daily Values	Calcium	% Daily Values	Iron	% Daily Values
8 g.	3%	4 g.	18%	3 g.	4 g.	2250 i.u.	45%	138 mg.	230%	80 mg.	8%	1.44 mg.	8%
9 g.	3%	5 g.	21%	3 g.	5 g.	2500 i.u.	50%	132 mg.	220%	80 mg.	8%	1.44 mg.	8%
7 g.	2%	3 g.	13%	3 g.	2 g.	500 i.u.	10%	48 mg.	80%	20 mg.	2%	1.08 mg.	8%
3 g.	1%	2 g.	8%	1 g.	1 g.	100 i.u.	2%	15 mg.	25%	20 mg.	2%	N/S	0%
2 g.	1%	1 g.	3%	1 g.	1 g.	N/S	0%	17 mg.	28%	20 mg.	2%	N/S	0%
2 g.	1%	1 g.	3%	1 g.	1 g.	N/S	0%	21 mg.	35%	20 mg.	2%	N/S	0%
8 g.	3%	2 g.	9%	5 g.	1 g.	22000 i.u.	440%	6 mg.	10%	20 mg.	2%	.36 mg.	2%
3 g.	1%	2 g.	7%	1 g.	1 g.	N/S	0%	27 mg.	45%	N/S	0%	.36 mg.	2%
2.5 g.	1%	1.5 g.	6%	1 g.	1 g.	N/S	0%	36 mg.	60%	N/S	0%	.36 mg.	2%
4 g.	1%	2 g.	7%	1 g.	1 g.	100 i.u.	2%	9 mg.	15%	40 mg.	4%	.36 mg.	2%
5 g.	2%	3 g.	12%	1 g.	1 g.	N/S	0%	2.4 mg.	4%	20 mg.	2%	.36 mg.	2%
4 g.	1%	2 g.	7%	0 g.	2 g.	2500 i.u.	50%	15 mg.	25%	60 mg.	6%	1.8 mg.	10%
0.5 g.	0%	0 g.	0%	0 g.	0.3 g.	100 i.u.	2%	N/S	0%	N/S	0%	N/S	0%
4 g.	1%	1 g.	5%	0 g.	1 g.	1750 i.u.	35%	9 mg.	15%	20 mg.	2%	N/S	0%
23 g.	8%	3 g.	10%	2 g.	3 g.	200 i.u.	4%	6 mg.	10%	N/S	0%	.72 mg.	4%
3 g.	1%	1 g.	3%	2 g.	1 g.	200 i.u.	4%	4.8 mg.	8%	20 mg.	2%	.36 mg.	2%
1 g.	0%	N/S	0%	1 g.	0 g.	N/S	0%	4.8 mg.	8%	N/S	0%	N/S	0%
3 g.	1%	1 g.	5%	2 g.	0 g.	N/S	0%	1.2 mg.	2%	N/S	0%	N/S	0%
3 g.	1%	2 g.	9%	0 g.	1 g.	1500 i.u.	30%	4.8 mg.	8%	40 mg.	4%	.72 mg.	4%
5 g.	2%	2 g.	8%	1 g.	1 g.	400 i.u.	8%	6 mg.	6%	20 mg.	2%	.72 mg.	4%
4 g.	1%	2 g.	7%	1 g.	1 g.	400 i.u.	8%	9 mg.	15%	20 mg.	2%	.72 mg.	4%
2 g.	1%	1 g.	3%	1 g.	0 g.	100 i.u.	2%	4.8 mg.	8%	20 mg.	2%	.36 mg.	2%
13 g.	4%	1 g.	5%	2 g.	2 g.	N/S	0%	2.4 mg.	4%	20 mg.	2%	2.7 mg.	15%
5 g.	2%	2 g.	8%	1 g.	1 g.	N/S	0%	1.2 mg.	2%	N/S	0%	.36 mg.	2%
4 g.	1%	1 g.	5%	1 g.	1 g.	5000 i.u.	100%	27 mg.	45%	40 mg.	4%	.72 mg.	4%
6 g.	2%	1 g.	4%	4 g.	1 g.	N/S	0%	42 mg.	70%	20 mg.	2%	.36 mg.	2%
4 g.	1%	2 g.	7%	1 g.	0 g.	N/S	0%	2.4 mg.	4%	20 mg.	2%	.72 mg.	4%

Food	Weight Per Serving	Calories	Calories from Fat	Fat	% Daily Values	Saturated Fat	% Daily Values	Cholesterol	% Daily Values	Sodium	% Daily Values
lettuce, iceberg, (1 1/2 cup)	89 g.	10	0	0 g.	0%	0 g.	0%	0 mg.	0%	10 mg.	0%
lettuce, looseleaf, 1 1/2 cup)	85 g.	15	0	0 g.	0%	0 g.	0%	0 mg.	0%	10 mg.	0%
lettuce, romaine, (1 1/2 cup)	84 g.	15	0	0 g.	0%	0 g.	0%	0 mg.	0%	5 mg.	0%
mung bean sprouts, raw	52 g.	15	0	0 g.	0%	0 g.	0%	0 mg.	0%	0 mg.	0%
mung bean sprouts, stir-fried	62 g.	30	0	0 g.	0%	0 g.	0%	0 gm.	0%	5 mg.	0%
mushroom, shiitake, steamed	72 g.	40	0	0 g.	0%	0 g.	0%	0 mg.	0%	0 mg.	0%
mushrooms, common (5 med.)	84 g.	20	0	0 g.	0%	0 g.	0%	0 mg.	0%	0 mg.	0%
mustard greens, cooked	70 g.	10	0	0 g.	0%	0 g.	0%	0 mg.	0%	10 mg.	0%
okra, slices cooked	80 g.	25	0	0 g.	0%	0 g.	0%	0 mg.	0%	0 mg.	0%
onion, cooked, chopped	105 g.	30	0	0 g.	0%	0 g.	0%	0 mg.	0%	0 mg.	0%
onion, raw, chopped	80 g.	27	0	0 g.	0%	0 g.	0%	0 mg.	0%	0 mg.	0%
parsley, chopped (1/2 cup)	30 g.	10	0	0 g.	0%	0 g.	0%	0 mg.	0%	15 mg.	1%
pea pods (snow peas) cooked	80 g.	35	0	0 g.	0%	0 g.	0%	0 mg.	0%	0 mg.	0%
pea pods (snow peas) raw	72 g.	30	0	0 g.	0%	0 g.	0%	0 mg.	0%	0 mg.	0%
peas, cooked from frozen	80 g.	60	0	0 g.	0%	0 g.	0%	0 mg.	0%	70 mg.	3%
peas, cooked from raw	80 g.	70	0	0 g.	0%	0 g.	0%	0 mg.	0%	0 mg.	0%
peas, raw	72 g.	60	0	0 g.	0%	0 g.	0%	0 mg.	0%	0 mg.	0%
potato, baked (med. size)	148 g.	160	0	0 g.	0%	0 g.	0%	0 mg.	0%	10 mg.	0%
potato, boiled (med. size)	136 g.	120	0	0 g.	0%	0 g.	0%	0 mg.	0%	5 mg.	5%
potato, mashed w/ milk/butter	105 g.	110	0	4.5 g.	7%	3 g.	15%	15 mg.	4%	310 mg.	13%
potato, mashed w/milk	105 g.	81	0	.5 g.	1%	N/S	0%	2 mg.	0%	318 mg.	13%
pumpkin, cooked	123 g.	25	0	0 g.	0%	0 g.	0%	0 mg.	0%	0 mg.	0%
radicchio, raw shredded	20 g.	5	0	0 g.	0%	0 g.	0%	0 mg.	0%	0 mg	0%
red radishes (7)	85 g.	15	0	0 g.	0%	0 g.	0%	0 mg.	0%	0 mg.	0%
rutabaga cube, cooked	85 g.	35	0	0 g.	0%	0 g.	0%	0 mg.	0%	15 mg.	1%
spaghetti squash, cooked/baked	78 g.	25	0	0 g.	0%	0 g.	0%	0 mg.	0%	N/S	0%
spinach, cooked	90 g.	20	0	0 g.	0%	0 g.	0%	0 mg.	0%	65 mg.	3%

Carbohydrates	% Daily Values	Fiber	% Daily Values	Sugars- Natural and Added	Protein	Vitamin A	% Daily Values	Vitamin C	% Daily Values	Calcium	% Daily Values	Iron	% Daily Values
2 g.	1%	1 g.	2%	1 g.	1 g.	300 i.u.	30%	3.6 mg.	6%	20 mg.	2%	.36 mg.	2%
3 g.	1%	2 g.	6%	1 g.	1 g.	1500 i.u.	30%	15 mg.	25%	60 mg.	6%	1.08 mg.	6%
2 g.	1%	2 g.	6%	N/S	1 g.	2250 i.u.	45%	21 mg.	35%	40 mg.	4%	1.08 mg.	6%
3 g.	1%	1 g.	4%	1 g.	2 g.	N/S	0%	6 mg.	10%	N/S	0%	.36 mg.	2%
7 g.	2%	2 g.	8%	3 g.	3 g.	N/S	0%	9 mg.	15%	N/S	0%	1.08 mg.	6%
10 g.	3%	2 g.	6%	1 g.	1 g.	N/S	0%	N/S	0%	N/S	0%	.36 mg.	2%
4 g.	1%	1 g.	4%	1 g.	2 g.	0 i.u.	0%	N/S	0%	N/S	0%	1.08 mg.	6%
1 g.	0%	1 g.	6%	0 g.	2 g.	200 i.u.	4%	18 mg.	30%	60 mg.	6%	.36 mg.	2%
6 g.	2%	2 g.	8%	2 g.	2 g.	500 i.u.	10%	12 mg.	20%	60 mg.	6%	.36 mg.	2%
6.5 g.	2%	1.5 g.	6%	4 g.	1 g.	0 i.u.	0%	6 mg.	10%	30 mg.	3%	N/S	0%
6 g.	2%	1.5 g.	6%	4 g.	1 g.	N/S	0%	6 mg.	10%	20 mg.	2%	N/S	0%
2 g.	1%	1 g.	5%	1 g.	1 g.	1500 i.u.	30%	42 mg.	70%	40 mg.	4%	1.8 mg.	10%
6 g.	2%	2 g.	9%	3 g.	3 g.	100 i.u.	2%	36 mg.	60%	40 mg.	4%	1.44 mg.	8%
5 g.	2%	2 g.	8%	3 g.	2 g.	100 i.u.	2%	42 mg.	70%	40mg.	4%	1.44 mg.	8%
11 g.	4%	4 g.	18%	4 g.	4 g.	500 iu.	10%	9 mg.	15%	20 mg.	2%	1.08 mg.	6%
12 g.	4%	4 g.	18%	5 g.	4 g.	500 i.u.	10%	12 mg.	20%	20 mg.	2%	1.08 mg.	6%
11 g.	4%	4 g.	15%	4 g.	4 g.	500 i.u.	10%	30 mg.	50%	20 mg.	2%	1.08 mg.	6%
37 g.	12%	4 g.	14%	2 g.	3 g.	0 i.u.	0%	18 mg.	30%	20 mg.	2%	1.8 mg.	10%
27 g.	9%	2 g.	10%	1 g.	3 g.	0 i.u.	0%	18 mg.	30%	N/S	0%	.36 mg.	2%
18 g.	6%	2 g.	6%	1 g.	2 g.	200 i.u	4%	6 mg.	10%	20 mg.	2%	.36 mg.	2%
18 g.	6%	2 g.	6%	1 g.	2 g.	N/S	0%	7 mg.	12%	20 mg.	2%	N/S	0%
6 g.	2%	2 g.	8%	4 g.	1 g.	13500 i.u.	270%	6 mg.	10%	20 mg.	2%	.72 mg.	4%
1 g.	0%	N/S	0%	N/S	0 g.	N/S	0%	1.2 mg.	2%	N/S	0%	N/S	0%
3 g.	1%	1 g.	5%	2 g.	1 g.	0 i.u.	0%	18 mg.	30%	20 mg.	2%	.36 mg.	2%
7 g.	2%	2 g.	6%	3 g.	1 g.	500 i.u.	10%	15 mg.	25%	40 mg.	4%	.36 mg.	2%
5 g.	2%	1 g.	4%	3 g.	1 g.	100 i.u.	2%	2.4 mg.	4%	20 mg.	2%	.36 mg.	2%
3 g.	1%	2 g.	9%	N/S	3 g.	7500 i.u.	150%	9 mg.	15%	100 mg.	10%	3.6 mg.	20%

Food	Weight Per Serving	Calories	Calories from Fat	Fat	% Daily Values	Saturated Fat	% Daily Values	Cholesterol	% Daily Values	Sodium	% Daily Values
spinach, raw (1 1/2 cups)	84 g.	20	0	0 g.	0%	0 g.	0%	0 mg.	0%	65 mg.	3%
squash, winter, baked/mashed	121 g.	45	5	1 g.	1%	0 g.	0%	0 mg.	0%	0 mg.	0%
sweet potato (1 med. baked)	130 g.	130	0	0 g.	0%	0 g.	0%	0 mg.	0%	15 mg.	1%
tomato (1 med.)	148 g.	30	0	0 g.	0%	0 g.	0%	0 mg.	0%	15 mg.	1%
tomato sauce (1/4 cup)	62 g.	20	0	0 g.	0%	0 g.	0%	0 mg.	0%	190 mg.	8%
tomatoes, stewed, no salt	128 g.	35	0	0 g.	0%	0 g.	0%	0 mg.	0%	20 mg.	1%
turnip cubes, cooked	78 g.	15	0	0 g.	0%	0 g.	0%	0 mg.	0%	40 mg.	2%
turnip greens, cooked	72 g.	15	0	0 g.	0%	0 g.	0%	0 mg.	0%	20 mg.	1%
watercress sprigs (10)	25 g.	5	0	0 g.	0%	0 g.	0%	0 mg.	0%	10 mg.	0%
zucchini (1/2 med. raw)	98 g.	20	0	0 g.	0%	0 g.	0%	0 mg.	0%	0 mg.	0%
zucchini, cooked	90 g.	20	0	0 g.	0%	0 g.	0%	0 mg.	0%	0 mg.	0%
SEA VEGETABLES (uncooked portions)											
agar-agar flakes, raw (1 Tbsp.)	2.5 g.	10	0	0 g.	0%	0 g.	0%	0 mg.	0%	10 mg.	0%
alaria, raw (1/2 cup)	10 g.	25	0	0 g.	0%	0 g.	0%	0 mg.	0%	420 mg.	18%
arame, raw (1/2 cup)	10 g.	30	0	0 g.	0%	0 g.	0%	0 mg.	0%	120 mg.	5%
dulse (1/2 cup)	10 g.	25	0	0 g.	0%	0 g.	0%	0 mg.	0%	170 mg.	7%
hiziki, raw (1/2 cup)	10 g.	30	0	0 g.	0%	0 g.	0%	0 mg.	0%	160 mg.	7%
kelp, Atlantic (1/2 cup)	10 g.	25	0	0 g.	0%	0 g.	0%	0 mg.	0%	450 mg.	19%
kombu, raw (3 1/2 inch piece)	3.3 g.	10	0	0 g.	0%	0 g.	0%	0 mg.	0%	90 mg.	4%
nori, raw (1 sheet)	2.5 g.	10	0	0 g.	0%	0 g.	0%	0 mg.	0%	5 mg.	0%
wakame flakes, raw (1/2 cup)	10 g.	25	0	0 g.	0%	0 g.	0%	0 mg.	0%	720 mg.	30%
wakame, raw (1/2 cup)	10 g.	25	0	0 g.	0%	0 g.	0%	0 mg.	0%	660 mg.	28%
FRUIT, fresh/cooked (1/2 cup or as noted)											
apple (1 med.)	154 g.	90	5	0.5 g.	15%	0 g.	0%	0 mg.	0%	0 mg.	0%
applesauce (1/2 cup)	122 g.	50	0	0 g.	0%	0 g.	0%	0 mg.	0%	0 mg.	0%
apricots (2)	71 g.	35	0	0 g.	0%	0 g.	0%	0 mg.	0%	0 mg.	0%
Asian pears (1)	122 g.	50	0	0 g.	0%	0 g.	0%	0 mg.	0%	0 mg.	0%

Carbohydrates	% Daily Values	Fiber	% Daily Values	Sugars- Natural and Added	Protein	Vitamin A	% Daily Values	Vitamin C	% Daily Values	Calcium	% Daily Values	Iron	% Daily Values
3 g.	1%	2 g.	9%	N/S	2 g.	5500 i.u.	110%	24 mg.	40%	80 mg.	8%	2.7 mg.	15%
11 g.	4%	3 g.	14%	3 g.	1 g.	4500 i.u.	90%	12 mg.	20%	20 mg.	2%	.36 mg.	2%
32 g.	11%	4 g.	16%	15 g.	2 g.	28500 i.u.	570%	30 mg.	3%	40 mg.	4%	.72 mg.	4%
7 g.	2%	2 g.	7%	14 g.	1 g.	1000 i.u.	20%	27 mg.	45%	N/S	0%	.72 mg.	4%
5 g.	2%	1 g.	5%	3 g.	1 g.	300 i.u.	6%	2.4 mg.	4%	N/S	0%	.72 mg.	4%
8 g.	3%	2 g.	8%	4 g.	1 g.	750 i.u.	15%	18 mg.	30%	40 mg.	4%	1.08 mg.	6%
4 g.	1%	2 g.	6%	1 g.	1 g.	N/S	0%	9 mg.	15%	20 mg.	2%	N/S	0%
3 g.	1%	2 g.	9%	0 g.	1 g.	4000 i.u.	80%	21 mg.	35%	100 mg.	10%	.72 mg.	4%
0 g.	0%	0 g.	0%	0 g.	1 g.	1250 i.u.	25%	12 mg.	20%	40 mg.	4%	N/S	0%
4 g.	1%	2 g.	7%	2 g.	1 g.	200 i.u.	4%	15 mg.	25%	20 mg.	2%	.36 mg.	2%
4 g.	1%	1 g.	5%	2 g.	1 g.	300 i.u.	6%	4.8 mg.	8%	20 mg.	2%	.26 mg.	2%
2 g.	1%	2 g.	9%	0 g.	0 g.	N/S	0%	0 mg.	0%	20 mg.	2%	N/S	1%
4 g.	1%	4 g.	17%	0 g.	2 g.	750 i.u.	15%	0 mg.	0%	100 mg.	10%	1.8 mg.	10%
7 g.	2%	7 g.	28%	0 g.	1 g.	500 i.u.	10%	0 mg.	0%	100 mg.	10%	.72 mg.	4%
4 g.	1%	4 g.	17%	0 g.	2 g.	100 i.u.	2%	0 mg.	0%	20 mg.	2%	3.6 mg.	20%
6 g.	2%	6 g.	24%	0 g.	0 g.	N/S	0%	0 mg.	0%	100 mg.	10%	.72 mg.	4%
4 g.	1%	4 g.	17%	0 g.	2 g.	100 i.u.	2%	0 mg.	0%	100 mg.	10%	4.5 mg.	25%
2 g.	1%	1 g.	4%	0 g.	0 g.	N/S	0%	0 mg.	0%	20 mg.	2%	0 i.u.	0%
1 g.	0%	1 g.	4%	0 g.	1 g.	400 i.u.	8%	6 mg.	10%	N/S	0%	N/S	0%
4 g.	1%	4 g.	17%	0 g.	2 g.	300 i.u.	6%	0 mg.	0%	80 mg.	8%	2.7 mg.	15%
4 g.	1%	4 g.	17%	0 g.	1 g.	400 i.u.	8%	0 mg.	0%	80 mg.	8%	1.44 mg.	8%
24 g.	8%	4 g.	17%	18 g.	0 g.	100 i.u.	0%	9 mg.	15%	20 mg.	2%	.36 mg.	2%
14 g.	5%	1 g.	6%	12 g.	0 g.	N/S	0%	1.2 mg.	2%	N/S	0%	N/S	0%
8 g.	3%	2 g.	7%	6 g.	1 g.	1750 i.u.	35%	6 mg.	10%	0 mg.	0%	.36 mg.	2%
13 g.	4%	4 g.	18%	9 g.	1 g.	N/S	0%	4.8 mg.	8%	N/S	0%	N/S	0%

Food	Weight Per Serving	Calories	Calories from Fat	Fat	% Daily Values	Saturated Fat	% Daily Values	Cholesterol	% Daily Values	Sodium	% Daily Values
avocado (1/3 med.)	55 g.	90	80	9 g.	13%	1.5 g.	7%	0 mg.	0%	5 mg.	0%
banana (1 med.)	126 g.	120	5	0.5 g.	1%	0 g.	0%	0 mg.	0%	0 mg.	0%
blueberries	72 g.	40	0	0 g.	0%	0 g.	0%	0 mg.	0%	0 mg.	0%
cantaloupe (1/4 med.)	134 g.	45	0	0 g.	0%	0 g.	0%	0 mg.	0%	10 mg.	1%
carambola (1)	127 g.	40	0	0 g.	0%	0 g.	0%	0 mg.	0%	0 mg.	0%
cherries, sweet (10)	72 g.	50	5	0.5 g.	0%	0 g.	0%	0 mg.	0%	0 mg.	0%
cranberries, raw	48 g.	25	0	0 g.	0%	0 g.	0%	0 mg.	0%	0 mg.	0%
grapefruit (1/2 med.)	154 g.	45	0	0 g.	0%	0 g.	0%	0 mg.	0%	0 mg.	0%
grapes, seedless	80 g.	60	0	0 g.	0%	0 g.	0%	0 mg.	0%	0 mg.	0%
guava (1)	90 g.	45	5	0.5 g.	0%	0 g.	0%	0 mg.	0%	0 mg.	0%
honeydew melon (1/10 med.)	134 g.	45	0	0 g.	0%	0 g.	0%	0 mg.	0%	15 mg.	1%
kiwifruit (2 med.)	148 g.	90	5	0.5 g.	1%	0 g.	0%	0 mg.	0%	5 mg.	0%
kumquat (4)	76 g.	50	0	0 g.	0%	0 g.	0%	0 mg.	0%	0 mg.	0%
lemon (1 med.)	58 g.	15	0	0 g.	0%	0 g.	0%	0 mg.	0%	0 mg.	0%
lime (1 med.)	67 g.	20	0	0 g.	0%	0 g.	0%	0 mg.	0%	0 mg.	0%
lychees (1/2 cup)	95 g.	60	0	0 g.	0%	0 g.	0%	0 mg.	0%	0 mg.	0%
mango (1/2 whole)	104 g.	70	0	0 g.	0%	0 g.	0%	0 mg.	0%	0 mg.	0%
nectarine (1 med.)	140 g.	70	5	0.5 g.	1%	0 g.	0%	0 mg.	0%	0 mg.	0%
orange (1 med.)	131 g.	60	0	0 g.	0%	0 g.	0%	0 mg.	0%	0 mg.	0%
papaya (1/2 whole)	152 g.	60	0	0 g.	0%	0 g.	0%	0 mg.	0%	0 mg.	0%
passion fruit (1)	18 g.	15	0	0 g.	0%	0 g.	0%	0 mg.	0%	5 mg.	0%
peach (1 med.)	87 g.	35	0	0 g.	0%	0 g.	0%	0 mg.	0%	0 mg.	0%
pear (1 med.)	166 g.	100	5	0.5 g.	1%	0 g.	0%	0 mg.	0%	0 mg.	0%
persimmon, Japanese (1 lg.)	168 g.	120	0	0 g.	0%	0 g.	0%	0 mg.	0%	0 mg.	0%
pineapple chunks	78 g.	40	0	0 g.	0%	0 g.	0%	0 mg.	0%	0 mg.	0%
plantain, cooked (1/2 cup)	90 g.	0	0	0 g.	0%	0 g.	0%	0 mg.	0%	0 mg.	0%
plums (2 med.)	132 g.	70	5	1 g.	1%	0 g.	0%	0 mg.	0%	0 mg.	0%

Carbohydrates	% Daily Values	Fiber	% Daily Values	Sugars- Natural and Added	Protein	Vitamin A	% Daily Values	Vitamin C	% Daily Values	Calcium	% Daily Values	Iron	% Daily Values
4 g.	1%	3 g.	13%	0 g.	1 g.	300 i.u.	6%	4.8 mg.	8%	N/S	0%	.72 mg.	4%
29 g.	10%	3 g.	12%	23 g.	1 g.	100 i.u.	2%	12 mg.	20%	N/S	0%	.36 mg.	2%
10 g.	3%	2 g.	8%	8 g.	0 g.	100 i.u.	2%	9 mg.	15%	N/S	0%	N/S	0%
11 g.	4%	1 g.	4%	10 g.	1 g.	4500 i.u.	90%	54 mg.	90%	20 mg.	2%	.36 mg.	2%
10 g.	3%	3 g.	14%	9 g.	1 g.	750 i.u.	15%	27 mg.	45%	N/S	0%	.36 mg.	2%
12 g.	4%	1 g.	5%	11 g.	1 g.	200 i.u.	4%	5 mg.	8%	20 mg.	2%	.36 mg.	2%
6 g.	2%	2 g.	8%	4 g.	0 g.	N/S	0%	6 mg.	10%	N/S	0%	N/S	0%
12 g.	4%	2 g.	8%	10 g.	1 g.	400 i.u.	4%	60 mg.	100%	20 mg.	2%	.36 mg.	2%
14 g.	5%	N/S	0%	14 g.	1 g.	100 i.u.	2%	9 mg.	15%	N/S	0%	.36 mg.	2%
11 g.	4%	5 g.	19%	5 g.	1 g.	750 i.u.	15%	168 mg.	280%	20 mg.	2%	.36 mg.	2%
12 g.	4%	1 g.	3%	12 g.	1 g.	100 i.u.	2%	36 mg.	60%	N/S	0%	0 mg.	0%
22 g.	7%	5 g.	20%	17 g.	1 g.	300 i.u.	6%	108 mg.	180%	40 mg.	4%	.72 mg.	4%
12 g.	4%	5 g.	20%	13 g.	1 g.	200 i.u.	4%	27 mg.	45%	40 mg.	4%	.36 mg.	2%
5 g.	2%	2 g.	6%	4 g.	1 g.	0 i.u.	0%	30 mg.	50%	20 mg.	2%	.36 mg.	2%
7 g.	2%	2 g.	8%	1 g.	0 g.	0 i.u.	0%	18 mg.	30%	20 mg.	2%	.36 mg.	2%
16 g.	5%	1 g.	5%	14 g.	1 g.	N/S	0%	66 mg.	110%	N/S	0%	.36 mg.	2%
18 g.	6%	2 g.	7%	15 g.	1 g.	4000 i.u	80%	30 mg.	50%	20 mg.	2%	N/S	0%
17 g.	6%	2 g.	9%	14 g.	1 g.	100 i.u.	2%	9 mg.	15%	N/S	0%	.36 mg.	2%
15 g.	5%	3 g.	12%	14 g.	1 g.	100 i.u.	2%	70 mg.	115%	N/S	0%	N/S	0%
15 g.	5%	3 g.	11%	9 g.	1 g.	400 i.u.	8%	96 mg.	160%	40 mg.	4%	N/S	0%
4 g.	1%	2 g.	7%	2 g.	0 g.	100 i.u.	2%	4.8 mg.	8%	N/S	0%	.36 mg.	2%
10 g.	3%	1.5 g.	7%	8 g.	0.5 g.	500 i.u.	10%	6 mg.	10%	N/S	0%	N/S	0%
25 g.	8%	4 g.	16%	17 g.	1 g.	0 i.u.	0%	6 mg.	10%	20 mg.	2%	.36 mg.	0%
31 g.	10%	6 g.	24%	25 g.	1 g.	3500 i.u.	70%	12 mg.	20%	20 mg.	2%	.36 mg.	2%
10 g.	3%	1 g.	4%	9 g.	0 g.	N/S	0%	12 mg.	20%	N/S	0%	.36 mg.	2%
24 g.	8%	2 g.	7%	4 g.	1 g.	750 i.u.	15%	9 mg.	15%	N/S	0%	.36 mg.	2%
17 g.	6%	2 g.	8%	13 g.	1 g.	400 i.u.	8%	12 mg.	20%	0 mg.	0%	0 mg.	0%

Food	Weight Per Serving	Calories	Calories from Fat	Fat	% Daily Values	Saturated Fat	% Daily Values	Cholesterol	% Daily Values	Sodium	% Daily Values
pomegranate (1)	154 g.	100	0	0 g.	0%	0 g.	0%	0 mg.	0%	0 mg.	0%
quince (1)	92 g.	50	0	0 g.	0%	0 g.	0%	0 mg.	0%	0 mg.	0%
raspberries, red	62 g.	30	0	0 g.	0%	0 g.	0%	0 mg.	0%	0 mg.	0%
strawberries (8)	72 g.	45	5	0.5 g.	0%	0 g.	0%	0 mg.	0%	0 mg.	0%
tamarinds (1)	2 g.	5	0	0 g.	0%	0 g.	0%	0 mg.	0%	0 mg.	0%
tangerine (2 med.)	168 g.	70	0	0 g.	0%	0 g.	0%	0 mg.	0%	0 mg.	0%
watermelon (2 cup diced)	280 g.	90	10	1 g.	2%	0 g.	0%	0 mg.	0%	5 mg.	0%
dried (1/4 cup or as noted)											
apple rings, packed	40 g.	100	0	0 g.	0%	0 g.	0%	0 mg.	0%	35 mg.	1%
apricots (10 halves)	35 g.	80	0	0 g.	0%	0 g.	0%	0 mg.	0%	0 mg.	0%
apricots (1/4 cup)	33 g.	80	0	0 g.	0%	0 g.	0%	0 mg.	0%	0 mg.	0%
dates (5 med.)	42 g.	110	0	0 g.	0%	0 g.	0%	0 mg.	0%	0 mg.	0%
dates, chopped 1/4 cup	44 g.	120	0	0 g.	0%	0 g.	0%	0 mg.	0%	0 mg.	0%
figs (2)	37 g.	100	0	0 g.	0%	0 g.	0%	0 mg.	0%	0 mg.	0%
papaya (2 pieces)	46 g.	120	0	0 g.	0%	0 g.	0%	0 mg.	0%	10 mg.	0%
peaches (3 halves)	39 g.	90	0	0 g.	0%	0 g.	0%	0 mg.	0%	0 mg.	0%
pear (2 halves)	35 g.	90	0	0 g.	0%	0 g.	0%	0 mg.	0%	0 mg	0%
prunes (5 small)	42 g.	100	0	0 g.	0%	0 g.	0%	0 mg.	0%	0 mg.	0%
raisins (unpacked)	36 g.	110	0	0 g.	0%	0 g.	0%	0 mg.	0%	10 mg.	0%
juice (3/4 cup)											
apple	170 g.	80	0	0 g.	0%	0 g.	0%	0 mg.	0%	5 mg.	0%
grape	190 g.	120	0	0 g.	0%	0 g.	0%	0 mg.	0%	5 mg.	0%
orange, fresh	170 g.	80	0	0 g.	0%	0 g.	0%	0 mg.	0%	0 mg.	0%
orange, reconstituted	187 g.	80	0	0 g.	0%	0 g.	0%	0 mg.	0%	0 mg.	0%
pineapple	188 g.	100	0	0 g.	0%	0 g.	0%	0 mg.	0%	0 mg.	0%
prune	192 g.	140	0	0 g.	0%	0 g.	0%	0 mg.	0%	0 mg.	0%

Carbohydrates	% Daily Values	Fiber	% Daily Values	Sugars- Natural and Added	Protein	Vitamin A	% Daily Values	Vitamin C	% Daily Values	Calcium	% Daily Values	Iron	% Daily Values
27 g.	9%	1 g.	4%	21 g.	1 g.	N/S	0%	9 mg.	15%	N/S	0%	.36 mg.	2%
14 g.	5%	2 g.	7%	12 g.	0 g.	N/S	0%	15 mg.	25%	20 mg.	2%	.72 mg.	4%
7 g.	2%	3 g.	11%	6 g.	1 g.	100 i.u.	2%	15 mg.	25%	20 mg.	2%	.36 mg.	2%
10 g.	3%	3 g.	12%	8 g.	1 g.	0 i.u.	0%	84 mg.	140%	20 mg.	0%	.72 mg.	4%
1 g.	0%	N/S	0%	N/S	0 g.	N/S	0%	N/S	0%	N/S	0%	N/S	0%
19 g.	6%	4 g.	15%	15 g.	1 g.	300 i.u.	30%	54 mg.	90%	20 mg.	2%	0 mg.	0%
20 g.	7%	1 g.	6%	19 g.	2 g.	100 i.u.	20%	27 mg.	45%	20 mg.	2%	.36 mg.	2%
26 g.	9%	3 g.	14%	22 g.	0 g.	N/S	0%	1.2 mg.	2%	N/S	0%	.72 mg.	4%
22 g.	7%	3 g.	13%	18 g.	1 g.	2500 i.u.	50%	1.2 mg.	2%	20 mg.	2%	1.8 mg.	10%
20 g.	7%	3 g.	12%	17 g.	1 g.	2250 i.u.	45%	1.2 mg.	2%	20 mg.	2%	1.44 mg.	8%
31 g.	10%	3 g.	13%	28 g.	1 g.	N/S	0%	0 mg.	0%	20 mg.	2%	.36 mg.	2%
33 g.	11%	3 g.	13%	29 g.	1 g.	N/S	0%	0 mg.	0%	20 mg.	2%	.36 mg.	2%
24 g.	8%	3 g.	14%	21 g.	1 g.	N/S	0%	N/S	0%	60 mg.	6%	.72 mg.	4%
30 g.	10%	5 g.	21%	18 g.	2 g.	400 i.u.	8%	36 mg.	60%	80 mg.	8%	.36 mg.	2%
24 g.	8%	3 g.	13%	20 g.	1 g.	750 i.u.	15%	2.4 mg.	4%	20 mg.	2%	1.44 mg.	8%
24 g.	8%	3 g.	11%	18 g.	1 g.	N/S	0%	2.4 mg.	4%	20 mg.	2%	.72 mg.	4%
26 g.	9%	3 g.	12%	18 g.	1 g.	750 i.u.	15%	1.2 mg.	2%	20 mg.	2%	1.08 mg.	6%
28 g.	9%	2 g.	10%	26 g.	1 g.	N/S	0%	2.4 mg.	4%	20 mg.	2%	1.08 mg.	6%
20 g.	7%	0 g.	0%	19 g.	0 g.	N/S	0%	1.2 mg.	2%	20 mg.	2%	.72 mg.	4%
28 g.	9%	0 g.	0%	28 g.	1 g.	N/S	0%	N/S	0%	20 mg.	2%	.36 mg.	2%
18 g.	6%	0 g.	0%	17 g.	1 g.	300 i.u.	6%	84 mg.	140%	20 mg.	2%	.36 mg.	2%
20 g.	7%	0 g.	0%	20 g.	1 g.	100 i.u.	2%	72 mg.	120%	20 mg.	2%	.36 mg.	2%
26 g.	9%	0 g.	0%	26 g.	1 g.	N/S	0%	21 mg.	35%	40 mg.	4%	.36 mg.	2%
34 g.	11%	2 g.	8%	25 g.	1 g.	N/S	0%	9 mg.	15%	20 mg.	2%	2.7 mg.	15%

Food	Weight Per Serving	Calories	Calories from Fat	Fat	% Daily Values	Saturated Fat	% Daily Values	Cholesterol	% Daily Values	Sodium	% Daily Values
MEAT (3 oz. roasted/broiled/braised or as noted)											
Beef											
beef hotdog (1)	57 g.	180	150	16 g.	25%	7 g.	35%	35 mg.	12%	590 mg.	24%
bottom round	85 g.	190	70	8 g.	12%	2.5 g.	14%	80 mg.	27%	45 mg.	2%
brisket	85 g.	330	240	27 g.	41%	11 g.	53%	80 mg.	27%	50 mg.	2%
chuck blade roast	85 g.	220	110	12 g.	19%	5 g.	24%	90 mg.	30%	60 mg.	3%
ground extra lean	85 g.	230	120	13 g.	21%	5 g.	26%	85 mg.	28%	70 mg.	3%
ground lean	85 g.	240	130	15 g.	23%	6 g.	30%	85 mg.	29%	75 mg.	3%
ground regular	85 g.	250	150	17 g.	26%	7 g.	33%	85 mg.	29%	80 mg.	3%
short ribs, lean	85 g.	250	140	15 g.	24%	7 g.	33%	80 mg.	26%	50 mg.	2%
tenderloin steak	85 g.	180	80	9 g.	13%	3 g.	16%	0 mg.	0%	55 mg.	2%
top sirloin steak	85 g.	170	60	6 g.	9%	2.5 g.	12%	75 mg.	25%	55 mg.	2%
Pork											
ham, canned reg.	85 g.	140	60	7 g.	11%	2.5 g.	12%	35 mg.	12%	910 mg.	38%
ham, canned extra lean	85 g.	120	35	4 g.	6%	1.5 g.	7%	25 mg.	9%	970 mg.	40%
ham, whole fresh	85 g.	130	40	4.5 g.	7%	1.5 g.	8%	45 mg.	16%	1130 mg.	47%
loin chop	85 g.	180	80	8 g.	13%	3 g.	15%	65 mg.	22%	55 mg.	2%
shoulder, lean	85 g.	200	100	11 g.	18%	4 g.	20%	75 mg.	26%	65 mg.	3%
spareribs, lean	85 g.	200	100	12 g.	18%	4 g.	21%	75 mg.	24%	55 mg.	2%
tenderloin	85 g.	170	70	8 g.	12%	3 g.	14%	65 mg.	22%	45 mg.	2%
tipless tenderloin	85 g.	140	35	4 g.	6%	1.5 g.	7%	65 mg.	22%	50 mg.	2%
Lamb											
chop, arm trimmed	85 g.	170	70	8 g.	12%	3 g.	15%	80 mg.	26%	70 mg.	3%
leg of lamb	85 g.	160	60	7 g.	10%	2.5 g.	12%	75 mg.	25%	60 mg.	2%
Game Meats											
buffalo	85 g.	120	20	2 g.	3%	1 g.	4%	70 mg.	23%	50 mg.	2%
venison	85 g.	130	25	2.5 g.	4%	1 g.	5%	95 mg.	32%	45 mg.	2%

Carbohydrates	% Daily Values	Fiber	% Daily Values	Sugars- Natural and Added	Protein	Vitamin A	% Daily Values	Vitamin C	% Daily Values	Calcium	% Daily Values	Iron	% Daily Values
1 g.	0%	0 g.	0%	1 g.	7 g.	0 i.u.	0%	15 mg.	25%	20 mg.	2%	.72 mg.	4%
0 g.	0%	0 g.	0%	0 g.	27 g.	0 i.u.	0%	0 mg.	0%	0 mg.	0%	2.7 mg.	15%
0 g.	0%	0 g.	0%	0 g.	20 g.	0 i.u.	0%	0 mg.	0%	0 mg.	0%	1.8 mg.	10%
0 g.	0%	0 g.	0%	0 g.	26 g.	0 i.u.	0%	0 mg.	0%	20 mg.	2%	2.7 mg.	15%
0 g.	0%	0 g.	0%	0 g.	24 g.	0 i.u.	0%	0 mg.	0%	0 mg.	0%	2.7 mg.	15%
0 g.	0%	0 g.	0%	0 g.	24 g.	0 i.u.	0%	0 mg.	0%	0 mg.	0%	1.8 mg.	10%
0 g.	0%	0 g.	0%	0 g.	23 g.	0 i.u.	0%	0 mg.	0%	0 mg.	0%	2.7 mg.	15%
0 g.	0%	0 g.	0%	0 g.	26 g.	0 i.u.	0%	0 mg.	0%	0 mg.	0%	2.7 mg.	15%
0 g.	0%	0 g.	0%	0 g.	24 g.	0 i.u.	0%	0 mg.	0%	0 mg.	0%	2.7 mg.	15%
0 g.	0%	0 g.	0%	0 g.	26 g.	0 i.u.	0%	0 mg.	0%	0 mg.	0%	2.7 mg.	0%
0 g.	0%	0 g.	0%	0 g.	18 g.	0 i.u.	0%	18 mg.	30%	0 mg.	0%	1.08 mg.	6%
0 g.	0%	0 g.	0%	0 g.	18 g.	0 i.u.	0%	24 mg.	40%	0 mg.	0%	.72 mg.	4%
0 g.	0%	0 g.	0%	0 g.	21 g.	0 i.u.	0%	0 mg.	0%	0 mg.	0%	.72 mg.	4%
0 g.	0%	0 g.	0%	0 g.	24 g.	0 i.u.	0%	0 mg.	0%	20 mg.	0%	.72 mg.	4%
0 g.	0%	0 g.	0%	0 g.	22 g.	0 i.u.	0%	0 mg.	0%	20 mg.	0%	1.44 mg.	8%
0 g.	0%	0 g.	0%	0 g.	22 g.	0 i.u.	0%	1.2 mg.	0%	20 mg.	2%	1.08 mg.	6%
0 g.	0%	0 g.	0%	0 g.	24 g.	0 i.u.	0%	0 mg.	0%	20 mg.	2%	1.08 mg.	6%
0 g.	0%	0 g.	0%	0 g.	24 g.	0 i.u.	0%	0 mg.	0%	0 mg.	0%	1.08 mg.	6%
0 g.	0%	0 g.	0%	0 g.	24 g.	0 i.u.	0%	0 mg.	0%	20 mg.	2%	1.8 mg.	10%
0 g.	0%	0 g.	0%	0 g.	24 g.	0 i.u.	0%	0 mg.	0%	0 mg.	0%	1.8 mg.	10%
0 g.	0%	0 g.	0%	0 g.	24 g.	N/S	0%	N/S	0%	N/S	0%	2.7 mg.	15%
0 g.	0%	0 g.	0%	0 g.	26 g.	N/S	0%	N/S	0%	N/S	0%	3.6 mg.	20%

Food	Weight Per Serving	Calories	Calories from Fat	Fat	% Daily Values	Saturated Fat	% Daily Values	Cholesterol	% Daily Values	Sodium	% Daily Values
venison sausage	85 g.	270	220	24 g.	37%	10 g.	51%	50 mg.	16%	830 mg.	35%
water buffalo	85 g.	110	15	1.5 g.	2%	0.5 g.	3%	50 mg.	17%	50 mg.	2%

POULTRY (3 oz. cooked/roasted or as noted)

chicken

Food	Weight Per Serving	Calories	Calories from Fat	Fat	% Daily Values	Saturated Fat	% Daily Values	Cholesterol	% Daily Values	Sodium	% Daily Values
breast, no skin	85 g.	140	25	3 g.	5%	1 g.	4%	70 mg.	24%	65 mg.	3%
breast, w/ skin	85 g.	170	60	7 g.	10%	2 g.	9%	70 mg.	24%	60 mg.	3%
drumstick, no skin	85 g.	150	45	5 g.	7%	1.5 g.	6%	80 mg.	26%	80 mg.	3%
drumstick, w/ skin	85 g.	180	90	10 g.	15%	2.5 g.	13%	75 mg.	26%	75 mg.	3%
wing, no skin	85 g.	170	60	7 g.	11%	2 g.	10%	70 mg.	24%	80 mg.	3%
wing, w/ skin	85 g.	250	150	17 g.	26%	4.5 g.	23%	70 mg.	24%	70 mg.	3%

turkey

Food	Weight Per Serving	Calories	Calories from Fat	Fat	% Daily Values	Saturated Fat	% Daily Values	Cholesterol	% Daily Values	Sodium	% Daily Values
dark meat, no skin	85 g.	160	60	6 g.	9%	2 g.	10%	70 mg.	24%	65 mg.	3%
ground turkey	85 g.	200	100	11 g.	17%	3 g.	14%	85 mg.	29%	90 mg.	4%
turkey hotdog (1)	45 g.	100	70	8 g.	12%	2.5 g.	13%	50 mg.	16%	640 mg.	27%
turkey sausage	85 g.	190	130	14 g.	21%	5 g.	24%	70 mg.	23%	570 mg.	24%
white meat, no skin	85 g.	120	10	1 g.	2%	0 g.	0%	75 mg.	24%	50 mg.	2%

FISH/SEAFOOD (3 oz. or quantities as noted, baked, broiled, steamed, or boiled)

Food	Weight Per Serving	Calories	Calories from Fat	Fat	% Daily Values	Saturated Fat	% Daily Values	Cholesterol	% Daily Values	Sodium	% Daily Values
blue crab	85 g.	90	15	1.5 g.	2%	0 g.	0%	85 mg.	28%	240 mg.	10%
catfish	85 g.	130	60	7 g.	11%	1.5 g.	8%	55 mg.	18%	70 mg.	3%
clams (12 small)	54 g.	80	10	1 g.	2%	0 g.	0%	35 mg.	12%	60 mg.	3%
cod	85 g.	90	5	0.5 g.	1%	0 g.	0%	45 mg.	16%	65 mg.	3%
haddock	85 g.	100	5	1 g.	1%	0 g.	0%	65 mg.	21%	75 mg.	3%
halibut	85 g.	20	25	2.5 g.	4%	0 g.	0%	35 mg.	12%	60 mg.	2%
lobster	85 g.	80	5	0.5 g.	1%	0 g.	0%	60 mg.	20%	320 mg.	13%
mackerel	85 g.	220	140	15 g.	23%	3.5 g.	18%	65 mg.	21%	70 mg.	3%
mahi-mahi	85 g.	70	5	1 g.	1%	0 g.	0%	20 mg.	7%	70 mg.	3%
ocean perch	85 g.	100	15	2 g.	3%	0 g.	0%	45 mg.	15%	80 mg.	3%

Carbohydrates	% Daily Values	Fiber	% Daily Values	Sugars- Natural and Added	Protein	Vitamin A	% Daily Values	Vitamin C	% Daily Values	Calcium	% Daily Values	Iron	% Daily Values
1 g.	0%	0 g.	0%	1 g.	10 g.	N/S	0%	18 mg.	30%	20 mg.	2%	1.44 mg.	8%
0 g.	0%	0 g.	0%	0 g.	23 g.	N/S	0%	N/S	0%	20 mg.	2%	1.8 mg.	10%
0 g.	0%	0 g.	0%	0 g.	26 g.	N/S	0%	0 mg.	0%	20 mg.	2%	.72 mg.	4%
0 g.	0%	0 g.	0%	0 g.	25 g.	100 i.u.	2%	0 mg.	0%	20 mg.	2%	1.08 mg.	6%
0 g.	0%	0 g.	0%	0 g.	24 g.	100 i.u.	2%	0 mg.	0%	20 mg.	2%	1.08 mg.	6%
0 g.	0%	0 g.	05%	0 g.	23 g.	100 i.u.	2%	0 mg.	0%	20 mg.	2%	1.08 mg.	6%
0 g.	0%	0 g.	0%	0 g.	26 g.	100 i.u.	2%	0 mg.	0%	20 mg.	2%	1.08 mg.	6%
0 g.	0%	0 g.	0%	0 g.	23 g.	100 i.u.	2%	0 mg.	0%	20 mg.	2%	1.08 mg.	6%
0 g.	0%	0 g.	0%	0 g.	24 g.	0 i.u.	0%	0 mg.	0%	20 mg.	2%	1.8 mg.	10%
0 g.	0%	0 g.	0%	0 g.	23 g.	0 i.u.	0%	0 mg.	0%	20 mg.	2%	1.8 mg.	10%
1 g.	0%	0 g.	0%	1 g.	6 g.	0 i.u.	0%	0 mg.	0%	40 mg.	4%	.72 mg.	4%
0 g.	0%	0 g.	0%	N/S	19 g.	0 i.u.	0%	0 mg.	0%	20 mg.	2%	1.44 mg.	8%
0 g.	0%	0 g.	0%	0 g.	26 g.	0 i.u.	0%	0 mg.	0%	20 mg.	2%	1.44 mg.	8%
0 g.	0%	0 g.	0%	0 g.	17 g.	0 i.u.	0%	2.4 mg.	4%	80 mg.	8%	.72 mg.	4%
0 g.	0%	0 g.	0%	0 g.	16 g.	0 i.u.	0%	1.2 mg.	2%	0 mg.	0%	.72 mg.	4%
3 g.	1%	0 g.	0%	1 g.	14 g.	300 i.u.	6%	12 mg.	20%	40 mg.	4%	.36 mg.	2%
0 g.	0%	0 g.	0%	0 g.	19 g.	0 i.u.	0%	1.2 mg.	2%	20 gm.	2%	.36 mg.	2%
0 g.	0%	0 g.	0%	0 g.	21 g.	100 i.u.	2%	0 mg.	0%	40 mg.	4%	1.08 mg.	6%
0 g.	0%	0 g.	0%	0 g.	23 g.	200 i.u.	4%	0 mg.	0%	60 mg.	6%	1.08 mg.	6%
1 g.	0%	0 g.	0%	0 g.	17 g.	100 i.u.	2%	0 mg.	0%	60 mg.	6%	.36 mg.	6%
0 g.	0%	0 g.	0%	0 g.	20 g.	200 i.u.	4%	0 mg.	0%	20 mg.	2%	1.44 mg.	6%
0 g.	0%	0 g.	0%	0 g.	16 g.	N/S	0%	N/S	0%	N/S	0%	N/S	0%
0 g.	0%	0 g.	0%	0 g.	20 g.	0 i.u.	0%	1.2 mg.	2%	100 mg.	10%	1.08 mg.	6%

Food	Weight Per Serving	Calories	Calories from Fat	Fat	% Daily Values	Saturated Fat	% Daily Values	Cholesterol	% Daily Values	Sodium	% Daily Values
orange roughy	85 g.	80	5	1 g.	1%	0 g.	0%	20 mg.	7%	70 mg.	3%
oysters	85 g.	140	35	4 g.	6%	1 g.	4%	85 mg.	28%	180 mg.	8%
Pacific rockfish	85 g.	100	15	1.5 g.	3%	0 g.	0%	35 mg.	12%	65 mg.	3%
pollock	85 g.	100	10	1 g.	2%	0 g.	0%	75 mg.	26%	95 mg.	4%
rainbow trout	85 g.	130	45	5 g.	8%	1.5 g.	7%	60 mg.	20%	50 mg.	2%
salmon	85 g.	150	60	7 g.	11%	1 g.	5%	60 mg.	20%	50 mg.	2%
shrimp	85 g.	80	10	1 g.	1%	0 g.	0%	165 mg.	55%	190 mg.	8%
sole/flounder	85 g.	100	10	1.5 g.	2%	0 g.	0%	60 mg.	19%	90 mg.	4%
swordfish	85 g.	130	40	4.5 g.	7%	1 g.	6%	45 mg.	14%	100 mg.	4%
tuna, canned/ water	85 g.	100	5	0.5 g.	1%	0 g.	0%	25 mg.	9%	290 mg.	12%
tuna, fresh yellowfin	85 g.	120	10	1 g.	2%	0 g.	0%	50 mg.	16%	40 mg.	2%
whiting	85 g.	100	15	1.5 g.	2%	0 g.	0%	70 mg.	24%	110 mg.	5%
BEANS (1/2 cup cooked or as noted)											
anasazi beans	86 g.	110	0	0 g.	0%	0 g.	0%	0 mg.	0%	0 mg.	0%
azuki beans	85 g.	110	0	0 g.	0%	0 g.	0%	0 mg.	0%	0 mg.	0%
black beans	86 g.	110	0	0 g.	0%	0 g.	0%	0 mg.	0%	0 mg.	0%
blackeyed peas	85 g.	110	0	0 g.	0%	0 g.	0%	0 mg.	0%	0 mg.	0%
chickpeas/garbanzo	82 g.	130	20	2 g.	3%	0 g.	0%	0 mg.	0%	5 mg.	0%
great northerns	88 g.	100	0	0 g.	0%	0 g.	0%	0 mg.	0%	0 mg.	0%
kidney beans	88 g.	110	0	0 g.	0%	0 g.	0%	0 mg.	0%	0 mg.	0%
lentils, green	99 g.	110	0	0 g.	0%	0 g.	0%	0 mg.	0%	0 mg.	0%
lentils, red	131 g.	120	0	0 g.	0%	0 g.	0%	0 mg.	0%	15 mg.	1%
lima beans	94 g.	110	0	0 g.	0%	0 g.	0%	0 mg.	0%	0 mg.	0%
mung beans	86 g.	110	0	0 g.	0%	0 g.	0%	0 mg.	0%	0 mg.	0%
navy beans	91 g.	130	5	0.5 g.	1%	0 g.	0%	0 mg.	0%	0 mg.	0%
pinto beans	85 g.	120	0	0 g.	0%	0 g.	0%	0 mg.	0%	0 mg.	0%
refried beans	127 g.	135	13	1.5 g.	2%	0.5 g.	2%	0 mg.	0%	537 mg.	22%

Carbohydrates	% Daily Values	Fiber	% Daily Values	Sugars- Natural and Added	Protein	Vitamin A	% Daily Values	Vitamin C	% Daily Values	Calcium	% Daily Values	Iron	% Daily Values
0 g.	0%	0 g.	0%	0 g.	16 g.	100 i.u.	2%	0 mg.	0%	40 mg.	4%	.36 mg.	2%
8 g.	3%	0 g.	0%	0 g.	16 g.	400 i.u.	8%	12 mg.	20%	20 mg.	2%	8.1 mg.	45%
0 g.	0%	0 g.	0%	0 g.	20 g.	200 i.u.	4%	0 mg.	0%	20 mg.	2%	.36 mg.	2%
0 g.	0%	0 g.	0%	0 g.	21 g.	0 i.u.	0%	0 mg.	0%	60 mg.	6%	.36 mg.	2%
0 g.	0%	0 g.	0%	0 g.	19 g.	0 i.u.	0%	1.2 mg.	2%	80 mg.	8%	.36 mg.	2%
0 g.	0%	0 g.	0%	0 g.	22 g.	0 i.u.	0%	0 mg.	0%	20 mg.	2%	.72 mg.	4%
0 g.	0%	0 g.	0%	0 g.	18 g.	200 i.u.	4%	2.4 mg.	4%	40 mg.	4%	2.7 mg.	15%
0 g.	0%	0 g.	0%	0 g.	21 g.	0 i.u.	0%	1.2 mg.	2%	20 mg.	2%	.36 mg.	2%
0 g.	0%	0 g.	0%	0 g.	22 g.	100 i.u.	2%	1.2 mg.	2%	N/S	0%	.72 mg.	4%
0 g.	0%	0 g.	0%	0 g.	22 g.	0 i.u.	0%	0 mg.	0%	N/S	0%	1.44 mg.	8%
0 g.	0%	0 g.	0%	0 g.	26 g.	100 i.u.	2%	1.2 mg.	2%	20 mg.	2%	.72 mg.	4%
0 g.	0%	0 g.	0%	0 g.	20 g.	100 i.u.	2%	0 mg.	0%	60 mg.	6%	.36 mg.	2%
20 g.	7%	7 g.	30%	2 g.	8 g.	0 i.u.	0%	N/S	0%	20 mg.	2%	1.8 mg.	10%
20 g.	7%	5 g.	21%	2 g.	8 g.	0 i.u.	0%	N/S	0%	20 mg.	2%	2.7 mg.	15%
20 g.	7%	7 g.	30%	2 g.	8 g.	0 i.u.	0%	N/S	0%	20 mg.	2%	2.7 mg.	15%
18 g.	6%	6 g.	22%	3 g.	7 g.	0 i.u.	0%	N/S	0%	20 mg.	2%	1.8 mg.	10%
22 g.	7%	5 g.	20%	1 g.	7 g.	0 i.u.	0%	1.2 mg.	2%	40 mg.	4%	2.7 mg.	15%
19 g.	6%	6 g.	25%	2 g.	7 g.	0 i.u.	0%	1.2 mg.	2%	60 mg.	6%	1.8 mg.	10%
20 g.	7%	6 g.	23%	2 g.	8 g.	0 i.u.	0%	1.2 mg.	2%	20 mg.	2%	2.7 mg.	15%
20 g.	7%	8 g.	31%	2 g.	9 g.	0 i.u.	0%	1.2 mg.	2%	20 mg.	2%	3.6 mg.	20%
22 g.	7%	6 g.	22%	2 g.	9 g.	0 i.u.	0%	N/S	0%	40 mg.	4%	.72 mg.	4%
20 g.	7%	7 g.	26%	3 g.	7 g.	0 i.u.	0%	N/S	0%	20 mg.	2%	2.7 mg.	15%
20 g.	7%	6 g.	23%	2 g.	8 g.	0 i.u.	0%	N/S	0%	20 mg.	2%	2.7 mg.	15%
24 g.	8%	8 g.	32%	2 g.	8 g.	0 i.u.	0%	1.2 mg.	2%	60 mg.	6%	2.7 mg.	15%
22 g.	7%	7 g.	29%	2 g.	7 g.	0 i.u.	0%	1.2 mg.	2%	40 mg.	4%	1.8 mg.	10%
23 g.	8%	7 g.	27%	2 g.	8 g.	0 i.u.	0%	8 mg.	13%	60 mg.	6%	2.5 mg.	12%

Food	Weight Per Serving	Calories	Calories from Fat	Fat	% Daily Values	Saturated Fat	% Daily Values	Cholesterol	% Daily Values	Sodium	% Daily Values
soybeans	86 g.	150	70	8 g.	12%	1 g.	6%	0 mg.	0%	0 mg.	0%
split peas	98 g.	120	0	0 g.	0%	0 g.	0%	0 mg.	0%	0 mg.	0%
tempeh (3 oz.)	85 g.	170	60	7 g.	10%	1 g.	5%	0 mg.	0%	5 mg.	0%
tofu, White Wave™ firm (3 oz.)	90 g.	90	50	6 g.	9%	1 g.	4%	0 mg.	0%	10 mg.	0%
tofu, White Wave™ reduced fat (3 oz.)	91 g.	90	35	4 g.	6%	0 g.	0%	0 mg.	0%	5 mg.	0%
tofu, Mori-Nu™ silken soft (1/3 box: 3.5 oz.)	99 g.	53	25	3 g.	4.5%	0.5 g.	2%	0 mg.	0%	7 mg.	0%
tofu, Mori-Nu™ silken firm (1/3 box: 3.5 oz.)	99 g.	60	24	2.5 g.	4%	0.5 g.	2%	0 mg.	0%	33 mg.	1%
tofu, Mori-Nu™ silken extra firm (1/3 box: 3.5 oz.)	99 g.	53	19	2 g.	3%	0.5 g.	2%	0 mg.	0%	63 mg.	2.5%
EGGS											
egg white (1)	33 g.	15	0	0 g.	0%	0 g.	0%	N/S	0%	55 mg.	2%
egg yolk (1)	17 g.	60	45	5 g.	8%	1.5 g.	8%	215 mg.	71%	5 mg.	0%
egg, large raw	50 g.	70	45	5 g.	8%	1.5 g.	8%	215 mg.	71%	65 mg.	3%
egg, fried in butter	46 g.	95	63	7 g.	11%	2 g.	10%	215 mg.	71%	160 mg.	7%
egg omelet	59 g.	90	60	7 g.	10%	2 g.	9%	205 mg.	69%	160 mg.	7%
egg, poached	50 g.	70	45	5 g.	8%	1.5 g.	8%	210 mg.	71%	60 mg.	3%
egg, scrambled w/milk/butter	61 g.	100	70	7 g.	11%	2 g.	11%	215 mg.	72%	170 mg.	7%
NUTS/SEEDS (1/3 cup whole/ 2 Tbsp. nut butter)											
almond butter	32 g.	200	170	19 g.	29%	2 g.	9%	0 mg.	0%	0 mg.	0%
almonds	47 g.	280	220	24 g.	38%	2.5 g.	12%	0 mg.	0%	5 mg.	0%
brazil nuts	46 g.	300	280	31 g.	47%	7 g.	37%	0 mg.	0%	0 mg.	0%
cashew butter	32 g.	190	140	16 g.	24%	3 g.	16%	0 mg.	0%	0 mg.	0%
cashews, roasted	45 g.	260	190	21 g.	32%	4 g.	21%	0 mg.	0%	5 mg.	0%
chestnuts	48 g.	90	5	0.5 g.	1%	0 g.	0%	0 mg.	0%	0 mg.	0%
coconut, dried	26 g.	170	150	17 g.	26%	15 g.	74%	0 mg.	0%	10 mg.	0%
hazelnuts/filberts	45 g.	280	250	28 g.	43%	2 g.	10%	0 mg.	0%	0 mg.	0%
macadamia nuts	44 g.	310	290	33 g.	50%	5 g.	24%	0 mg.	0%	0 mg.	0%
peanut butter, chunky	32 g.	190	140	16 g.	24%	3 g.	15%	0 mg.	0%	5 mg.	0%

Carbohydrates	% Daily Values	Fiber	% Daily Values	Sugars- Natural and Added	Protein	Vitamin A	% Daily Values	Vitamin C	% Daily Values	Calcium	% Daily Values	Iron	% Daily Values
9 g.	3%	5 g.	21%	3 g.	14 g.	0 i.u.	0%	1.2 mg.	2%	80 mg.	8%	4.5 mg.	25%
21 g.	7%	8 g.	33%	3 g.	8 g.	0 i.u.	0%	N/S	0%	20 mg.	2%	1.44 mg.	8%
14 g.	5%	1.2 g.	9%	4 g.	16 g.	500 i.u.	10%	N/S	0%	80 mg.	8%	1.8 mg.	10%
1 g.	0%	1 g.	2%	N/S	10 g.	N/S	0%	N/S	0%	100 mg.	10%	1.8 mg.	10%
4 g.	2%	2 g.	6%	N/S	10 g.	N/S	0%	N/S	0%	40 mg.	4%	1.44 mg.	8%
2.5 g.	1%	N/S	0%	N/S	4.5 g.	N/S	0%	N/S	0%	30 mg.	3%	.8 mg.	4.5%
2.5 g.	1%	N/S	0%	N/S	6.5 g.	N/S	0%	N/S	0%	30 mg.	3%	1.08 mg.	6%
2.5 g.	1%	N/S	0%	N/S	8 g.	N/S	0%	N/S	0%	35.5 mg.	3.5%	1.08 mg.	6%
0 g.	0%	0 g.	0%	0 g.	4 g.	0 i.u.	0%	0 mg.	0%	N/S	0%	N/S	0%
0 g.	0%	0 g.	0%	0 g.	3 g.	300 i.u.	6%	0 mg.	0%	20 mg.	2%	.72 mg.	4%
1 g.	0%	0 g.	0%	1 g.	6 g.	300 i.u.	6%	0 mg.	0%	20 mg.	2%	.72 mg.	4%
1 g.	0%	0 g.	0%	1 g.	6 g.	400 i.u.	8%	0 mg.	0%	20 mg.	2%	.72 mg.	4%
1 g.	0%	0 g.	0%	0 g.	6 g.	400 i.u.	8%	0 mg.	0%	20 mg.	2%	.72 mg.	4%
1 g.	0%	0 g.	0%	1 g.	6 g.	300 i.u.	6%	0 mg.	0%	20 mg.	2%	.72 mg.	4%
1 g.	0%	0 g.	0%	1 g.	7 g.	400 i.u.	8%	N/S	0%	40 mg.	4%	.72 mg.	4%
7 g.	2%	1 g.	5%	3 g.	5 g.	0 i.u.	0%	0 mg.	0%	80 mg.	8%	1.08 mg.	6%
10 g.	3%	5 g.	20%	3 g.	9 g.	0 i.u.	0%	0 mg.	0%	100 mg.	10%	1.8 mg.	10%
6 g.	2%	3 g.	11%	1 g.	7 g.	0 i.u.	0%	0 mg.	0%	80 mg.	8%	1.44 mg.	8%
9 g.	3%	1 g.	3%	2 g.	6 g.	0 i.u.	0%	0 mg.	0%	20 mg.	2%	1.44 mg.	8%
15 g.	5%	1 g.	5%	3 g.	7 g.	0 i.u.	0%	0 mg.	0%	20 mg.	2%	2.7 mg.	15%
21 g.	7%	5 g.	21%	5 g.	1 g.	0 i.u.	0%	18 mg.	30%	N/S	0%	.36 mg.	2%
6 g.	2%	4 g.	17%	2 g.	2 g.	0 i.u.	0%	0 mg.	0%	N/S	0%	.72 mg.	4%
7 g.	2%	3 g.	11%	2 g.	6 g.	0 i.u.	0%	0 mg.	0%	80 mg.	8%	1.44 mg.	8%
6 g.	2%	4 g.	16%	2 g.	4 g.	0 i.u.	0%	0 mg.	0%	40 mg.	4%	1.08 mg.	6%
7 g.	2%	2 g.	8%	3 g.	8 g.	0 i.u.	0%	0 mg.	0%	20 mg.	2%	.72 mg.	4%

Food	Weight Per Serving	Calories	Calories from Fat	Fat	% Daily Values	Saturated Fat	% Daily Values	Cholesterol	% Daily Values	Sodium	% Daily Values
peanuts, dry roasted	48 g.	280	220	24 g.	37%	3.5 g.	17%	0 mg.	0%	0 mg.	0%
pecans	36 g.	240	220	24 g.	37%	2 g.	10%	0 mg.	0%	0 mg.	0%
pine nuts	40 g.	230	220	24 g.	38%	4 g.	19%	0 mg.	0%	30 mg.	1%
pistachio nuts	42 g.	240	180	20 g.	31%	2.5 g.	13%	0 mg.	0%	0 mg.	0%
pumpkin seeds, rstd	21 g.	90	35	4 g.	6%	1 g.	4%	0 mg.	0%	0 mg.	0%
sesame seeds, hulled	48 g.	280	210	23 g.	36%	3.5 g.	17%	0 mg.	0%	15 mg.	1%
sesame seeds, whole	48 g.	270	210	24 g.	36%	3.5 g.	17%	0 mg.	0%	5 mg.	0%
sesame tahini	30 g.	180	160	18 g.	27%	2.5 g.	12%	0 mg.	0%	5 mg.	0%
sunflower seeds	48 g.	270	210	24 g.	36%	2.5 g.	12%	0 mg.	0%	0 mg.	0%
walnuts	33 g.	210	180	20 g.	31%	2 g.	9%	0 mg.	0%	0 mg.	0%
DAIRY (1 cup milk, yogurt & non-dairy alternatives and 1½ oz. cheese, or as noted)											
cream, half & half (2 Tbsp.)	30 ml.	30	30	3.5 g.	5%	2 g.	11%	10 mg.	4%	10 mg.	1%
cream, heavy (2 Tbsp.)	30 ml.	100	100	11 g.	17%	7 g.	34%	40 mg.	14%	10 mg.	0%
cream, light (2 Tbsp.)	30 ml.	90	80	9 g.	14%	6 g.	29%	35 mg.	11%	10 mg.	0%
cream, sour (2 Tbsp.)	29 ml.	60	50	6 g.	9%	3.5 g.	19%	15 mg.	4%	15 mg.	1%
milk, 1% - vit. A added	240 ml.	100	20	2.5 g.	4%	1.5 g.	7%	10 mg.	3%	115 mg.	5%
milk, 2% - vit A added	240 ml.	110	40	4.5 g.	7%	2.5 g.	14%	15 mg.	6%	115 mg.	5%
milk, goat	240 ml.	160	80	9 g.	14%	6 g.	30%	25 mg.	9%	115 mg.	5%
milk, nonfat dry (2 Tbsp.)	15 g.	50	0	0 g.	0%	0 g.	0%	5 mg.	1%	80 mg.	3%
milk, skim - vit A added	240 ml.	80	0	0 g.	0%	0 g.	0%	5 mg.	1%	115 mg.	5%
milk, whole	240 ml.	140	70	8 g.	12%	4.5 g.	24%	30 mg.	10%	110 mg.	5%
yogurt cheese (2 Tbsp.)	30 ml.	30	10	1 g.	1%	0.5 g.	3%	5 mg.	1%	25 mg.	1%
yogurt, goat	227 g.	130	50	6 g.	10%	5 g.	24%	28 gm.	9%	120 mg.	5%
yogurt, lowfat	227 g.	140	30	3.5 g.	5%	2.5 g.	11%	15 mg.	5%	160 mg.	7%
yogurt, nonfat	227 g.	130	0	0 g.	0%	0 g.	0%	5 mg.	1%	170 mg.	7%
yogurt, whole milk	227 g.	140	70	7 g.	11%	5 g.	24%	30 mg.	10%	105 mg.	4%

Carbohydrates	% Daily Values	Fiber	% Daily Values	Sugars- Natural and Added	Protein	Vitamin A	% Daily Values	Vitamin C	% Daily Values	Calcium	% Daily Values	Iron	% Daily Values
10 g.	3%	4 g.	15%	2 g.	11 g.	0 i.u.	0%	0 mg.	0%	20 mg.	2%	1.08 mg.	6%
6 g.	2%	3 g.	11%	2 g.	3 g.	0 i.u.	0%	1.2 mg.	2%	20 mg.	2%	.72 mg.	4%
8 g.	3%	4 g.	17%	2 g.	5 g.	0 i.u.	0%	0 mg.	0%	N/S	0%	1.08 mg.	6%
10 g.	3%	5 g.	18%	3 g.	9 g.	200 i.u.	2%	3.6 mg.	6%	60 mg.	6%	2.7 mg.	15%
11 g.	4%	8 g.	30%	1 g.	4 g.	0 i.u.	0%	0 mg.	0%	20 mg.	2%	.72 mg.	4%
6 g.	2%	6 g.	25%	1 g.	10 g.	0 i.u.	0%	0 mg.	0%	60 mg.	6%	1.44 mg.	8%
11 g.	4%	6 g.	22%	1 g.	8 g.	0 i.u.	0%	0 mg.	0%	450 mg.	45%	5 mg.	27%
5 g.	2%	3 g.	11%	1 g.	6 g.	0 i.u.	0%	0 mg.	0%	40 mg.	4%	.72 mg.	4%
9 g.	3%	5 g.	20%	2 g.	11 g.	0 i.u.	0%	0 mg.	0%	60 mg.	6%	3.6 mg.	20%
6 g.	2%	2 g.	6%	1 g.	5 g.	0 i.u.	0%	0 mg.	0%	40 mg.	4%	.72 mg.	4%
1 g.	0%	0 g.	0%	1 g.	1 g.	100 i.u.	2%	0 mg.	0%	40 mg.	4%	N/S	0%
1 g.	0%	0 g.	0%	1 g.	1 g.	400 i.u.	8%	0 mg.	0%	20 mg.	2%	N/S	0%
1 g.	0%	0 g.	0%	1 g.	1 g.	300 i.u.	6%	0 mg.	0%	20 mg.	2%	N/S	0%
1 g.	0%	0 g.	0%	1 g.	1 g.	200 i.u.	4%	0 mg.	0%	40 mg.	4%	N/S	0%
11 g.	4%	0 g.	0%	11 g.	7 g.	500 i.u.	10%	2.4 mg.	4%	300 mg.	30%	N/S	0%
11 g.	4%	0 g.	0%	11 g.	8 g.	500 i.u.	10%	2.4 mg.	4%	300 mg.	30%	N/S	0%
10 g.	3%	0 g.	0%	10 g.	8 g.	400 i.u.	8%	2.4 mg.	4%	300 mg.	30%	N/S	0%
8 g.	3%	0 g.	0%	8 g.	5 g.	N/S	0%	1.2 mg.	2%	20 mg.	20%	N/S	0%
11 g.	4%	0 g.	0%	11 g.	8 g.	500 i.u.	10%	2.4 mg.	4%	300 mg.	30%	N/S	0%
11 g.	4%	0 g.	0%	11 g.	7 g.	300 i.u.	6%	2.4 mg.	4%	250 mg.	25%	N/S	0%
3 g.	1%	0 g.	0%	3 g.	3 g.	N/S	0%	0 mg.	0%	100 mg.	10%	N/S	0%
10 g.	3%	0 g.	0%	7 g.	8 g.	N/S	0%	1.2 mg.	2%	240 mg.	24%	N/S	0%
16 g.	5%	0 g.	0%	16 g.	12 g.	100 i.u.	2%	2.4 mg.	4%	400 mg.	40%	.36 mg.	2%
17 g.	6%	0 g.	0%	17 g.	13 g.	N/S	0%	2.4 mg.	4%	450 mg.	45%	.36 mg.	2%
11 g.	4%	0 g.	0%	11 g.	8 g.	300 i.u.	6%	2.4 mg.	4%	250 mg.	25%	N/S	0%

Food	Weight Per Serving	Calories	Calories from Fat	Fat	% Daily Values	Saturated Fat	% Daily Values	Cholesterol	% Daily Values	Sodium	% Daily Values
Non-Dairy Alternatives (1 cup or as noted)											
almond milk											
Almond Mylk (Wholesome & Hearty™)	240 ml.	80	40	4 g.	6%	0 g.	0%	0 mg.	0%	190 g.	8%
homemade	240 ml.	91	58	6.5 g.	10%	0.5 g.	3%	0 mg.	0%	8 mg.	0%
amasake, Grainaissance Amazake™											
almond	237 ml.	200	35	4 g.	7%	.5 g.	2%	0 mg.	0%	20 mg.	1%
almond light	237 ml.	110	20	2 g.	3%	0 g.	0%	0 mg.	0%	75 mg.	3%
plain	237 ml.	150	0	0 g.	0%	0 g.	0%	0 mg.	0%	20 mg.	1%
plain light	237 ml.	90	0	0 g.	0%	0 g.	0%	0 mg.	0%	75 mg.	3%
rice milk											
EdenRice ™	240 ml.	110	25	3 g.	4%	0.5 g.	2%	0 mg.	0%	85 mg.	4%
Rice Dream™ beverage	240 ml.	120	18	2 g.	3%	0 g.	0%	0 mg.	0%	80 mg.	3.5%
Rice Dream™ enriched	240 ml.	120	20	2 g.	3%	0 g.	0%	0 mg.	0%	90 mg.	4%
Westbrae Rice Drink™	240 ml.	100	25	3 g.	5%	0.5 g.	0%	0 mg.	0%	70 mg.	3%
rice/soy milk											
EdenBlend™	240 ml.	120	30	3 g.	4%	0.5 g.	2%	0 mg.	0%	85 mg.	4%
soymilk											
Edensoy™ Extra	240 ml.	130	45	5 g.	8%	0.5 g.	2%	0 mg.	0%	100 mg.	4%
Edensoy™ plain	240 ml.	130	35	4 g.	6%	0.5 g.	2%	0 mg.	0%	105 mg.	4%
Westsoy™ plain	240 ml.	140	45	5 g.	8%	1 g.	5%	0 mg.	0%	140 mg.	6%
Westsoy™ plain lite	240 ml.	100	20	2 g.	3%	0.5 g.	2%	0 mg.	0%	120 mg.	5%
soy yogurt											
White Wave™ vanilla (6 oz.)	171 g.	140	25	2.5 g.	4%	0 g.	0%	0 mg.	0%	45 mg.	2%
Cheeses (1 1/2 oz. cheese, 1/2 cup fresh or cottage cheese, or as noted)											
blue cheese	43 g.	150	110	12 g.	19%	8 g.	40%	30 mg.	11%	590 mg.	25%
brick	43 g.	160	110	13 g.	19%	8 g.	40%	30 mg.	13%	240 mg.	10%
brie	43 g.	140	110	12 g.	18%	7 g.	37%	45 mg.	14%	270 mg.	11%

Carbohydrates	% Daily Values	Fiber	% Daily Values	Sugars- Natural and Added	Protein	Vitamin A	% Daily Values	Vitamin C	% Daily Values	Calcium	% Daily Values	Iron	% Daily Values
6 g.	3%	2 g.	8%	6 g.	2 g.	100 i.u.	2%	N/S	0%	N/S	0%	.36 mg.	2%
7.5 g.	2.5%	1.5 g.	5.5%	5 g.	2.5 g.	0 i.u	0%	N/S	0%	40 mg.	4%	1.52 mg.	8.5%
35 g.	12%	5 g.	20%	31 g.	4 g.	0 i.u.	0%	0 mg.	0%	40 mg.	4%	1.44 mg.	8%
20 g.	7%	2 g.	8%	19 g.	2 g.	0 i.u.	0%	0 mg.	0%	0 mg.	0%	.36 mg.	2%
34 g.	11%	4 g.	16%	30 g.	3 g.	0 i.u.	0%	0 mg.	0%	20 mg.	2%	1.08 mg.	6%
20 mg.	7%	2 g.	8%	19 g.	2 g.	0 i.u.	0%	0 mg.	0%	0 mg.	0%	.36 mg.	2%
21 g.	7%	0 g.	0%	16 g.	1 g.	0 i.u.	0%	0 mg.	0%	40 mg.	4%	.36 mg.	2%
25 g.	8.5%	0 g.	0%	11 g.	1 g.	0 i.u.	0%	0 mg.	0%	20 mg.	2%	.36 mg.	2%
25 g.	8.5%	0 g.	0%	11 g.	1 g.	500 i.u.	10%	0 mg.	0%	300 mg.	30%	0 mg.	0%
18 g.	6%	0 g.	0%	18 g.	1 g.	500 i.u.	10%	0 mg.	0%	250 mg.	25%	0 mg.	0%
16 g.	5%	0 g.	0%	12 g.	7 g.	0 i.u.	0%	0 mg.	0%	20 mg.	2%	1.08 mg.	6%
12 g.	4%	0 g.	0%	7 g.	9 g.	1500 i.u.	30%	0 mg.	0%	20 mg.	2%	1.8 mg.	10%
13 g.	4%	0 g.	0%	7 g.	10 g.	0 i.u.	0%	0 mg.	0%	80 mg.	8%	1.8 mg.	10%
18 g.	6%	0 g.	0%	12 g.	5 g.	0 i.u.	0%	0 mg.	0%	20 mg.	2%	.36 mg.	2%
15 g.	5%	0 g.	0%	10 g.	3 g.	0 i.u.	0%	0 mg.	0%	20 mg.	2%	.36 mg.	2%
23 g.	8%	1 g.	4%	10 g.	6 g.	0 i.u.	0%	0 mg.	0%	20 mg.	2%	1.44 mg.	8%
1 g.	0%	0 g.	0%	1 g.	9 g.	300 i.u.	6%	0 mg.	0%	200 mg.	20%	N/S	0%
1 g.	0%	0 g.	0%	1 g.	10 g.	500 i.u.	10%	0 mg.	0%	300 mg.	30%	.36 mg.	2%
0 g.	0%	0 g.	0%	0 g.	9 g.	300 i.u.	6%	0 mg.	0%	80 mg.	8%	.36 mg.	2%

Food	Weight Per Serving	Calories	Calories from Fat	Fat	% Daily Values	Saturated Fat	% Daily Values	Cholesterol	% Daily Values	Sodium	% Daily Values
camembert	43 g.	130	90	10 g.	16%	7 g.	33%	30 mg.	10%	360 mg.	15%
cheddar cheese	43 g.	170	130	14 g.	22%	9 g.	45%	45 mg.	15%	260 mg.	11%
cheddar, Cabot VitaLait™	43 g.	105	60	7 g.	10%	4.5 g.	23%	23 mg.	7.5 %	255 mg.	10.5%
colby	43 g.	170	120	14 g.	21%	9 g.	43%	40 mg.	13%	260 mg.	11%
cottage cheese, creamed	105 g.	110	45	4.5 g.	7%	3 g.	15%	15 mg.	5%	430 mg.	18%
cream cheese (2 Tbsp.)	29 g.	100	90	10 g.	16%	6 g.	32%	30 mg.	11%	85 mg.	4%
edam	43 g.	150	110	12 g.	18%	7 g.	37%	40 mg.	13%	410 mg.	17%
feta	43 g.	110	80	9 g.	14%	6 g.	32%	40 mg.	13%	470 mg.	20%
goat cheddar	43 g.	190	140	15 g.	23%	10 g.	52%	45 mg.	15%	150 mg.	6%
gorgonzola	43 g.	170	120	13 g.	21%	8 g.	41%	35 mg.	12%	770 mg.	32%
gruyere	43 g.	180	120	14 g.	21%	8 g.	40%	45 mg.	16%	140 mg.	6%
monterrey jack	43 g.	160	120	13 g.	20%	8 g.	41%	40 mg.	13%	230 mg.	9%
mozzarella, part skim	43 g.	120	70	7 g.	11%	4.5 g.	23%	25 mg.	8%	220 mg.	9%
mozzarella, whole milk	43 g.	120	80	9 g.	14%	6 g.	28%	35 mg.	11%	160 mg.	7%
Parmesan (2 Tbsp.)	12 g.	60	35	4 g.	6%	2.5 g.	12%	10 mg.	3%	230 mg.	10%
provolone	43 g.	150	100	11 g.	36%	7 g.	36%	30 mg.	10%	370 mg.	16%
ricotta (1/2 cup)	123 g.	170	90	10 g.	15%	6 g.	30%	40 mg.	13%	150 mg.	6%
romano (2 Tbsp.)	12 g.	50	30	3.5 g.	5%	2 g.	11%	15 mg.	4%	150 mg.	6%
Swiss cheese	43 g.	160	110	12 g.	18%	8 g.	38%	40 mg.	13%	110 mg.	5%
Non-Dairy Cheese Alternatives											
Soya Kaas™ cheddar style	43 g.	105	68	7.5 g.	11.5%	1 g.	4%	0 mg.	0%	375 mg.	16%
Soya Kaas™ mozzarella style	43 g.	105	69	7.5 g.	11.5%	1 g.	4%	0 mg.	0%	285 mg.	12%
Soyco™ soy parmesan (2 Tbsp.)	14 g.	35	15	1.5 g.	2.5%	0.5 g.	2%	0 mg.	0%	220 mg.	9%
FATS/OILS (1 Tbsp.)											
butter	14 g.	100	100	11 g.	18%	7 g.	36%	30 mg.	10%	115 mg.	5%
canola oil	14 g.	120	120	14 g.	21%	1 g.	5%	0 mg.	0%	0 mg.	0%
corn oil	14 g.	120	120	14 g.	22%	2 g.	9%	0 mg.	0%	0 mg.	0%

Carbohydrates	% Daily Values	Fiber	% Daily Values	Sugars- Natural and Added	Protein	Vitamin A	% Daily Values	Vitamin C	% Daily Values	Calcium	% Daily Values	Iron	% Daily Values
0 g.	0%	0 g.	0%	0 g.	8 g.	400 i.u.	8%	0 mg.	0%	150 mg.	15%	N/S	0%
1 g.	0%	0 g.	0%	1 g.	11 g.	500 i.u.	10%	0 mg.	0%	300 mg.	30%	.36 mg.	2%
1 g.	0%	0 g.	0%	0 g.	12 g.	500 i.u.	10%	0 mg.	0%	300 mg.	30%	N/S	0%
1 g.	0%	0 g.	0%	1 g.	10 g.	400 i.u.	8%	0 mg.	0%	300 mg.	30%	.36 mg.	2%
3 g.	1%	0 g.	0%	3 g.	13 g.	200 i.u.	4%	0 mg.	0%	60 mg.	6%	N/S	0%
1 g.	0%	0 g.	0%	1 g.	2 g.	400 i.u.	8%	0 mg.	0%	20 mg.	2%	.36 mg.	2%
1 g.	0%	0 g.	0%	1 g.	11 g.	400 i.u.	8%	0 mg.	0%	300 mg.	30%	.36 mg.	2%
2 g.	1%	0 g.	0%	2 g.	6 g.	200 i.u.	4%	0 mg.	0%	200 mg.	20%	.36 mg.	2%
1 g.	0%	0 g.	0%	1 g.	13 g.	750 i.u.	15%	0 mg.	0%	400 mg.	40%	.72 mg.	4%
0 g.	0%	0 g.	0%	0 g.	10 g.	500 i.u.	10%	0 mg.	0%	200 mg.	20%	N/S	0%
0 g.	0%	0 g.	0%	0 g.	13 g.	500 i.u.	10%	0 mg.	0%	450 mg.	45%	N/S	0%
0 g.	0%	0 g.	0%	N/S	10 g.	400 i.u.	8%	0 mg.	0%	300 mg.	30%	.36 mg.	2%
1 g.	0%	0 g.	0%	1 g.	12 g.	300 i.u.	6%	0 mg.	0%	300 mg.	30%	N/S	0%
1 g.	0%	0 g.	0%	1 g.	8 g.	300 i.u.	6%	0 mg.	0%	200 mg.	20%	N/S	0%
0 g.	0%	0 g.	0%	0 g.	5 g.	100 i.u.	2%	0 mg.	0%	150 mg.	15%	N/S	0%
1 g.	0%	0 g.	0%	1 g.	11 g.	300 i.u.	6%	0 mg.	0%	300 mg.	30%	.36 mg.	2%
6 g.	2%	0 g.	0%	6 g.	14 g.	500 i.u.	10%	0 mg.	0%	350 mg.	35%	.72 mg.	4%
0 g.	0%	0 g.	0%	0 g.	4 g.	100 i.u.	2%	0 mg.	0%	150 mg.	15%	N/S	0%
1 g.	0%	0 g.	0%	1 g.	12 g.	400 i.u.	8%	0 mg.	0%	400 mg.	40%	N/S	0%
1 g.	1%	0 g.	0%	0 g.	9 g.	N/S	0%	N/S	0%	N/S	0%	N/S	0%
1 g.	1%	0 g.	0%	0 g.	9 g.	N/S	0%	N/S	0%	N/S	0%	N/S	0%
1 g.	0%	0.5 g.	2%	0 g.	5 g.	250 i.u.	5%	0 mg.	0%	20 mg.	2%	N/S	0%
0 g.	0%	0 g.	0%	0 g.	0 g.	400 i.u.	0%	0 mg.	0%	0 mg.	0%	0 mg.	0%
0 g.	0%	0 g.	0%	0 g.	0 g.	0 i.u.	0%	0 mg.	0%	0 mg.	0%	0 mg.	0%
0 g.	0%	0 g.	0%	0 g.	0 g.	0 i.u.	0%	0 mg.	0%	0 mg.	0%	0 mg.	0%

Food	Weight Per Serving	Calories	Calories from Fat	Fat	% Daily Values	Saturated Fat	% Daily Values	Cholesterol	% Daily Values	Sodium	% Daily Values
flax seed oil	14 g.	120	120	14 g.	22%	1 g.	5%	0 mg.	0%	0 mg.	0%
margarine, stick & soft tub*	14 g.	100	100	11 g.	17%	2 g.	10%	0 mg.	0%	135 mg.	6%
mayonnaise	14 g.	100	100	11 g.	17%	1.5 g.	8%	10 mg.	3%	80 mg.	3%
olive oil	14 g.	120	120	14 g.	22%	2 g.	9%	0 mg.	0%	0 mg.	0%
peanut oil	14 g.	120	120	14 g.	22%	2 g.	12%	0 mg.	0%	0 mg.	0%
safflower hi-oleic oil	14 g.	120	120	14 g.	22%	1 g.	4%	0 mg.	0%	0 mg.	0%
safflower oil	14 g.	120	120	14 g.	22%	1.5 g.	6.5%	0 mg.	0%	0 mg.	0%
sesame oil	14 g.	120	120	14 g.	21%	2 g.	10%	0 mg.	0%	0 mg.	0%
Spectrum Spread™	14 g.	90	90	11 g.	17%	0.5 g.	3%	0 mg.	0%	85 mg.	0%
salad dressing (2 Tbsp.)											
Caesar, Newman's Own™	31 g.	150	140	16 g.	25%	1.5 g.	8%	3 mg.	1%	450 mg.	19%
French, Ayla's Fat-Free™	30 g.	10	0	0 g.	0%	0 g.	0%	0 mg.	0%	150 mg.	0%
French, typical	31 g.	130	120	13 g.	20%	3 g.	15%	0 mg.	0%	430 mg.	18%
Honey Mustard, Caesar Cardini™	30 g.	140	120	13 g.	20%	1.5 g.	8%	0 mg.	0%	195 mg.	7%
Italian, Pritikin™	31 g.	20	0	0 g.	0%	0 g.	0%	0 mg.	0%	115 mg.	5%
Lime Dill, Caesar Cardini™	30 g.	130	120	15 g.	23%	2 g.	10%	0 mg.	0%	195 mg.	7%
Miso Sesame, Simply Delicious™	30 g.	90	80	10 g.	16%	1 g.	4%	0 mg.	0%	210 mg.	8%
Oil & Vinegar, Newman's Own™	27 g.	150	150	16 g.	25%	2.5 g.	13%	0 mg.	0%	150 mg.	6%
Ranch, Newman's Own™	29 g.	180	170	19 g.	29%	3 g.	15%	5 mg.	2%	170 mg.	7%
Raspberry Vinaigrette, Annie's™	30 g.	110	80	9 g.	14%	0.5 g.	3%	0 mg.	0%	70 mg.	3%
Russian, Ayla's Fat-Free™	30 g.	10	0	0 g.	0%	0 g.	0%	0 mg.	0%	140 mg.	6%
Thousand Island, Hain™	31 g.	110	80	9 g.	14%	1.5 g.	8%	1 mg.	1%	180 mg.	8%
Tofu Poppyseed, Simply Delicious™	30 g.	90	80	8 g.	12%	1 g.	4%	0 mg.	0%	240 mg.	0%
SWEETS (1 Tbsp. or as noted)											
barbados molasses	20 g.	60	0	0 g.	0%	0 g.	0%	0 mg.	0%	0 mg.	0%
barley malt	21 g.	60	0	0 g.	0%	0 g.	0%	0 mg.	0%	0 mg.	0%
blackstrap molasses	20 g.	50	0	0 g.	0%	0 g.	0%	0 mg.	0%	10 mg.	0%

*margarines contain significant amounts of trans-fatty acids

Carbohydrates	% Daily Values	Fiber	% Daily Values	Sugars- Natural and Added	Protein	Vitamin A	% Daily Values	Vitamin C	% Daily Values	Calcium	% Daily Values	Iron	% Daily Values
0 g.	0%	0 g.	0%	0 g.	0 g.	0 i.u.	0%	0 mg.	0%	0 mg.	0%	0 mg.	0%
0 g.	0%	0 g.	0%	0 g.	0 g.	500 i.u.	10%	0 mg.	0%	0 mg.	0%	0 mg.	0%
0 g.	0%	0 g.	0%	0 g.	0 g.	N/S	0%	0 mg.	0%	N/S	0%	0 mg.	0%
0 g.	0%	0 g.	0%	0 g.	0 g.	0 i.u.	0%	0 mg.	0%	0 mg.	0%	0 mg.	0%
0 g.	0%	0 g.	0%	0 g.	0 g.	0 i.u.	0%	0 mg.	0%	0 mg.	0%	0 mg.	0%
0 g.	0%	0 g.	0%	0 g.	0 g.	0 i.u.	0%	0 mg.	0%	0 mg.	0%	0 mg.	0%
0 g.	0%	0 g.	0%	0 g.	0 g.	0 i.u.	0%	0 mg.	0%	0 mg.	0%	0 g.	0%
0 g.	0%	0 g.	0%	0 g.	0 g.	0 i.u.	0%	0 mg.	0%	0 mg.	0%	0 mg.	0%
0 g.	0%	0 g.	0%	0 g.	0 g.	0 i.u.	0%	0 mg.	0%	0 mg.	0%	0 mg.	0%
1 g.	0%	0 g.	0%	1 g.	1 g.	0 i.u.	0%	0 mg.	0%	0 mg.	0%	0 mg.	0%
3 g.	1%	0 g.	0%	2 g.	0 g.	100 i.u.	2%	1.8 mg.	3%	0 mg.	0%	0 mg.	0%
5 g.	2%	0 g.	0%	5 g.	0 g.	0 i.u.	0%	0 mg.	0%	0 mg.	0%	0 mg.	0%
4 g.	2%	1 g.	4%	2 g.	0 g.	0 i.u.	0%	0 mg.	0%	0 mg.	0%	0 mg.	0%
5 g.	2%	0 g.	0%	3 g.	0 g.	0 i.u.	0%	0 mg.	0%	0 mg.	0%	0 mg.	0%
1 g.	2%	1 g.	4%	0 g.	0 g.	0 i.u.	0%	0 mg.	0%	0 mg.	0%	0 mg.	0%
4 g.	2%	0 g.	0%	0 g.	0 g.	0 i.u.	0%	0 mg.	0%	0 mg.	0%	0 mg.	0%
1 g.	0%	0 g.	0%	1 g.	0 g.	0 i.u.	0%	0 mg.	0%	0 mg.	0%	0 mg.	0%
2 g.	1%	0 g.	0%	1 g.	1 g.	100 i.u.	0%	0 mg.	0%	0 mg.	0%	.36 mg.	2%
8 g.	3%	0 g.	0%	7 g.	0 g.	0 i.u.	0%	0 mg.	0%	0 mg.	0%	0 mg.	0%
3 g.	1%	0 g.	0%	2 g.	0 g.	0 i.u.	0%	1.8 mg.	3%	N/S	0%	0 mg.	0%
6 g.	2%	0 g.	0%	4 g.	0 g.	0 i.u.	0%	0 mg.	0%	0 mg.	0%	0 mg.	0%
6 g.	2%	0 g.	0%	0 g.	0 g.	0 i.u.	0%	0 mg.	0%	0 mg.	0%	0 mg.	0%
14 g.	5%	0 g.	0%	13 g.	0 g.	0 i.u.	0%	0 mg.	0%	60 mg.	6%	.72 mg.	4%
14 g.	5%	0 g.	0%	8 g.	1 g.	0 i.u.	0%	0 mg.	0%	N/S	0%	N/S	0%
12 g.	4%	0 g.	0%	9 g.	0 g.	0 i.u.	0%	0 mg.	0%	200 mg.	20%	3.6 mg.	20%

Food	Weight Per Serving	Calories	Calories from Fat	Fat	% Daily Values	Saturated Fat	% Daily Values	Cholesterol	% Daily Values	Sodium	% Daily Values
brown rice syrup	15 g.	43	0	0 g.	0%	0 g.	0%	0 mg.	0%	5 mg.	0%
brown sugar, packed	14 g.	50	0	0 g.	0%	0 g.	0%	0 mg.	0%	5 mg.	0%
date sugar	12 g.	30	0	0 g.	0%	0 g.	0%	0 mg.	0%	0 mg.	0%
FruitSource™	14 g.	44	0	0 g.	0%	0 g.	0%	0 mg.	0%	0 mg.	0%
honey	21 g.	60	0	0 g.	0%	0 g.	0%	0 mg.	0%	0 mg.	0%
jam, strawberry	20 g.	50	0	0 g.	0%	0 g.	0%	0 mg.	0%	0 mg.	0%
jelly, fruit juice sweetened	19 g.	40	0	0 g.	0%	0 g.	0%	0 mg.	0%	5 mg.	0%
jelly, grape	18 g.	50	0	0 g.	0%	0 g.	0%	0 mg.	0%	5 mg.	0%
maple syrup	20 g.	50	0	0 g.	0%	0 g.	0%	0 mg.	0%	0 mg.	0%
white sugar	12 g.	50	0	0 g.	0%	0 g.	0%	0 mg.	0%	0 mg.	0%
Sport Energy Bars											
PowerBar™ Apple/Cinnamon	65 g.	225	23	2.5 g.	4%	0.5 g.	3%	0 mg.	0%	90 mg.	4%
PowerBar™ Chocolate	65 g.	225	18	2 g.	3%	0.5 g.	3%	0 mg.	0%	90 mg.	4%
PowerBar™ Malt/Nut	65 g.	225	23	2.5 g.	4%	0.5 g.	3%	0 mg.	0%	90 mg.	4%
Stoker™ Apple Oat	75 g.	252	27	3 g.	5%	0 g.	0%	0 mg.	0%	21 mg.	2%
Stoker™ Real Cocoa	75 g.	252	27	3 g.	5%	0 g.	0%	0 mg.	0%	60 mg.	2%
MISCELLANEOUS CONDIMENTS											
guacamole w/ tomatoes (2 Tbsp.)	29 g.	35	30	3 g.	5%	N/S	0%	0 mg.	0%	55 mg.	2%
ketchup (1 Tbsp.)	15 g.	0	0	0 g.	0%	0 g.	0%	0 mg.	0%	180 mg.	8%
gomasio: Eden Sesame Shake™ (1/2 tsp.)	1.5 g.	10	5	0.5 g.	1%	0 g.	0%	0 mg.	0%	40 mg.	2%
miso, barley (1 Tbsp.)	16 g.	20	10	1 g.	1%	0 g.	0%	0 mg.	0%	760 mg.	32%
miso, brown rice(1 Tbsp.)	16 g.	25	10	1 g.	1%	0 g.	0%	0 mg.	0%	810 mg.	34%
miso, soybean (1 Tbsp.)	16 g.	30	15	1.5 g.	2%	0 g.	0%	0 mg.	0%	600 mg.	25%
miso, white shiro(1 Tbsp.)	16 g.	30	10	1 g.	1%	0 g.	0%	0 mg.	0%	410 mg.	17%
mustard, prepared (1 Tbsp.)	16 g.	10	5	0.5 g.	1%	0 g.	0%	0 mg.	0%	200 mg.	8%
olives, green (3)	12 g.	15	15	1.5 g.	2%	0 g.	0%	0 mg.	0%	280 mg.	12%
olives, ripe large (3)	14 g.	15	15	1.5 g.	2%	0 g.	0%	0 mg.	0%	120 mg.	5%

Carbohydrates	% Daily Values	Fiber	% Daily Values	Sugars- Natural and Added	Protein	Vitamin A	% Daily Values	Vitamin C	% Daily Values	Calcium	% Daily Values	Iron	% Daily Values
10.5 g.	3.5%	0 g.	0%	5 g.	0 g.	0 i.u.	0%	0 mg.	0%	0 mg.	0%	0 mg.	0%
13 g.	4%	0 g.	0%	13 g.	0 g.	0 i.u.	0%	0 mg.	0%	20 mg.	2%	.36 mg.	2%
9 g.	3%	0 g.	0%	9 g.	0 g.	0 i.u.	0%	0 mg.	0%	N/S	0%	N/S	0%
11 g.	3.5%	0 g.	0%	7 g.	0 g.	0 i.u.	0%	0 mg.	0%	N/S	0%	N/S	0%
17 g.	6%	0 g.	0%	17 g.	0 g.	0 i.u.	0%	N/S	0%	N/S	0%	N/S	0%
14 g.	5%	0 g.	0%	14 g.	0 g.	0 i.u.	0%	2.4 mg.	4%	0 mg.	0%	.36 mg.	2%
10 g.	3%	0 g.	0%	10 g.	0 g.	0 i.u.	0%	0 mg.	0%	0 mg.	0%	0 mg.	0%
13 g.	4%	0 g.	0%	13 g.	0 g.	0 i.u.	0%	0 mg.	0%	0 mg.	0%	0 mg.	0%
13 g.	4%	0 g.	0%	13 g.	0 g.	0 i.u.	0%	0 mg.	0%	20 mg.	2%	.36 mg.	2%
12 g.	4%	0 g.	0%	12 g.	0 g.	0 i.u.	0%	0 mg.	0%	0 mg.	0%	0 mg.	0%
42 g.	14%	3 g.	13%	14 g.	10 g.	0 i.u.	0%	60 mg.	100%	300 mg.	30%	6.3 mg.	35%
42 g.	14%	3 g.	13%	14 g.	10 g.	0 i.u.	0%	60 mg.	100%	300 mg.	30%	6.5%	35%
42 g.	14%	3 g.	13%	18 g.	10 g.	0 i.u.	0%	60 mg.	100%	300 mg.	30%	6.5 mg.	35%
50 g.	15%	4 g.	16%	21 g.	10 g.	100 i.u.	2%	60 mg.	100%	420 mg.	42%	6.5 mg.	35%
46 g.	15%	4 g.	16%	16 g.	10 g.	100 i.u.	2%	60 mg.	100%	420 mg.	42%	6.5 mg.	35%
2 g.	1%	1 g.	2%	N/S	0 g.	200 i.u.	4%	3.6 mg.	6%	N/S	0%	.36 mg.	2%
4 g.	1%	0 g.	0%	2 g.	0 g.	200 i.u.	4%	2.4 mg.	4%	N/S	0%	N/S	0%
0 g.	0%	0 g.	0%	0 g.	<1 g.	0 i.u.	0%	0 mg.	0%	N/S	0%	0 mg.	0%
2 g.	0%	1 g.	4%	N/S	2 g.	N/S	0%	1.2 mg.	2%	N/S	0%	.72 mg.	4%
3 g.	1%	1 g.	4%	N/S	2 g.	N/S	0%	1.2 mg.	2%	N/S	0%	.36 mg.	2%
2 g.	0%	1 g.	4%	N/S	3 g.	N/S	0%	2.4 mg.	4%	20 mg.	2%	.72 mg.	4%
5 g.	2%	1 g.	4%	3 g.	2 g.	N/S	0%	N/S	0%	N/S	0%	N/S	0%
1 g.	0%	N/S	0%	N/S	1 g.	N/S	0%	0 mg.	0%	20 mg.	2%	.36 mg.	2%
0 g.	0%	0 g.	0%	N/S	0 g.	N/S	0%	N/S	0%	N/S	0%	.36 mg.	2%
1 g.	0%	0 g.	0%	N/S	0 g.	100 i.u.	2%	N/S	0%	20 mg.	2%	.36 mg.	2%

Food	Weight Per Serving	Calories	Calories from Fat	Fat	% Daily Values	Saturated Fat	% Daily Values	Cholesterol	% Daily Values	Sodium	% Daily Values
pickles, dill (4 slices)	24 g.	5	0	0 g.	0%	0 g.	0%	0 mg.	0%	310 mg.	13%
pickles, dill low salt (4)	24 g.	5	0	0 g.	0%	0 g.	0%	0 mg.	0%	0 mg.	0%
salsa (hot sauce) (2 Tbsp.)	30 g.	15	0	0 g.	0%	0 g.	0%	0 mg.	0%	260 mg.	11%
salt, sea (1/2 tsp.)	3 g.	0	0	0 g.	0%	0 g.	0%	0 mg.	0%	1150 mg.	48%
tamari soy sauce (1 Tbsp.)	15 g.	10	0	0 g.	0%	0 g.	0%	0 mg.	0%	940 mg.	39%
umeboshi plum paste (1 Tbsp.)	15 g.	5	0	0 g.	0%	0 g.	0%	0 mg.	0%	1410 mg.	59%
vinegar, apple cider (1 Tbsp.)	14 g.	7	0	0 g.	0%	0 g.	0%	0 mg.	0%	55 mg.	0%
vinegar, balsamic (1 Tbsp.)	15 g.	5	0	0 g.	0%	0 g.	0%	0 mg.	0%	0 mg.	0%
vinegar, red wine (1 Tbsp.)	15 g.	0	0	0 g.	0%	0 g.	0%	0 mg.	0%	0 mg.	0%
vinegar, white wine (1 Tbsp.)	15 g.	0	0	0 g.	0%	0 g.	0%	0 mg.	0%	90 mg.	4%
MISCELLANEOUS SNACKS (1 cup popcorn or 1 oz. chips and pretzels (approx. 18 pieces)											
popcorn (air-popped)	8 g.	30	N/S	0 g.	0%	0 g.	0%	0 mg.	0%	0 mg.	0%
popcorn (oil-popped)	11 g.	60	30	3 g.	5%	0.5 g.	3%	0 mg.	0%	5 mg.	4%
potato chip, w/salt (17)	28 g.	150	90	10 g.	15%	3 g.	16%	0 mg.	0%	170 mg.	7%
potato chips, no salt (17)	28 g.	150	90	10 g.	15%	3 g.	16%	0 mg.	0%	0 mg.	0%
pretzels, typical thick Dutch	30 g.	110	10	1 g.	2%	0 g.	0%	0 mg.	0%	510 mg.	21%
pretzels, Newman's Own Organic (17)	30 g.	110	10	1.5 g.	2%	0 g.	0%	0 mg.	0%	350 mg.	15%
pretzels, Newman's Own Organic no/salt (17)	30 g.	110	10	1.5 g.	2%	0 g.	0%	0 mg.	0%	105 mg.	4%
tortilla chips, typical (1 oz.)	30 g.	150	71	8 g.	12%	1.5 g.	8%	0 mg.	0%	158 mg.	7%
tortilla chips, Guiltless Gourmet™, no oil/ w/salt	28 g.	110	10	1 g.	1%	0 g.	0%	0 mg.	0%	160 mg.	7%
tortilla chips, Guiltless Gourmet™, no oil/ no salt	28 g.	110	10	1 g.	1%	0 g.	0%	0 mg.	0%	26 mg.	1%

Percent (%) Daily Values are based on a 2,000 calorie diet. Your daily values may be higher or lower based on your calorie needs:

	Calories:	**2000**	**2500**
Total Fat	Less than	65 g.	80 g.
Saturated Fat	Less than	20 g.	25 g.
Cholesterol	Less than	300 mg.	300 mg.
Sodium	Less than	2,400 mg.	2,400 mg.
Total Carbohydrate		300 mg.	375 mg.
Dietary Fiber		25 g.	30 g.

Calories per gram: Fat- 9 calories   Carbohydrate-4 calories   Protein- 4 calories
RDI for vitamin A: 5000 i.u., **vitamin C:** 60 mg., **calcium:** 1000 mg., **iron:** 18 mg.

Carbohydrates	% Daily Values	Fiber	% Daily Values	Sugars- Natural and Added	Protein	Vitamin A	% Daily Values	Vitamin C	% Daily Values	Calcium	% Daily Values	Iron	% Daily Values
1 g.	0%	0 g.	0%	N/S	0 g.	100 i.u.	2%	N/S	0%	N/S	0%	N/S	0%
1 g.	0%	0 g.	0%	N/S	0 g.	100 i.u.	2%	N/S	0%	N/S	0%	N/S	0%
2 g.	1%	1 g.	5%	2 g.	N/S	200 i.u.	4%	N/S	0%	20 mg.	2%	N/S	0%
0 g.	0%	0 g.	0%	0 g.	0 g.	0 i.u.	0%	0 mg.	0%	N/S	0%	0 mg.	0%
1 g.	0%	0 g.	0%	N/S	2 g.	N/S	0%	N/S	0%	N/S	0%	.36 mg.	2%
1 g.	0%	0 g.	0%	N/S	0 g.	N/S	0%	N/S	0%	N/S	0%	.36 mg.	2%
2 g.	1%	0 g.	0%	0 g.	0 g.	N/S	0%	N/S	0%	N/S	0%	N/S	0%
2 g.	1%	0 g.	0%	2 g.	0 g.	0 i.u.	0%	0 mg.	0%	0 mg.	0%	.36 mg.	2%
0 g.	0%	0 g.	0%	0 g.	0 g.	0 i.u.	0%	0 mg.	0%	0 mg.	0%	N/S	0%
0 g.	0%	0 g.	0%	0 g.	0 g.	0 i.u.	0%	0 mg.	0%	0 mg.	0%	N/S	0%
6 g.	2%	1 g.	5%	N/S	1 g.	N/S	0%	0 mg.	0%	N/S	0%	.36 mg.	2%
6 g.	2%	1 g.	4%	N/S	1 g.	N/S	0%	0 mg.	0%	N/S	0%	.36 mg.	2%
15 g.	5%	1 g.	5%	1 g.	2 g.	N/S	0%	9 mg.	15%	N/S	0%	.36 mg.	2%
15 g.	5%	1 g.	5%	1 g.	2 g.	N/S	0%	9 mg.	15%	N/S	0%	.36 mg.	2%
24 g.	8%	1 g.	4%	1 g.	3 g.	N/S	0%	N/S	0%	20 mg.	2%	1.44 mg.	8%
24 g.	8%	1 g.	3%	1 g.	2 g.	N/S	0%	N/S	0%	N/S	0%	N/S	0%
24 g.	8%	1 g.	3%	1 g.	2 g.	N/S	0%	N/S	0%	N/S	0%	N/S	0%
19 g.	6%	2 g.	8%	N/S	2 g.	N/S	0%	0 mg.	0%	46 mg.	5%	.46 mg.	2.5%
22 g.	7%	3 g.	12%	N/S	3 g.	100 i.u.	2%	4.8 mg.	8%	100 mg.	10%	1.08 mg.	6%
22 g.	7%	3 g.	12%	N/S	3 g.	100 i.u.	2%	4.8 mg.	8%	100 mg.	10%	1.08 mg.	6%

N/S: Indicates that the amount of a particular nutrient present in a serving is insignificant. **Calories from Fat:** when the food contains less than 5 calories from fat. **Saturated Fat:** when the food contains less than 0.5 grams of total fat per serving and if no claims are made about fat or cholesterol content and if no claims asre made about calories from fat. **Cholesterol:** when the food contains less than 2 mg. cholesterol per serving and makes no claim about fat, fatty acids or cholesterol. **Dietary Fiber:** when a serving contains less than 1 gram of dietary fiber. **Sugars:** when a serving contains less than 1 gram of sugar and no claims are made about sweeteners, sugars, or sugar alcohol content. **Vitamins and minerals:** when a serving contains less than 2% of the Recommended Daily Intake (RDI).

Bibliography

American Health Magazine. New York, NY, issues 1992-1994.

Bailey, Janet. *Keeping Food Fresh.* New York: Harper & Row. 1989.

Belleme, Jan & John. *Cooking With Japanese Foods.* Garden City Park, NY: Avery Publishing Group, Inc. 1993.

Bon Appétit Magazine. Los Angeles, CA, issues 1989-1994.

Brody, Jane. *Jane Brody's Good Food Book.* New York: Bantam Books. 1985.

Brody, Jane. *Jane Brody's Nutrition Book.* New York: Bantam Books. 1982.

Cheney, Susan Jane. *Breadtime Stories.* Berkeley, CA: Ten Speed Press. 1990.

Colbin, Annemarie. *Food And Healing.* New York: Ballantine Books. 1986.

Cooking Light Magazine. Birmingham, AL, issues 1988-1994.

East West Journal. *Shopper's Guide to Natural Foods.* Garden City Park: Avery Publishing Group. 1987.

East West Journal Magazine. Brookline Village, MA, issues 1988-1991.

Eating Well Magazine. Charlotte, VT, issues 1990-1994.

Environmental Nutrition Newsletter. New York, NY, issues 1990-1994.

Freeland-Graves, Jeanne & Peckham, Gladys C. *Foundations of Food Preparation,* 5th Ed. New York: Macmillan Publishing Co. 1987.

Gelles, Carol. *The Complete Whole Grain Cookbook.* New York: Donald I. Fine, Inc. 1989

Greenstein, George. *Secrets of a Jewish Baker.* Freedom, CA: The Crossing Press. 1993.

Hazan, Giuliano. *The Classic Pasta Cookbook.* New York: Dorling Kindersley, Inc. 1993.

HSUS News. (Humane Society of the United States) Washington, D.C., issues 1988-1994.

Humane Society of the U.S. *The Humane Consumer And Producer Guide.* Washington, D.C.: The Humane Society of the U.S. 1993.

Igoe, Robert S. *Dictionary of Food Ingredients*: Second Edition. New York: Van Nostrand Reinhold. 1989.

Jacobson, Michael. *Safe Food: Eating Wisely In A Risky World.* Los Angeles: Living Planet Press. 1991.

Jones, Marjorie Hurt. *The Allergy Self-Help Cookbook*. Emmaus, PA: Rodale Press. 1984.

Lewis, Richard. *Food Additives Handbook*. New York: Van Nostrand Reinhold. 1989.

McGee, Harold. *On Food and Cooking*. New York: Collier Books. 1984.

Merinoff, Linda. *The Glorious Noodle*. New York: Poseidon Press. 1986.

National Academy of Sciences. *Diet and Health*. Washington, D.C.: National Academy Press. 1989.

National Academy of Sciences. *Alternative Agriculture*. Washington, D.C.: National Academy Press. 1989.

Natural Health: The Guide To Well-Being Magazine. Brookline Village, MA, issues 1991-1994.

Nutrition Action Health Letter. Washington, D.C., issues 1988-1994.

Ornish, M.D., Dean. *Dr. Dean Ornish's Program for Reversing Heart Disease*. New York: Ballantine Books. 1990.

Rosso, Julee & Lukins, Sheila. *The New Basics Cookbook*. New York: Workman Publishing Co. 1989.

Rosso, Julee. *Great Good Food*. New York: Crown Publishers. 1993.

Strauss, Sandra C. *Fancy Fruits and Extraordinary Vegetables*. Mamaroneck, NY: Hastings House. 1992.

University of California, *Berkeley Wellness Newsletter*. New York, New York, issues 1988-1994.

Vegetarian Gourmet Magazine. Montrose, PA, issues 1992-1993.

Vegetarian Times Magazine. Oak Park, IL, issues 1988-1994.

Whitney, Eleanor & Hamilton, Eva May Nunnelley. *Understanding Nutrition*: Fourth Edition. St. Paul: West Publishing Co. 1987.

Wood, Rebecca. *The Whole Foods Encyclopedia*. New York: Prentice-Hall Press. 1988.

Woteki, Catherine E. & Thomas, Paul R. *Eat For Life*. Washington, D.C. National Academy Press. 1992.

Special thanks to Spectrum Naturals, Inc., especially Rees Moorman, for detailed information on fats and oils.

Index

S

saccharin, 320-321

safflower oil

    high oleic, 302-303, 358

    regular, 290, 302, 358

salmonella, 233, 236

sardines, 196, 274

scarlet runner beans, 220

sea palm, 136

sea vegetables, 132-137

    cooking guides, 132-133

    nutrition, 132

    see specific varieties

semolina flour, 87, 328

sesame seeds, 249-250, 274, 352

    black sesame seeds, 250

    calcium content, 249

    gomasio (sesame salt), 250

    hulling of, 249

    oil, 303, 358

    sesame butter, 250

    sesame rice pasta, 107

    tahini, 250, 352

serrano peppers, 119

sev, 77, 110

sherry vinegar, 121

shiitake mushrooms, 123, 124, 125, 336

shoyu, 224-225

shrimp , 201, 202, 203, 204, 206, 274, 348

soba, 108, 332

sodium, 4, 14

soldier beans, 220

somen, 108

sorbitol, 321

sorghum, 58-59

    cracked, 59

    molasses, 58, 320

    whole grain, 59

sorrel, 121

sour cream, 263-264

soy

    black soybeans, 222

    cheese, 276, 356

    flour, 73, 84, 328

    grits, 222

    milk, 274, 275, 354

    miso, 222-223

    oil, 303-304

    soy protein isolate, 227

    soy sauce, 223-225

    tempeh, 225-226, 274, 348

    texturized vegetable protein (TVP), 226-227

    tofu, 227-231, 274

    yellow soybeans, 222

soymilk, 274-275, 335

soy sauce, 223-225

    common soy sauce, 223

    low sodium shoyu, 224

    shoyu, 224-225

    tamari, 224-224

spaghetti squash, 127, 128, 336

spelt

    bread, 97

    flakes, 59, 326

    flour, 73, 84-85, 328

    pasta, 107, 332

    whole grain, 59, 326

split peas, 216, 348

sprouts, 97, 130-131

    bread, yeasted, 97

    cooking guidelines, 131

    how to sprout, 131

    nutrition, 130, 332, 326

squashes, 114, 127-128, 338

stevia, 321

straw mushrooms, 124

sugars, refined/unrefined, 322-323

    brown sugar, 322, 360

    demarara sugar, 322

    evaporated cane juice, 322-323

    muscovado sugar, 323

    simple sugars, 306-307

        fructose, 307

        glucose, 307

        lactose, 306

        maltose, 307

        sucrose, 307

    turbinado sugar, 323

    unrefined sugar, 322

    which sugar best to use, 306

    white sugar, 322, 360

sulfites/sulfur dioxide, 141, 150-151, 201, 320

sunflower seeds, 250-251, 274, 352

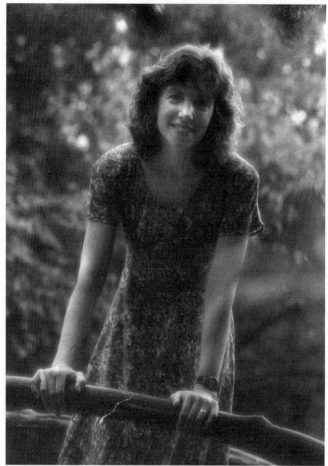
photo by Jed Share

Margaret M. Wittenberg is a nationally recognized lecturer, researcher, writer, cooking teacher, and consultant with over 20 years experience promoting good food and optimum health. Her previous book, *Experiencing Quality: A Shopper's Guide to Whole Foods,* has been used by natural foods stores throughout the country as a reference and training guide. She lives in the Texas Hill Country.

**The Crossing Press
publishes a full
selection of cookbooks.**

**To receive our current
catalog, please call toll-free,
800-777-1048.**